Basic Science for

Modern Cosmetic Dermatology

Basic Science for
Modern Cosmetic Dermatology

Chief Editors

Chakaravarthi Srinivas MD FRCP
Professor
Department of Dermatology
PSG Institute of Medical Sciences and Research
Coimbatore, India

Michèle Verschoore MD
L'Oréal Research and Innovation
Asnières, France

Assistant Editor

Claire Battie PharmD
L'Oréal Research and Innovation
Asnières, France

JAYPEE The Health Sciences Publisher

New Delhi | London | Philadelphia | Panama

Jaypee Brothers Medical Publishers (P) Ltd

Headquarters
Jaypee Brothers Medical Publishers (P) Ltd
4838/24, Ansari Road, Daryaganj
New Delhi 110 002, India
Phone: +91-11-43574357
Fax: +91-11-43574314
Email: jaypee@jaypeebrothers.com

Overseas Offices

J.P. Medical Ltd
83 Victoria Street, London
SW1H 0HW (UK)
Phone: +44-2031708910
Fax: +02-03-0086180
Email: info@jpmedpub.com

Jaypee-Highlights Medical Publishers Inc
City of Knowledge, Bld. 237, Clayton
Panama City, Panama
Phone: +1 507-301-0496
Fax: +1 507-301-0499
Email: cservice@jphmedical.com

Jaypee Medical Inc.
The Bourse
111 South Independence Mall East
Suite 835, Philadelphia, PA 19106, USA
Phone: +1 267-519-9789
Email: jpmed.us@gmail.com

Jaypee Brothers Medical Publishers (P) Ltd
17/1-B Babar Road, Block-B, Shaymali
Mohammadpur, Dhaka-1207
Bangladesh
Mobile: +08801912003485
Email: jaypeedhaka@gmail.com

Jaypee Brothers Medical Publishers (P) Ltd
Bhotahity, Kathmandu
Nepal
Phone: +977-9741283608
Email: kathmandu@jaypeebrothers.com

Website: www.jaypeebrothers.com
Website: www.jaypeedigital.com

Inquiries for bulk sales may be solicited at: jaypee@jaypeebrothers.com

Basic Science for **Modern Cosmetic Dermatology**

First Edition: **2015**

ISBN 978-93-5152-124-2

Printed at : Samrat Offset Pvt.Ltd.

Contributors

Chief Editors

Chakaravarthi Srinivas MD FRCP
Professor, Department of Dermatology
PSG Institute of Medical Sciences and Research, Coimbatore, India

Michèle Verschoore MD
L'Oréal Research and Innovation, Asnières, France

Assistant Editor

Claire Battie PharmD
L'Oréal Research and Innovation, Asnières, France

Contributing Authors

Frédéric Amaral PhD
L'Oréal Research and Innovation
Aulnay-sous-Bois, France

AK Bajaj MD
Bajaj Skin Clinic, Allahabad, India

Bruno A Bernard PhD
L'Oréal Research and Innovation, Asnières, France

Françoise Bernerd PhD
L'Oréal Research and Innovation
Aulnay-sous-Bois, France

Lionel Breton PhD
L'Oréal Research and Innovation
Aulnay-sous-Bois, France

Cécile Clavaud PhD
L'Oréal Research and Innovation
Aulnay-sous-Bois, France

Suzy Cointereau-Chardon
L'Oréal Research and Innovation
Chevilly-Larue, France

Stéphane Commo PhD
L'Oréal Research and Innovation
Aulnay-sous-Bois, France

José Cotovio PhD
L'Oréal Research and Innovation
Aulnay-sous-Bois, France

Mark Donovan PhD
L'Oréal Research and Innovation
Aulnay-sous-Bois, France

Frédéric Flament PhD
L'Oréal Research and Innovation
Chevilly-Larue, France

Kiran Godse MD FRCP
Department of Dermatology
D.Y. Patil Medical College and Hospital
Nerul, Navi Mumbai, India

Somesh Gupta MD DNB MNAMS
Department of Dermatology and Venereology
All India Institute of Medical Sciences, New Delhi, India

Prashant S Hegde PhD
L'Oréal Research and Innovation, Bengaluru, India

Virginie Hourblin
L'Oréal Research and Innovation
Aulnay-sous-Bois, France

Arun C Inamadar MD DVD FRCP
Department of Dermatology
SBMP Medical College, BLDE University, Bijapur, India

Hema Jerajani MD
Department of Dermatology
MGM Medical College and Hospital, Mumbai, India

Roland Jourdain
L'Oréal Research and Innovation
Aulnay-sous-Bois, France

Uday Khopkar MD
Department of Dermatology
KEM Hospital and Seth GS Medical College
Mumbai, India

Niti Khunger MD DDV DNB
Department of Dermatology
VM Medical College and Safdarjung Hospital
New Delhi, India

Muthuvel Kumaresan MD
Department of Dermatology
PSG Institute of Medical Science and Research
Coimbatore, India

Nina Madnani MD
P.D. Hinduja National Hospital and Medical
Research Centre, Mumbai, India

Namita Misra PhD
L'Oréal Research and Innovation, Mumbai, India

Asit Mittal MD
Department of Dermatology
RNT Medical College, Udaipur, India

Dominique Moyal PhD
L'Oréal Research and Innovation
Asnières, France

Stéphanie Nouveau PhD
L'Oréal Research and Innovation
Aulnay-sous-Bois, France

Christian Oresajo PhD
L'Oréal Research and Innovation, Clark, USA

Jean-Paul Ortonne MD
Department of Dermatology
University Hospital of Nice, Nice, France

Sathish B Pai MD DVD
Department of Dermatology
Kasturba Medical College, Manipal University
Manipal, India

Davinder Parsad MD
Department of Dermatology
Postgraduate Institute of Medical Education
and Research, Chandigarh, India

Thierry Passeron MD PhD
Department of Dermatology &
INSERM U1065, team 12, C3M
University Hospital of Nice, Nice, France

Christian Pellevoisin PhD
Episkin Academy
Lyon, France

Reena Rai MD
Department of Dermatology
PSG Institute of Medical Science and Research
Coimbatore, India

Narasimha Rao P MD DD PhD
Department of Dermatology
Bhaskar Medical College, Hyderabad, India

Nita Roy PhD
L'Oréal Research and Innovation, Bengaluru, India

Mukta Sachdev MD
Manipal Hospital, Bengaluru, India

Didier Saint-Léger DEA Pr Honoris Causa
TING S.A, Paris, France

Vinay Saraf MD DVD
Dr. B. Nanavati Hospital and Research Center
Mumbai, India

Abir Saraswat MD DNB
Indushree Skin Clinic, Lucknow, India

Suresh Talwar MD
Lucknow, India

Manoj K Tembhre
Department of Dermatology and Venereology
All India Institute of Medical Sciences
New Delhi, India

Amit Tewari PhD
L'Oréal Research and Innovation
Bengaluru, India

Maya Vedamurthy MD FIAD FRCP
RSV Skin and Laser Centre and Apollo Hospitals
Chennai, India

Shyam Verma MD MBBS DVD FRCP FAAD
Nirvana Skin Clinic, Vadodara, India

Anupama Wagle MD
L'Oréal Research and Innovation
Mumbai, India

Foreword

Dermatology is evolving and many subspecialties are gaining prominence. Amongst them is cosmetic dermatology. Cosmetic dermatology is not simple beauty care, but is based on science. This profusely illustrated book, edited by Dr Michèle Verschoore and Prof Chakaravarthi Srinivas, and co-authored by eminent French and Indian authors, fulfils a long felt need by very lucidly explaining the basic science behind cosmetic dermatology.

Deepak Parikh MD
Consultant Dermatologist
Professor and Head, Department of Pediatric Dermatology
Bai Jerbai Wadia Hospital for Children
Parel, Mumbai, India

Preface

Cosmetic Dermatology is an ancient medical specialty. For many centuries, medical doctors have identified esthetic skin disorders and advised the best preventive habits and appropriate cosmetics to correct those troubles. This medical specialty has been mainly inspired by empirical approaches and the observation, day after day, of the positive resolution of those disorders and the ensuing satisfaction of patients. During the second half of the twentieth century, tremendous progress has been made in developing new tools for examining and characterizing skin, mucous membranes, hair and nails.

More recently, outstanding advances in molecular biology, genomics and proteomics have paved the way for biological profiling of individuals according to their innate characteristics and to study the impact of their environment, cultural habits, etc. on their hair and skin.

Today, traditional cosmetic dermatology is enriched by this new basic science knowledge and cosmetic products are being developed using data inherited from tradition but also generated using scientific approaches to ensure efficacy and safety. Cosmetic Dermatology is a science which endeavors to define the most appropriate preventive measures for the protection of hair and skin, and this preventive approach is especially meaningful with increases in life expectancy.

This textbook is the fruit of intense dialog and work between renowned Indian dermatologists with expertise in Cosmetic Dermatology and international scientists known for their excellence in basic Cosmetic Science.

This textbook is aimed at readers who wish to have a broad overview of cosmetic dermatology including the most recent advances in basic Cosmetic Science. It will help each Indian practitioner to better apprehend the science behind modern cosmetics and guide him or her towards adapted cosmetic recommendations for each patient.

Each chapter was co-written by Indian experts and International experts, and this methodology has resulted in outstanding mutual understanding. I wish to thank all authors for this intensive work leading to this positive outcome.

I, on behalf of Prof Srinivas, Chief Editor of this book and all the authors, would like to express my sincere felicitations and gratitude to Claire Battie, Assistant Editor of this textbook, for her continuous scientific support and coordination.

We wish this book to be a guide for young scientists who devote their time to Hair and Skin Science in India. We also wish this textbook to be useful to practicing cosmetic dermatologists through its updated approach to Cosmetic Science.

Michèle Verschoore MD
L'Oréal Research and Innovation
Asnières, France

Preface

There is this story of a Camel which requests for a small space in the tent and the master obliges. Slowly but surely the camel creeps in and the space for the master is much reduced. Camel, you will agree with me is a bit large and a tiny corner will not suffice. Cosmetic Dermatology too has now occupied a major place in dermatologic practice. The master has two options, one is walk off in a huff or else try and tame the Camel and still remain the master.

There is every reason to pursue the path of integration and moving forward. The dilemma is, a rigorously trained dermatologist cannot wear the label of Cosmetologist alone. However, he/she can become a Dermato-cosmetologist akin to Dermatopathologist wherein the practice of cosmetology is not based on grandmother's (bless her soul) concoctions, or copies of recipes from nowhere by nobody. The practice of Cosmetology by the Dermatologist should be based on strong foundation and not whims, fairy tales and half-baked untested concoctions.

Beauty is regional just as food and dressing habits. What is good and acceptable elsewhere may not be ideal for Indian skin which differs from other types of skin. That Indians, themselves, which includes their skin lack homogeneity is another issue. Our problems need dedicated solution based on an understanding of basic principle of dermatology in general and Indian skin in particular. This book conceived by Dr Michèle Verschoore and ably assisted by Claire Battie in her capacity as Assistant Editor and the progress of which was monitored by Dr Ameet Valia and moulded by Professor Jean-Paul Ortonne, is our small time effort to breathe hardcore science into this subspeciality referred to as Cosmetology.

Chakaravarthi Srinivas MD FRCP
Professor, Department of Dermatology
PSG Institute of Medical Sciences and Research
Coimbatore, India

Contents

Chapter 1

General Introduction on Skin and Hair Physiologies

Michèle Verschoore, *L'Oréal Research and Innovation, Asnières, France*
Chakaravarthi Srinivas, *PSG Institute of Medical Sciences and Research, Coimbatore, India*
Asit Mittal, *RNT Medical College, Udaipur, India*

INTRODUCTION

Skin health and beauty science has been driven by innovative ingredients and new formulation technologies and, in a large part, by the tremendous advances in the knowledge of skin and hair physiology in the last 20 years.

Thanks to the cosmetic industry and dermatology researches, numerous programs allowed the structure and functions of the different compartments of skin and of hair to be deeper understood and a number of interaction processes to be deciphered. This chapter will briefly summarize the main features of skin and hair structure and functions. More elaborate data will be given in each chapter dedicated to specific aspects.

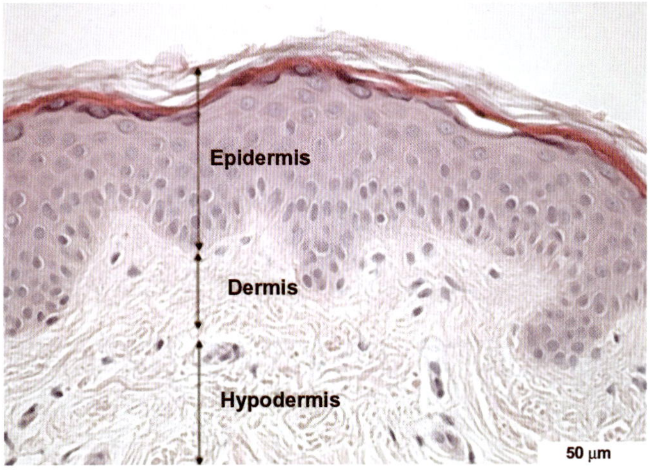

Figure 1: Histological section of human skin (HE staining, ×400) ©L'Oréal Research and Innovation

SKIN PHYSIOLOGY

Skin is a very large organ which represents the most extensive opening of the human body towards the external environment. In a 75 kg adult, skin weighs around 4 kg (excluding hypodermis), and covers a surface area of about 1.5–2 m^2. It forms a protective envelope and constitutes the first line of defense against external aggressions. Since skin regulates body temperature and fulfills barrier function, it is equipped with alarm, surveillance, exchange and adaptation systems. With a network of some 200,000 nerve endings, it is also the sensorial center of touch.

Skin is a complex structure, made up of various compartments. Basically, skin is composed of three superimposed tissue compartments: (1) epidermis; (2) dermis; and (3) hypodermis or subcutis (Fig. 1). Each compartment of the skin owns characteristic features and functions.[1-3]

These three compartments are anatomically and physiologically very different. The epidermis is the upper, stratified, very thin epithelial tissue, composed of different types of cell. Dermis is 20–40 times thicker and made up of a network of fibers and connective tissue stroma supporting a low population of cells. It is a resistant tissue which protects the body against mechanical injury and ensures the tensile and elastic properties of the skin. At last, hypodermis is the underlying general support of the skin.[4]

Epidermis

Epidermis is the outer compartment of the skin. Its thickness varies from 0.05 millimeter to 1.5 millimeter; the thinnest being found on the eyelids and the thickest on palm and soles. Although being the thinnest tissue of the skin, it plays a crucial role in forming the last barrier between the body and environment. Moreover, its outermost so-called horny layer or the stratum corneum is highly resistant to both physical and chemical assaults and protects against invasion by toxic agents, microorganisms and the impact of solar UV rays. Barrier function is provided by specific, tight architecture and continuous renewal epidermis also contributes to skin color. Hence, a better knowledge of this basic structure of the epidermis enables the practitioner to improve the appearance of patients' skin.

The epidermis is mainly composed of cells, 95% of which being keratinocytes at progressive stages of differentiation; other cells are melanocytes and Langerhans cells.

The anatomical particularity of epidermis lies in its structural organization in four distinct main layers. From bottom to top, the layers are named: stratum basale, stratum spinosum, stratum granulosum, and stratum corneum (SC) (Fig. 2). A fifth layer called the *stratum lucidum* can be distinguished between the stratum granulosum and the SC, but only in the thick skin of palms and soles. Keratinocytes originate from the lower layer where they divide and undergo progressive differentiation when moving upwards to the outer layers.

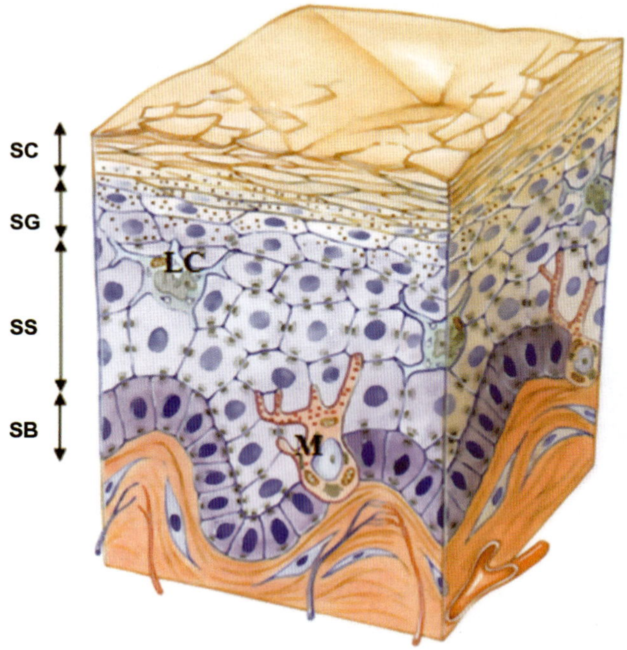

Figure 2: Schematic representation of human epidermis (×500) ©L'Oréal Research and Innovation
Abbreviations: SB, stratum basale; SS, stratum spinosum; SG, stratum granulosum; SC, stratum corneum; M, melanocytes; LC, Langerhans cells.

The stratum basale is made of one layer of small and highly active keratinocytes: basal cells. They replicate and give rise to all the other layers of epidermis where keratinization takes place along with migration upwards. This single cell layer of parent keratinocytes is attached to the dermal epidermal junction (DEJ) via hemi-desmosomes.

Above the stratum basale, the stratum spinosum consists of several layers of enlarging keratinocytes with numerous surface interconnections called desmosomes responsible for the "prickling" appearance of the cells. Desmosomes form a specific network ensuring the stability of this layer.

Above this layer, the stratum granulosum is composed of keratinocytes with two types of granules containing either keratin and keratohyalin or lipids.

Once they reach the SC, keratinocytes are fully differentiated, and become flat corneocytes, of a somewhat pentagonal shape of 40–50 μm in size, devoid of nuclei and surrounded by a tough envelope. As a last step of epidermal turnover, corneocytes are individually shed from the skin surface as a result of controlled action of proteolytic enzymes towards desmosomes. This normal physiological process is called desquamation and involves the degradation of intercellular lipid lamellar structure and definitive loss of intercellular connections. Cells of the SC (corneocytes) are the largest and most abundant within epidermis (more details in Chapter 8: -Stratum Corneum, Dry Skin, Xerosis and Moisturizers). SC thickness is made up of the stacking of 15–100 or more cell layers depending on body location and is the primary protective barrier from the external environment.

Keratinocytes take around 14 days to fully mature as they migrate from the basal layer to the SC; the dividing cells in the stratum basale replicate every 200–400 hours. The dead corneocytes are then shed from the horny layer within a further 14 days. This cell turnover rate of 28 days is dramatically shortened in keratinization disorders such as psoriasis, leading to a destructured and loose organization of the SC.

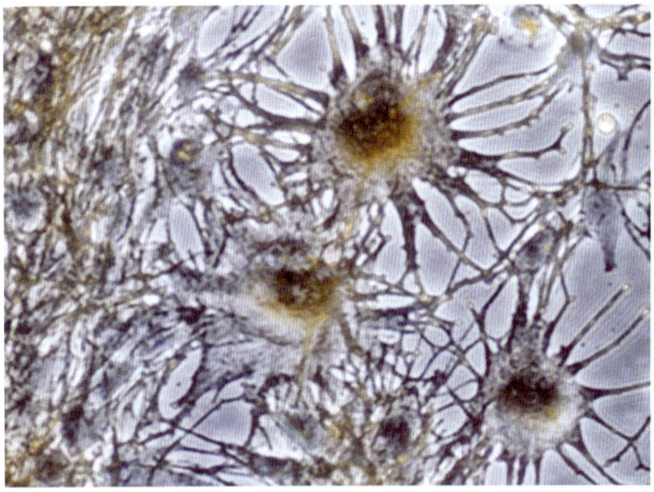

Figure 3: Melanocytes of pigmented skin (*in vitro* culture) observed under phase-contrast microscopy
©L'Oréal Research and Innovation

Other skin cells that can be found in the basal layer of the epidermis are melanocytes (Fig. 3). They produce a brown pigment, melanin, which is intended to protect the skin from the harmful effects of solar UV rays by absorbing their radiant energy. Melanocytes are characterized by their long extensions, dendrites, allowing the pigment to be transferred to neighboring keratinocytes. Stored in round cell structures called melanosomes, melanin is the major determinant of skin color (more details in Chapter 5: Physiology of Pigmentation: New Biological Concepts Associated with Skin and Hair Pigmentation). Since melanocytes account for 2–3% of epidermal cells, each melanocyte has to supply melanin to ca. 35 keratinocytes. Melanin production can be stimulated by sun exposure but also by various hormones such as melanocyte-stimulating hormone (MSH), adrenocorticotrophic hormone (ACTH), estrogens and progesterone. With aging, a decline is observed in the number of melanocytes populating the skin of an individual; their density decreases by 6–10% per decade.

In addition to keratinocytes and melanocytes, the epidermis contains Langerhans cells, most prominent in the stratum spinosum, which are responsible for the immunological function of the skin (see Fig. 4). Originating from the bone marrow, they serve as antigen-presenting cells. These highly dendritic cells capture and uptake foreign antigens that penetrate through the SC or that are generated from altered internal proteins. After processing them into small peptide fragments, they bind them to major histocompatibility complexes, and subsequently present them to lymphocytes for activation of the immune system. An example of activation of this immune system component is contact hypersensitivity.

Dermis

Dermis, 20–40 times thicker than epidermis, contributes to 3–4% of the total body weight. Its thickness varies from about 1 mm on the face to 4 mm on the back and thigh.

As compared to epidermis, dermis is a more complex structure composed of two layers:

1. The superficial papillary dermis (just below epidermis), interdigitated with the underside of the epidermis.
2. The deeper reticular dermis, making up about 90% of dermal thickness, and overlying the subcutaneous adipose tissue.

Composed of 80% water, elastin and collagen fibers embedded in a glycoprotein gel, dermis is a cushion tissue acting against mechanical stress. In contrast with epidermis, it is endowed with a rich vasculature providing nutritional and energy-rich elements to the epidermis and plays a primordial role in thermoregulation and healing.

Unlike epidermis, dermis contains a limited number of cells, mostly fibroblasts and some mast cells, histiocytes, leukocytes and melanocytes. Its structure results from interactions between the constituents of extracellular matrix (ECM) and fibroblasts. The latter are spindle-shaped cells which synthetize all the major constituents of the ECM: collagen, elastic fibers, and glycosaminoglycans (GAGs) etc. The latter composing what is generally called the "ground substance".

Dermal collagen forms a tight fibrillar network with a great tensile strength and thereby provides skin with a potential in extensibility and resistance to shear and other mechanical stress. Dermis mostly contains collagen type I and small amount of collagen type III. Collagen fibers are thought to change throughout life with a decrease in amount and deterioration of fibrillar architecture which is well correlated with changes in clinical appearance of ageing skin.

Although elastic fibers account for less than 1% of the weight of dermis, they nevertheless play a huge functional

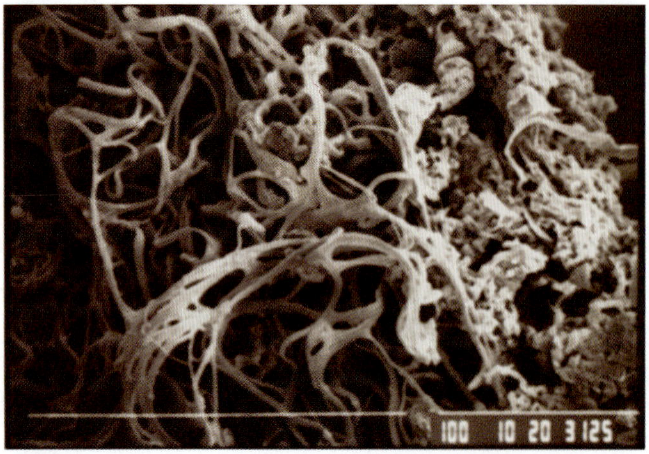

Figure 4: Human dermis visualized by scanning electonic microscopy (×500): elastin fibers network within the superficial dermis
©L'Oréal Research and Innovation

role by resisting to deformational forces and allow skin to recover its resting shape (Fig. 4). They consist of delicate, straight, branching fibers which supply and maintain the tonus of the skin. Some degradation of these fibers occurs during "normal" physiological events, such as growth, pregnancy, wound healing, but also in some chronic diseases and as a result of chronic sun exposures.

Embedding the fibrillar components of the dermis, the "ground substance" is a gel-like supporting matrix, composed of GAGs and proteoglycans (PGs) which trap water and contribute to maintain the dermal cohesion and structure. The decrease in both amount and nature of GAGs with chronic aging leads to a less swollen and less resistant skin.

In addition to nerve and sense endings, dermis also hosts blood and lymphatic vessels, hair follicles, sweat glands (eccrine and apocrine) and sebaceous glands.

Skin is innervated by about one million of nerve fibers; the densest concentrations are found in areas where sensation is paramount, such as face and hands. As skin may perceive a great number of sensations, including touch and temperature, various types of detectors ensure specific messages. Globally, sensory receptors can be divided into three groups: (1) mechanical; (2) thermal; and (3) nociceptive. When stimulated, they transmit the information through the spinal cord to central nervous system. Cutaneous feelings are significant in beauty care. In addition to efficiency, the success of cosmetics depends upon the pleasant feeling they can induce or be associated with and on the disappearance of unpleasant feelings induced by dryness, irritation or stinging. This explains why sensorial evaluation holds a growing place in beauty care.

Skin has also a rich blood supply. Blood vessels, made of arterioles, venules and capillaries, supply nutrition to the skin, but the skin vasculature is more elaborate than necessary for nutrition. Actually, these vessels play also an important role in temperature regulation. Indeed, dilation or contraction of arteriovenous anastomoses plays a direct role in skin thermoregulation. The changes in blood flow through the capillary loops help to control direct heat loss through the surface of the skin.

Dermal Epidermal Junction: Between Epidermis and Dermis

The DEJ is an undulating basement membrane that allows the epidermis to closely adhere to and interact with dermis. It forms an extensive interface composed of two layers, lamina lucida and lamina densa. Lamina lucida is thinner and lies directly beneath the basal layer of epidermal keratinocytes. The thicker lamina densa is in direct contact with the underlying dermis.

The DEJ is essential for skin cohesion. Apart from its cohesive role, DEJ also provides a dynamic interface between keratinocytes and fibroblasts, with strong interactions and back and forth signaling between the two cell types. In addition, this exchange zone allows the basal keratinocytes to be fed from dermal vessels.

Dermal epidermal junction alterations have been shown to occur as a result of several skin diseases, such as bullous pemphigoid and epidermolysis bullosa, as well as ageing where its undulation feature decrease, leading to a flattened DEJ. This emphasizes the crucial interactions between fibroblasts and keratinocytes.

Hypodermis

Hypodermis is a reservoir of energy; it sculpts the body and has a key role in regulating body temperature. Its thickness varies from 1 mm to 5 cm. The fat is stored in spherical cells, adipocytes, the volume of which depends on diet, age and physical activity (Fig. 5). Adipocytes synthesize, store and degrade fat, mostly under the form of triglycerides. The catabolism of this fat depends upon

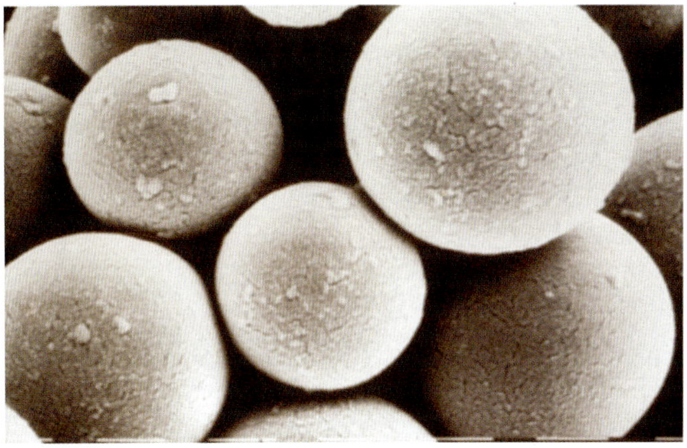

Figure 5: Observation of the hypodermis by electronic microscopy: visualization of adipocytes
©L'Oréal Research and Innovation

many factors, including nutrition, endocrine and nervous activity. With aging, fat redistribution occurs eventually resulting in sagging of facial features and increased storage in thigh and/or abdomen areas.

HAIR PHYSIOLOGY

Comparably to skin, the appearance of hair is often closely related to our perception of health and self-confidence.

There are estimated 5 million hair follicles on the body of an adult human, of which 100,000–120,000 cover the scalp, producing terminal hairs reaching a density of about 200 hairs/cm^2. The hair follicle can be viewed as an invagination of epidermis into dermis and hypodermis enclosing a small aggregate of dermal cells called dermal papilla in its deeper section. The follicles are dispersed in the dermis, the longest ones extending downwards into the adipose tissue, about 4 mm below the skin surface.

Hair has two principal parts: the shaft and the root (or hair follicle); the hair follicle is the site of intense biochemical and metabolic activity which leads to the development and growth of the hair shaft. Different compartments are located between the deepest parts of the root and the surface of the scalp. The dermal papilla, a pear-shaped mesenchymal condensate embedded into the matrix epithelium of the lower end of hair follicle, controls hair growth cycles and the size of the hair follicle and shaft.[5]

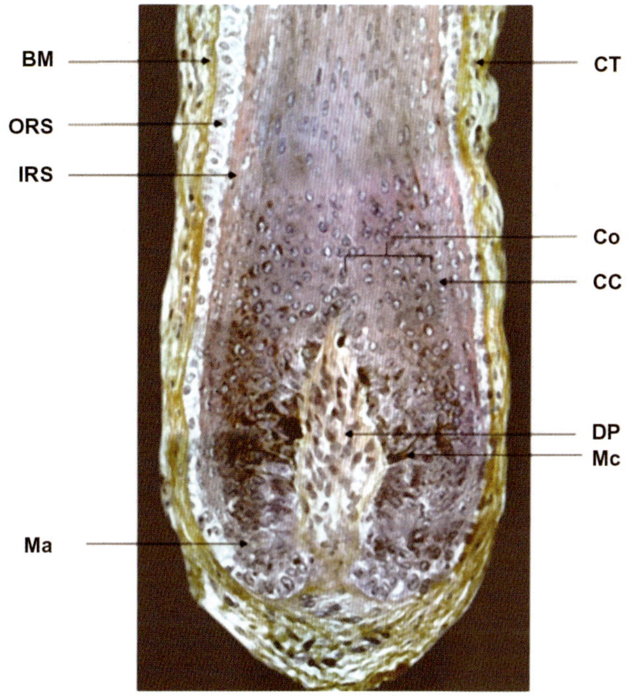

Figure 6: Hair bulb compartments (×400)
©L'Oréal Research and Innovation
Abbreviations: CC, cuticle; Co, cortex; CT, connective tissue; DP, dermal papilla; BM, basement membrane; IRS, inner root sheath; Ma, matrix ; Mc, melanocytes; ORS, outer root sheath.

Hair grows through division of epithelial matrix cells surrounding the dermal papilla, in the lower region of hair follicle called the hair bulb (Fig. 6).

The bulb includes two types of cell: keratinocytes at different states of differentiation and large dendritic melanocytes. From a critical level of the hair bulb (Auber line), the cells engage various programs of differentiation. Around the top of dermal papilla, the melanocytes synthesize melanin and transfer it to the hair shaft cortical cells, which give hair its color.

The hair shaft is formed in the center of the hair follicle through the maturation of keratinocytes which rapidly synthesize keratins. Then they lose their biological activity making these elongated, rigid and keratin-rich elements, which, assembled, shape. The shaft or hair fiber as a long cylinder of keratinized cells whose biochemical structure, ensures its remarkable resistance. The structure of the hair fiber is very complex, made up of three concentric compartments produced from three different cell types,

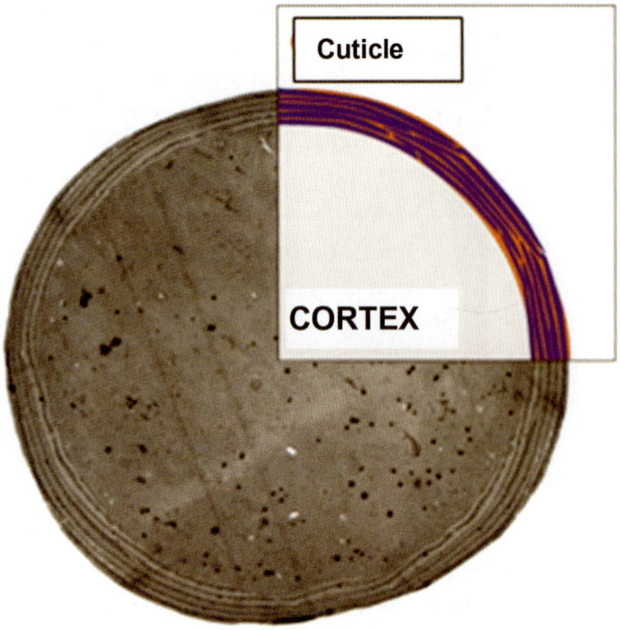

Figure 7: Cross-section of the hair shaft
©L'Oréal Research and Innovation

namely cuticle, cortical and medulla cells (Fig. 7). Medulla is in the center of hair, often discontinuous or absent in humans. The cortex which accounts for 80% of the fiber volume, gives hair its physical and mechanical properties. It is made up of spindle-shaped cells firmly inter-cemented containing highly cross-linked fibrillar keratin and melanin pigments responsible for hair color. These cortical cells are grouped in compact fascicles parallel to the axis of the hair. Finally, the cuticle is the hair's 7 outermost protective sheath, composed of 7–10 superimposed layers of unpigmented horny cells, resembling to some extent to the organization of the skin SC, with flat cells covering each other like roof tiles.[5]

In normal circumstances, hair production in each follicle follows a cyclic pattern, with three main phases (anagen, catagen and telogen) (more details in Chapter 12: New Insights in Hair Research). The hair fiber is produced in the anagen or active growth phase. Following the anagen phase, the follicle enters in catagen phase, a period of controlled regression of the follicle. Finally, the telogen phase corresponds to resting stage, before hair shedding and entering a new hair cycle.

A hair shaft grows by approximately 0.3–0.5 mm per day, or around 1.0–1.5 centimeters per month. But a variety of factors can affect the hair growth cycle, and cause temporary or permanent hair loss (alopecia). These influences are both of external and internal origins, such as medication, radiation, chemotherapy, chemical exposure, hormonal and nutritional factors, thyroid and immune system imbalance, skin diseases, physiological or psychological stress.[6]

SKIN AND HAIR DIVERSITY

Understanding the physiology of normal skin and hair is a key point to provide appropriate response to cosmetic problem. Understanding the skin and hair diversities will also enable the most suitable responses to be provided for alleviating cosmetic problems that are specific to ethnic backgrounds.

Skin Diversity

The color of the skin, among other criteria, is probably the most obvious pattern that differentiates individuals (see Chapter 4). The level of pigmentation varies with the amount and nature/quality of melanin packaged within melanosomes in epidermis.[7] Largest melanosomes with optimal content in black eumelanin are identified in dark skin whereas light skin harbors the smallest organelles and, furthermore, is more prone to contain poorly protective yellow to red pheomelanins. Distributed singly within the keratinocytes in dark skin, melanosomes are found as scattered clusters in light skin. They are identified in the outermost epidermal layers, i.e. the SC, in dark skin unlike in light skin. The increased eumelanin content provides protection against UV rays, albeit of a limited potential. Recent studies focused on the relationship between skin color types and UV-induced damage.[8,9] Using an objective tool to measure skin color, it was shown that all skin color types were sensitive to UV's with an inverse relationship between constitutive pigmentation and UV-induced DNA damage. A light to tan skins present higher risks of DNA damage than brown and dark skin types. It is thus of paramount importance to develop appropriate tests to better grasp problems specific to different skin photo-types.[10]

Apart from skin color, some other physiological differences do exist between different ethnicities. Girardeau et al.[11] showed that African DEJ is characterized by highly convoluted appearance, as compared to

Caucasian and that papillary dermis is more active in dark-skinned subjects likely explaining the delayed onset of skin aging signs among dark-skinned population.

Color and structure are related to the biomechanical properties of skin such as extensibility, elasticity and recovery. These differences are thought being linked at least partly to the UV protection afforded by endogenous melanin pigments to darker skin.

Dyspigmentation is a significant concern in some populations with dark skin including Asian, Hispanic, African and Indian populations. This type of skin indeed entails specific pigmentation patterns, which can be prevented or mitigated by cosmetic care. Disorders may range from uneven pigmentation encountered in normal skin to discoloration, post inflammatory hyperpigmentation and melasma. Appropriate cosmetics are being developed to address such conditions.

New tools are now available to better understand the diversity of skin. In particular, the development and availability of pigmented reconstructed skin models can bring new insights in the comprehension of different biological mechanisms.

Hair Diversity

Hair diversity, its style, color, shape and growth pattern is one of our most defining characteristics.

Hair shape is initially defined in the bulb of the follicle and not by the angle of emergence from the skin surface.[12] The shape of the hair shaft is then very diversified from straight to very curly.[13] A method was developed to classify hair in eight different shape patterns based on morphologic parameters, regardless of ethnic origin. The hair structural characteristics were analyzed according to four parameters related to hair curliness (curve diameter and curl index) and kinking of the hair (number of waves and number of twists).[14] The shape of hair fiber plays a role in the hair physical properties. For example, a study showed that fiber dimensions were linked to alterations of hair induced by shaking process. Hairs of a large cross-sectional area (Asian hairs in general) logically appear to be less breakable than those of a smaller cross-sectional area.[15]

There is also a great diversity in hair structure with age. Based upon the examination of very long hair (length > 4 m), a study has explored the natural ageing process of hair. The Asian woman involved in this study had no hair cut for 26 years and had carefully prevented her hair from chemical and environmental aggressions. The study showed that hair gradually changed from outside to inside. The cuticle was firstly degraded with loss of shine, smoothness and hydrophobic protection. Cortex then appeared degraded, leading to loss of mechanical resistance. Lastly, the keratin network was damaged with breakages and split ends. This model of hair degradation, indicating changes along the fiber, provides a model of the time-dependent damage process of human hair.[16]

Panhard et al. studied the diversity of hair greying depending on ethnic/geographical origin in 1,464 middle aged volunteers from various part of the world.[17] The age of onset of hair greying and its progression with age clearly differed with ethnic/geographical origins: subjects of Asian and African descent had less grey hair than those of the same age of Caucasian descent. For example, the frequency of hair greying in volunteers aged 45–65 years was 78% in the Indian subgroup, as compared to 43% in Sub-Saharan African, 62% in Japanese and 93% in French subgroups.

Some new investigations attempt to explain those observations at the biological level. Hair color is indeed one of the most conspicuous phenotypes in humans, ranging from black, brown, blond to red. This diversity arises mostly from the amount and ratio of the black-dark brown eumelanin and the reddish-brown pheomelanin. Recent studies by Commo et al. on the chemical composition of melanin pigments in hair of different ethnic origin and ages showed that eumelanin contents were significantly higher in African-American hairs, followed by East-Asian and Caucasian hairs.[18] The study also suggests that the production of eumelanin declines with age, possibly because of progressive loss of function, absence of expression of dopachrome tautomerase (TRP2) in the hair follicle melanocytes. Ultimately, a white hair, i.e. deprived of any pigment, shows a complete absence of melanocytes within the bulb.

CONCLUSION

Hair and skin physiologies are very similar irrespective of country and ethnic origins. However, differences in skin color, and cultural and environmental variations influence hair and skin physiologies and should therefore be taken into account when comparing scientific works performed in different parts of the world. Further works offering an increased knowledge of hair and skin physiologies in India are needed, towards an adequate understanding and evaluation of cosmetics and dermatologic treatments.

REFERENCES

1. Zhang XJ, Liu WD, He CD. Basic science for modern dermatology. Beijing: People's Medical Publishing House, 2001.
2. Liu W, Zhang HL. Skin science and efficacy evaluation of cosmetics. Beijing: Chemical Industry Publishing House, 2005.
3. Baran R, Maibach HI. Textbook of Cosmetic Dermatology, 3rd edition. UK: Taylor & Francis Group; 2005.
4. Chu D. In: Wolff K, Goldsmith LA, Katz SI, et al. Fitzpatrick's dermatology in general medicine. 7th edition. New York: McGraw Hill; 2008: pp. 57-66.
5. Wilkinson JD, Shaw, S. Skin tests, In: Bouillon C (Ed). 2nd edition. The Science of Hair Care. Marcel Dekker Inc., New York and Basel, 2005.
6. Bernard B. La vie révélée du follicule du cheveu humain. Medecine sciences. 2006;22:138-43.
7. Alaluf S, Adkins D, Barrett K, et al. Ethnic variation in melanin content and composition in photoexposed and photoprotected human skin. Pigment Cell Res. 2002;15:112-8.
8. Del Bino S, Sok J, Bessac E, et al. Relationship between skin response to ultraviolet exposure and skin color type. Pigment Cell Res. 2006;19:606-14.
9. Del Bino S, Sok J, Bernerd F. Assessment of ultraviolet-radiation-induced DNA damage within melanocytes in skin of different constitutive pigmentation. Br J Dermatol. 2013;168:1120-3.
10. Régnier M, Staquet MJ, Schmitt D, et al. Integration of Langerhans cells into pigmented reconstructed human epidermis. J Invest Dermatol. 1997;109:510-12.
11. Girardeau S, Mine S, Pageon H, et al. The Caucasian and African skin types differ morphologically and functionally in their dermal component. Exp Dermatol. 2009;18:704-11.
12. Thibaut S, Bernard BA. The biology of hair shape. Int J Dermatol. 2005;44:2-3.
13. Thibaut S, Gaillard O, Bouhanna P, et al. Human hair shape is programmed from the bulb. Brit J Derm. 2005;152:632-8.
14. Loussouarn G, Garcel AL, Lozano I, et al. Worldwide diversity of hair curliness: a new method of assessment. Int J Dermatol. 2007;46:2-6.
15. Galliano A, Saint Olive Baque C, Marty G, et al. Resistance of human hair cuticle after a shaking process in wet conditions: comparison between Chinese and Caucasian hair. Int J Cosm Sci. 2010;32:356-68.
16. Thibaut S, de Becker E, Bernard BA, et al. Chronological ageing of human hair keratin fibres. Int J Cosm Sci. 2010;32:422-34.
17. Panhard S, Lozano I, Loussouarn G. Greying of the human hair: a worldwide survey, revisiting the '50' rule of thumb. Br J Dermatol. 2012;167:865-73.
18. Commo S, Wakamatsu K, Lozano I, et al. Age-dependent changes in eumelanin composition in hairs of various ethnic origins. Int J Cosmet Sci. 2012;34:102-7.

Chapter 2

In Vivo Noninvasive Methods and Imaging Techniques for Investigating the Skin

Anupama Wagle, *L'Oréal Research and Innovation, Mumbai, India*
Uday Khopkar, *KEM Hospital and Seth GS Medical College Mumbai, India*

INTRODUCTION

The human skin is a complex structure that affords protection *vis à vis* the assaults from the external environment. Its outermost layer, the stratum corneum (SC), represents the true interface with the environment and is a clear example of the successful adaptation of a tissue. The stratum corneum is heterogeneous in structure and has been compared to a brick-wall model, in which non-continuous, essentially proteinaceous, terminally differentiated keratinocytes or corneocytes (bricks) are embedded into a continuous matrix of specialized lipids (mortar). The SC consists of 12–16 layers of flattened corneocytes which have a mean thickness of 1 μm and mean surface area of 1,000 μm^2 according to age.

The skin is a sensitive dynamic boundary. It offers protection from infection, ultraviolet rays and trauma. It is essential for controlling water and contributes to the synthesis of essential substances such as vitamin D and other major substances such as collagen, elastin, melanin, etc. The skin is also an important organ of social and sexual contact. Its perception, deeply rooted within cultures of all social groups, is largely driven by its appearance and associated structures. The present chapter deals with novel, non-invasive bioengineering methods of measuring and imaging as tools for evaluating all aspects of the skin. The advantage of bioengineering and imaging techniques is that almost all the properties of the living skin and their changes in healthy (aging) or in pathologic (e.g. dermatitis, psoriasis) conditions are now objectively measurable and quantifiable under non-invasive ways.

These non invasive methods are by nature objective, quantitative, and generally investigator independent, and can be calibrated and validated *in vivo* and/or *in vitro* on reconstructed skin models. If bioengineering measurements are properly performed under standard conditions, they can also lead to a harmonization of results/data and allow inter-laboratory and inter-observer comparisons to be made.

SKIN MOISTURE ASSESSMENT

Water plays an important role in the complex structure of the SC which influences its elasticity, tensile strength, barrier characteristics and electrical resistance. In the absence of water, the SC is an intrinsically rigid and brittle structure prone to cracking. The state of hydration of the SC is governed by three factors:

1. Water arising from the underlying epidermis.
2. Water loss due to evaporation from the surface.
3. Intrinsic ability of this horny layer to hold water.

The water content of the normal SC should be in the range of 10–20%. Under 10%, the skin looks dry, rough or may even show chaps. To keep the skin with proper moisture level, it is essential to maintain unaltered the physiological environment of skin and promote normal metabolic activity. Moisturizing cosmetic products increase the water content of the SC by their capacity to retain water, mimicking skin natural moisturizing factor (NMF), or by preventing uncontrolled water loss, by reinforcing the SC lipid content. Based on the various modes of action of cosmetics, different techniques can be used to evaluate skin moisturization.

Electrical Properties

The flow of an electrical current (μA range) through the skin surface is related to the water content of the SC. This directly affects the conductance and capacitance of the skin. However, these parameters are not linearly related to the water content of the skin and are affected by other factors such as the presence of ions, dipolar proteins as well as water bound to keratin.

Conductance Measurements[1,2]

The water present in the SC contains various solutes that conduct electrical current, a capacity used in equipments such as SKICON™. Skin conductance is measured as a high frequency current of 3.5 MHz passes through the skin, using electrodes consisting of a 2 mm diameter disk and a guard ring with an external diameter of 4 mm, creating a 1 mm distance between the inner and outer probe. When the probe is placed onto the measured area, a high-frequency current flows and measurement values are given in micro-Siemens units from 0 μs to 1999 μs.

Capacitance Measurements[2,3]

Skin capacitance, resulting from such a naturally dielectric medium, reflects its hydration state. The higher the water content, the higher the capacitance. Capacitance sensors can then record the dielectric constant of the skin which changes with water content.

The measuring probe (0.65 cm^2) consists of an interdigitated grid of gold covered electrodes. On the probe head, a thin piece of glass avoids direct galvanic contact between the electrode and skin the surface. An electric scattered field penetrates the very first layers of the skin up to 10–20 μm during measurement and the dielectric constant is determined. One track builds up a surplus of electrons (anode), the other a lack of electrons (cathode), creating an electric field. The repetition frequency varies from 1.15 MHz for a very dry medium to 0.95 MHz for a very hydrated medium, measurements being given in arbitrary units, from 0 AU to 120 AU.

The capacitance method is associated with a short measuring time (seconds) and good reproducibility. To date, the assessment of moisturizing cosmetic products is often performed using Corneometer™ (Courage & Khazaka, Köln, Germany).

Skin Capacitance Imaging (SCI)[4-6]

A special type of non-optical skin surface imaging called SkinChip™ has been developed (Fig. 1). This method is an

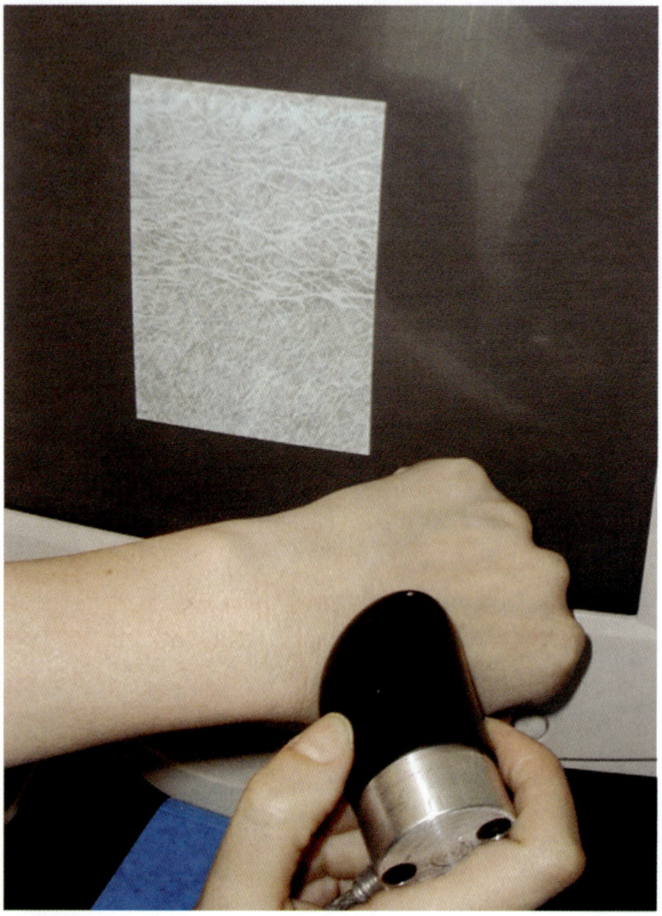

Figure 1: SkinChip™ measurement
©L'Oréal Research and Innovation/Catherine Olivry

application of the silicon image sensor (SIS) technology initially developed for recording fingerprints for security reasons. The sensor is composed of 92160 micro-capacitors dispersed onto a 18 x 12.8 mm sensor plate which measures skin capacitance every 50 μm. These micro-capacitors are protected by a thin silicon oxide layer and therefore closely applied to the skin surface for 5 seconds, a short and sufficient time for recording its capacitance profile.

The SCI images are acquired and displayed in real time on a computer screen where capacitance values are transformed into a range of 256 gray levels to form a non-optical image, where the darker pixels represent high capacitance and the clearer ones, a low capacitance value. The mean gray level of the image then represents the average skin surface hydration. This correlates well with

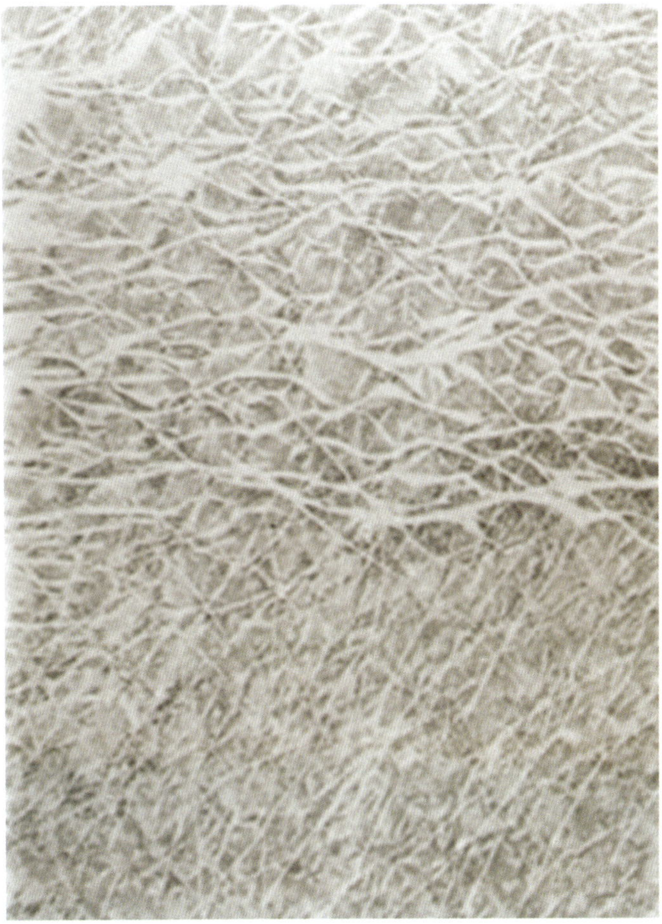

Figure 2: Visualization of a nonhydrated leg skin (upper part) versus hydrated skin (lower part) with Skinchip™ ©L'Oréal Research and Innovation

the average capacitance value of the Corneometer™. The latter averages the capacitance of the contact area while SkinChip™ not only displays a more detailed distribution histogram of the capacitance value but images the skin micro-relief (fine line and cross-line orientations) and its changes with aging. Treating skin with an efficient moisturizer results in a darker capacitance image of the skin with more regular micro-relief network (Fig. 2). Sweating can also be quantitatively measured and visualized.[6] Subcutaneous immunotherapy (SCIT) was also used to study numerous skin lesions: acne pustules and papules, warts, keratoses, pityriasis versicolor, nevi, psoriatic lesions, etc. In some cases, lesions, quite invisible to the naked eye can be easily detected by SCIT because of anhidrotic conditions.[7]

Transepidermal Water Loss[8-10]

Transepidermal water loss refers to the flux of water (in $g/m^2/h$) that continuously diffuses/evaporates from the skin toward the environment, not to be confused with sweat production. Since mostly governed by the structural organization of the SC (and its changes with various disorders) and its thickness, measuring TEWL provides crucial information on the state of the SC. A flaky, disorganized or thinned SC will invariably lead to elevated TEWL values. For example, in the case of specific dermatitis such as psoriasis or ichthyosis or other dry skin diseases, the water level is very low and TEWL is higher than normal. Since TEWL is linked to the hydration level of skin, it is often used together with measurement of water content in horny layer to evaluate the effect of moisturizing cosmetics and to assess and compare the effects of different skincare products.

Since SC quality greatly influences TEWL amplitude, any fluctuations of relative humidity and/or air temperature must be avoided during the measurement; a special room equipped with temperature and humidity control is needed to ensure reproducible results. Two techniques are available for measuring such an important parameter:

1. *Open-chamber technique*: The principle of Open-chamber device is based on Fick's diffusion law. It measures the gradient of water vapor evaporating from the skin surface using an open sensor placed perpendicular onto the skin surface. The probe consists of an open cylinder including two humidity and two thermal sensors located at different distances above the skin surface. From these measurements, the flux of water vapor can be calculated in $mg/cm^2/min$ or $g/m^2/hour$.
2. *Closed-chamber technique*: The difference from Open-chamber technique lies in the closed top of the measuring chamber. A cylindrical hood covers the skin to gather vapor evaporating from the skin surface. One temperature and humidity sensor is used to record the relative humidity. The change in vapor concentration is initially rapid and then gradually decreases as the humidity reaches near 100%. Closed-chamber method does not enable TEWL to be recorded continuously since skin evaporation decreases when the air in the closed chamber reaches water vapor saturation.

Spectroscopic Properties

Attenuated Total Reflectance Fourier Transform Infrared Spectroscopy (ATR-FTIR)[11]

This technique is directly used to estimate the skin surface water in vivo. The absorption for amide-I (1,645 cm^{-1}) is influenced by proteins and water while amide-II (1545 cm^{-1}) is restricted to proteins. The water content of the SC can thus be estimated by calculating the ratio between the two attenuation measurements (amide-I/amide-II= Moisture Factor). The depth of measurement varies slightly with the instrument and wavelength, generally considered a few μm below the surface.

Further improvement in this technique using O-H expansion/contraction at 2,100 cm^{-1} has been suggested. The water content of removed SC (using tape strippings) calculated through gravimetry shows good linearity up to 0.2 g H_2O/cm^2 and using such measurements, the estimated moisture content of the skin surface layers is about 9%.

Raman Spectroscopy [12,13]

In this method, the sample of interest is illuminated by a laser beam of a very narrow wavelength band. The electrical component of the electromagnetic field within the laser beam drives the electronic cloud of the molecules present in the sample. The driven and oscillating electronic cloud re-emits most of the collided laser light without energy loss, the only difference being the direction in which the photons are ejected from the molecules. This process is referred to as elastic scattering (Rayleigh scattering), where a very small amount of laser light scatters the ejected photons of a different energy from the injected photon, the difference in energy being released or taken up by the molecules. By measuring the intensity and energy of the re-emitted light of frequencies different than the laser frequency, a Raman spectrum can be obtained.

Raman spectroscopy is a truly non-invasive analytical technique for studying the composition of human SC at the molecular level. The monitoring of topically applied skin penetrating agents can be studied with time along with their interaction with skin components such as water, collagen, lipids, etc.

Near Infrared Spectroscopy[14,15]

The use of near infrared spectroscopy (NIR) to measure SC water content has been reported by de Rigal et al. in 1993. Water molecules have two distinct near infrared absorption bands at 1,450 nm and 1,940 nm. The authors measured the difference between peak absorption of the water molecule at 1,940 nm and the lowest absorption at 1,100 nm for skin and compared it with skin surface conductance and clinical signs. They found that the severity of dry skin more closely corresponded with the difference in absorbance than with skin surface conductance, indicating that NIR measurements extend beyond the SC.

SEBUM LEVEL MEASUREMENT

Sebaceous glands secrete sebum and excrete it onto the skin surface, where sebum diffuses and is emulsified with sweat to form a sebum film that keeps the skins surface smooth and glossy and also prevents water evaporation from the body. Sebum has the function of lubricating skin. Therefore, a certain amount of sebum is necessary for healthy skin, preventing the skin from becoming dry and from fissuring and chapping. Sebum also increases skin elasticity and its capacity to resist stress and insults from the surroundings. However, excess sebum not only results in shiny skin and a dark color, but also favors the development of acne and blemishes that affect the appearance of the skin. Excessive sebum secretion is indeed one major factor that fuels skin diseases such as acne and seborrheic dermatitis.

Some skincare products can alter the sebum level to maintain a normal sebum film. Monitoring sebum excretion on the skin surface may be helpful for studies on sebum-related diseases conducted by clinicians.[16] Accurately measuring the sebum level is of great value for evaluating the effect of these products, understanding the skin type on the face and preventing and mitigating seborrheic diseases. Researchers can choose the most appropriate method based upon the requirements of the study project and thoroughly consider the requirements of each method and the value of information generated by collected data.

Sebumeter

Sebumeter® (Courage & Khazaka, Germany), a commercial device, is now commonly used. It is based on the principle of photometer and measures the change in transmittance of an adhesive tape 0.1 mm thick. The higher the amount

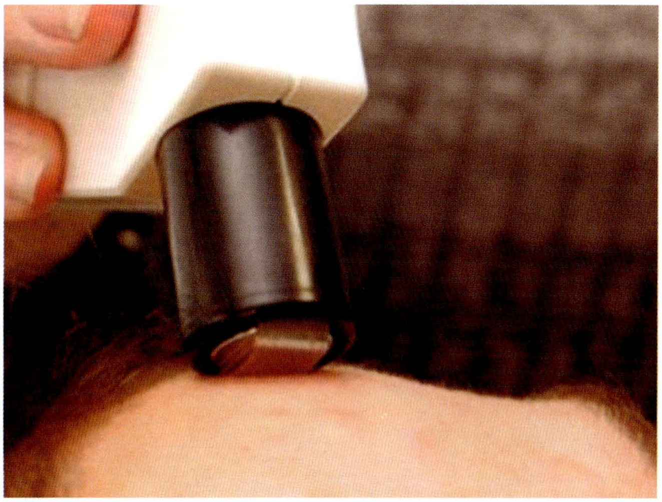

Figure 3: Sebumeter measurement
©L'Oréal Research and Innovation

of sebum absorbed by the adhesive tape, the greater the recorded increase in transmittance; thus, the content of skin sebum can be measured indirectly.[17] Sebumeter® has a probe with small volume and is convenient to use; it can measure the sebum at any site (Fig. 3). The result is expressed as µg sebum/cm² and the whole process takes 30 seconds.

Sebutape

Another measurement technique is Sebutape® (CuDerm Corporation, Dallas, USA), which also uses a special sebum-absorbing adhesive tape. However, unlike the above method, it is firstly used to remove fat from the skin area to be tested. The special tape is placed onto the skin. After a contact time of one hour, some transmittance spots may be observed. They correspond to excreting (active) follicles. Excreted sebum is gradually absorbed by the tape. After removing the tape, transmittance spots and their surface area can be measured with a simple image analysis software. The special sebum-absorbing tape is an oil-absorbing micropore film. Since fat does not scatter light, the micropore film becomes transparent when air in the micropores is replaced by absorbed fat. The design characteristics of the micropore film minimize the diffusion of fat on both sides of the micropore so that the outlets of active follicles create a distinct border. The size of the transparent zone can be used to detect the amount of sebum. To perform the measurement, the film is placed over a dark background for convenient visual evaluation and computer-assisted image analysis. The parameters measured with Sebutape include the amount of absorbed sebum, the number of sebum spots, and the largest and smallest sebum spots. Extraordinary large and fusional sebum spots are commonly seen in patients with seborrheic dermatitis. The evaluation must be conducted within 24 hours of removing the tape to avoid lateral spreading. If the sample cannot be assessed immediately, it is suggested to keep it under -30°C.

Other Methods

There are also gravimetric methods that are rarely used today because they are cumbersome and time consuming. They are based on the use of solvents (ethyl ether) to remove sebum from a cigarette paper pressed onto the skin surface for hours.

SKIN AGING ASSESSMENT

All living organisms are subjected to aging, a multifaceted process that differs for various organisms. In humans, it is a physiological process corresponding to a progressive loss in the homeostatic capacity of the organs and tissues. As for skin, two main processes are involved in aging. First, the intrinsic changes induced by chronological aging that progressively affect the skin structure, physiology and mecanobiology. Second, since skin is the organ most exposed to environmental conditions (e.g. sun exposure and related UVB and UVA rays), exposure will lead to deep changes at both cellular and molecular levels, in turn modifying the skin texture and appearance.

A major feature of skin aging is loss of its elasticity. Many different non-invasive instruments are available for evaluating the mechanical properties of the skin, based on various mechanical stresses including tensile, torsional, indentation or suction skin deformations.

Elasticity Measurement

Suction Method[18-20]

In this method, the skin is stretched perpendicularly to its plane by applying a given depression or suction. In the late 1980s, Courage & Khazaka Electronics developed an instrument based on the suction method called

Cutometer™. A negative pressure is applied to the surface of the skin, using a vacuum pump which draws the skin into the probe. This causes a vertical displacement of the skin to the plane, which is measured by a noncontact optical system. This optical system consists of a light source and a receiver, two glass prisms facing each other and leading the light from the transmitter to the receiver. The reduction in the infrared light beam, depending on the elevation of the skin, is recorded. It can also measure Stress time curve in which the vacuum is suddenly applied and released. From this curve, the pure elastic properties, elastic recovery and viscoelastic properties can be quantified. These have clearly been shown to be related to the degree of aging and skin laxity.

Torsion Method [21,22]

The measurement is performed parallel to the skin surface in order to give a stronger influence to the skin's upper layers (epidermis and dermis versus hypodermis). The most frequently used parameters are extensibility and torsion recovery. The commercial instrument is Twistometer® (or Torquemeter®, Diastron, UK) (Fig. 4). In the torsional method, a central disk is attached to the skin with adhesive tape and rotates under a predetermined torque. The amount of skin under test is limited by a stationary guard ring that is attached by adhesive tape. The gap between the central disk and the concentric guard ring is of critical importance. When measuring the upper layers of the skin, maximum sensitivity is achieved by restricting the gap to 1 mm. For studies of full skin thickness, the gap is increased to 5 mm, allowing the torsional forces to be applied to the deeper layers.

When a torque is applied onto the skin, an initial rapid rotation is followed by a slower exponential phase as the skin progressively resists the torsional forces. The initial rapid phase, which is referred as Ue, is a measure of the extensibility of the skin and has been demonstrated to be a useful measure of SC hydration. The slower phase is due to a creeping effect, which reflects the viscosity and plasticity of skin. When the torque is removed, a progressive recovery from the deformation allows the immediate or delayed recovery (skin elasticity) to be defined.

Sophisticated analysis algorithms have been applied to the curve data with a reported increase in the sensitivity of the method.

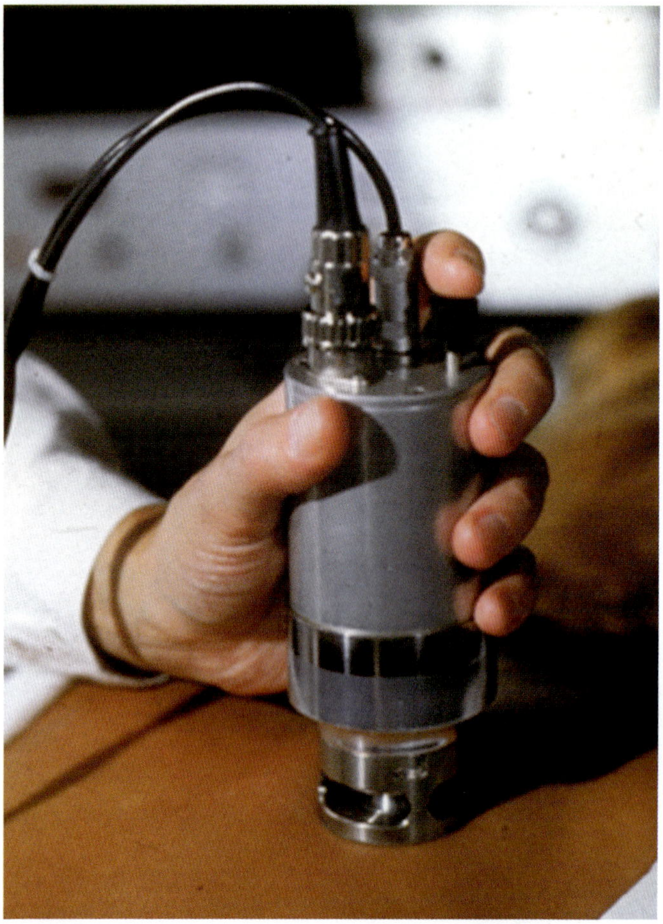

Figure 4: Twistometer®
©L'Oréal Research and Innovation/Stéphane Lefebvre

Indentation Method [23]

This method is based upon the traditional ballistometry principle of impacting an object at a constant force and measuring skin firmness by indentation and dynamic resilience (elasticity) through the degree of rebounds. The torsional ballistometer consists of a 25 cm long slim line probe. The probe contains a rigid low mass arm suspended at its balance point on a torsion wire. A ruby tipped stylus is fixed to one end. The arm is activated by a solenoid that elevates the probe tip from the test surface. When released, the arm oscillates around its balance position and the stylus bounces repeatedly on the test site, up to cessation. The position of the arm is monitored by an optical sensor.

The peak penetration depth of the probe tip provides indentation: the more the identation, the looser the skin. Greater numbers of rebounds imply higher skin elasticity.

Resonance Methods[24,25]

Measurement of resonance running time (RRT) has been shown to be inversely related to skin stiffness. The probe head contains two sensors that are placed on the skin. The first emits an acoustical shockwave and the other serves as a receiver. Shockwaves propagate differently through the skin according to the state of the elastic fibers and the moisture content. The time needed by the wave to travel from emitter to receiver is the recorded parameter.

Aged skin is characterized, among other symptoms, by profound changes in the orientation of collagen fibers in the dermis. In young skin, these fibers are very small and are oriented in all directions (isotropy). With age, the fibers thicken, with a preferential orientation (anisotropy). The degree of isotropy/anisotropy in dermis can be evaluated using the Reviscometer®. The propagation speed of the shockwave applied to the skin surface at different angles gives the degree of isotropy/anisotropy.

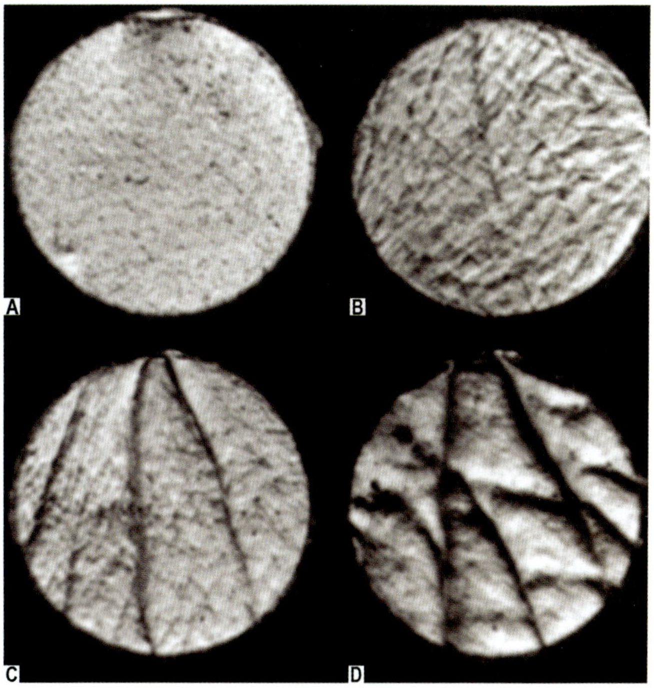

Figure 5: Prints of crow's feet wrinkles from four different ages (from A to D, A being the youngest)
©L'Oreal Research and Innovation

Skin Surface Microrelief

The skin surface is not perfectly flat, and is characterized by a special relief which probably reproduces the 3D organization of the deeper layers (Fig. 5). A simple examination with the naked eye, or with high microscopic magnification or by hand palpation can give qualitative information.

According to the technology used, the most frequent methods applied to the study of skin topography can be separated into four subgroups:

1. *Optical profilometry*:[26,27] Optical profilometry is a non-contact interferometric method for characterizing skin surface topography from skin silicone replicas. There are two set ups of this principle:

   a. Autofocusing system: In this system, a diode laser is focused on a point of the replica, the reflected part being focused on a detector which pilots the position of the focusing lens with a motor. When the object is moved, any relief variation loses focus and decreases the intensity of the light received by the detector. This would be followed by focusing lens repositioning at the convergence point of the light beam, and hence recording microrelief profile.

   b. Triangulation system: This method uses three reference points of the fixed source, a laser diode; the point of the surface to be analyzed whose height varies according to the local relief; the image of this point formed by an optical system on the detector plane. When the whole measurement system is displaced relative to the surface, the image formed on the detector changes position and the measurement of this position gives the height of the measured point relative to that of the previous image point.

2. *Mechanical profilometry*:[28] This technique is based on the linear displacement of a stylus along the surface of a skin replica. Its successive vertical movements (i.e. valleys and peaks) alter the voltage of the output signal, which is then digitized to display reconstructed 2D profiles and subsequent 3D images.

3. *Laser profilometry*:[29,30] It is an optical method based upon the amplification and reflection of light from the

skin replica, depending on the topography. It includes three different techniques. The first uses dynamic focusing, the laser beam being permanently focused on the specimen. The height of a point at its surface is deduced from the position of the mobile lens (Fig. 6). The other two are based upon the theory of triangulation (Fig. 7). Either single or double triangulation can be used. As the height of the specimen varies, the position of the light spot, reflected onto the detector, also varies, enabling the height of the specimen to be determined.

Common to these three techniques, the surface of the specimen is scanned by means of a table moved mechanically in X and Y axes. The recorded variable height (Z axis) therefore allows a 3D representation of the skin surface to be obtained.

4. *Interference fringe profilometry:*[29] This consists in calculating a phase image from interference fringe image projection, giving access to the altitude of each point. The fundamental principle of this system is based upon a projective Moire Profiler that projects the image of a reference grating onto the surface of the object under test. A CCD camera then acquires fringes that are later computerized (Fig. 8). By processing the Moire fringes of the surface of the object under test with the computer-added phase

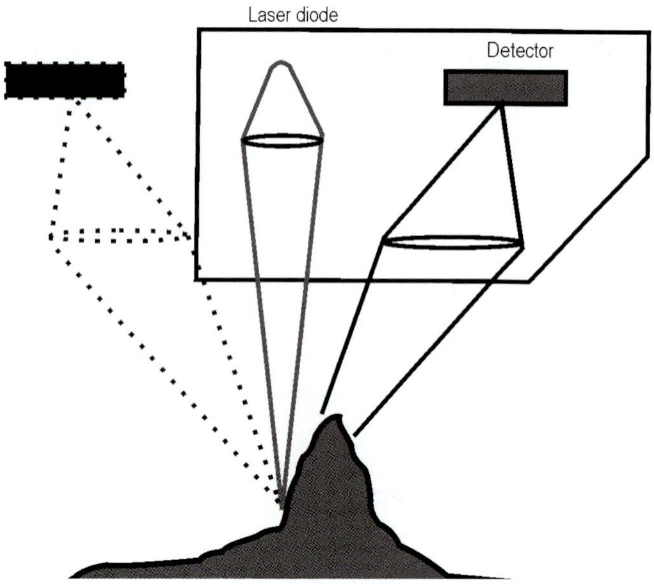

Figure 7: Surface measurement by double triangulation method ©L'Oréal Research and Innovation

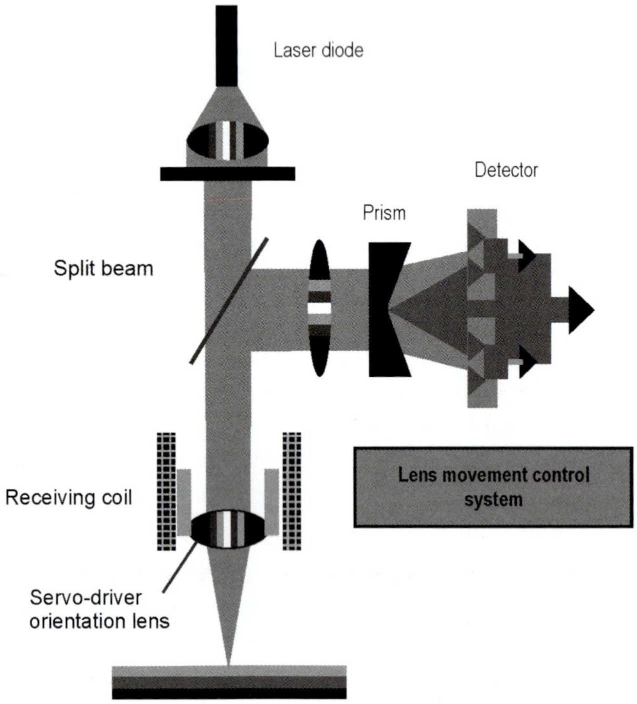

Figure 6: Principle of surface measurement by laser scanning ©L'Oréal Research and Innovation

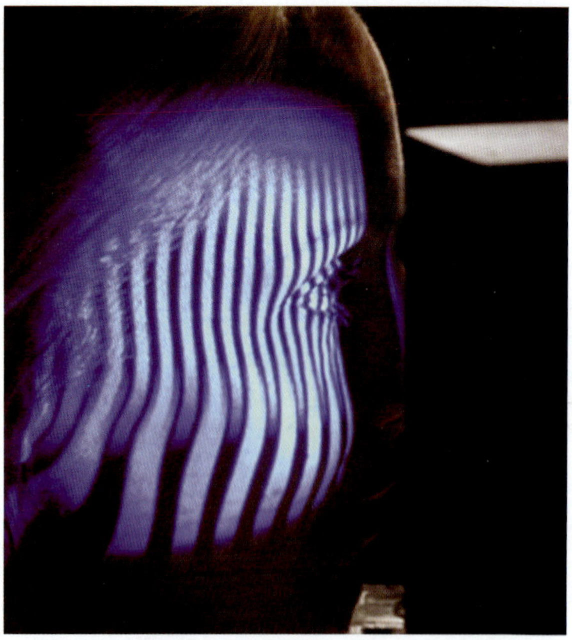

Figure 8: Fringe profilometry measurement © L'Oréal Research and Innovation/Isabelle Walter

shifting algorithm, the 3D shape information of the object can be obtained.

SKIN COLOR ASSESSMENT

Human skin is not an opaque surface. Rather, skin has depth and layers, and its appearance is in part determined by the relative proportion between reflected and absorbed light. The amount and color of reflected light is, in turn, determined by the nature and distribution of light absorbing molecules (chromophores) beneath the SC, particularly melanins, hemoglobin and carotenoids.

Facial skin normally allows more than 90% of light to penetrate its surface.[31] White light passing through the skin's transparent surface is scattered back toward the surface by dermal collagen, which acts essentially as a mirror within the skin. The color of light during its journey into the skin becomes modified by the various chromophores, and is reflected back toward the surface. This modified light color is then diffused by the SC, generating a variably luminous glow. Skin color measurements have extensive applications in the fields of skin cosmetology and the skin pigmentation disorders. The classification of skin color is not only helpful to distinguish ethnical-differences, but also to predict the extent of pigmentation and erythema after sunburn. People with darker skin are more likely to develop increased pigmentation after sun exposure, whereas those with lighter skin are more prone to exhibit sunburn.[32,33]

Tristimulus Colorimeter[34,35]

The most used reflectance spectrophotometers for skin color measurement are Chromameter CR™ series. The probe consists of a pulsed xenon arc lamp which illuminates the skin surface. The light reflected by the skin is described in absolute values in a 3D colorimetric system defined by Commission Internationale de l'Eclairage (CIE) that converts it into L*a*b*. The L* value, ranging from the black (0) to white scale (100), is mostly affected by melanin content: the higher the melanin content, the lower the L*. The a* value ranges from red to green region: the higher the a*, the redder the skin. The b* value mainly indicates the yellowness of skin (the higher the b*, the yellower the skin), but is also affected by melanin.

Full Band Reflectance Spectrometer[36]

This technique of skin color measurement is found in instruments like the derma spectrometer or Mexameter™. This skin is illuminated by a light-emitting diode (LED). The reflected light then passes through filters specific to three wavelengths, namely 568 nm (green light), 660 nm (red light) and 870 nm (in the near infrared range). The reflected light at these wavelengths is detected by a photodiode and a built-in microcomputer calculates erythema and melanin indexes.

SKIN IMAGING TECHNIQUES AND SYSTEMS

Most diagnoses in dermatology rely on visual/clinical examination of the skin, i.e. a non-invasive approach. Most physician diagnosis criteria include anatomic distribution, color, configuration and visible surface changes of a given lesion. In some cases, an invasive (and somewhat painful) punch biopsy has to be performed and further processed histologically to confirm a given diagnosis. In brief, there is a clear need for developing non-invasive methods providing a clear imaging of the skin surface and its deeper structures. Imaging modalities relevant to skin include various modifications of electromagnetic wave imaging (optical, infrared, nuclear magnetic resonance), acoustical wave imaging, mechanical wave imaging. Usually, tomographic images, i.e. 2D cross-sectional images are acquired by a medical imaging system. The 3D tissue volumes are usually imaged by acquiring stacks of consecutive 2D images.[37]

Polarized Imaging Technique[35,36,38,39]

Among the various attributes associated with skin beauty, skin radiance is paramount. The latter is an optical parameter amounted the light emitted from an object as a light source. Although this definition becomes rather vague when applied to the skin, many experiments were conducted to understand this aspect, most using the polarizing image system as an objective tool.

This system uses an instrument called Samba, initially developed by Bossa Nova Technologies™. It consists of an illumination unit equipped with linear polarizing filters and a high resolution digital camera equipped with liquid-crystal polarizer, the polarization angle of which can be electronically flipped from the direction

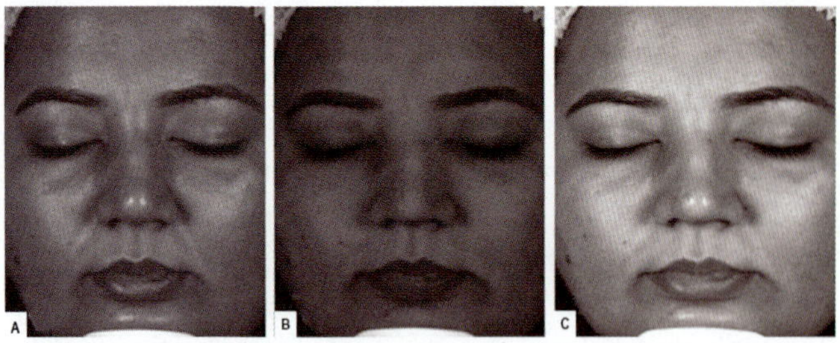

Figure 9: Polarized images using the Samba technique. **A,** P-image giving subsurface and surface reflection. **B,** C-image representing subsurface reflection. **C,** S-image derived by pixel subtraction of P- and C-images
©L'Oréal Research and Innovation

parallel (P) to the plane of polarization of the polarizing filters of the illumination unit to the one that is at 90° to this direction referring to the crossed (C) orientation. When the two polarizing filters are parallel, both the surface and subsurface reflections are present in the resulting image. However, when the two polarizing polarization filters are oriented in a cross-position, surface reflection is excluded and the subsurface reflection is only present in the crossed image (C-image). By subtracting the corresponding pixels in the C-image from those in the P-image, a surface reflectance S-image can be extracted (Fig. 9).

Dermascopy or Dermatoscopy[40-42]

It is a diagnostic technique used worldwide for identifying and diagnosing skin lesions. A dermascope is similar to a magnifying lens, having inbuilt features of an illuminated system, with increased magnification. Structures as deep as the reticular dermis can be assessed. Besides, it enables images to be recorded.

The working principle of dermascopy lies in the transillumination of a lesion with a high magnification to visualize subtle features. Incident light undergoes reflection, refraction, diffraction and absorption, all based on physical properties of the skin. Dermascopy can be done either by the contact technique, which uses non-polarized light source to illuminate the skin surface, or bye the non-contact technique, where a liquid interface is used between the skin and the lens to reduce surface reflection. In the latter, there is no contact of the lens with the skin; the cross-polarized lens absorbs all the scattered light and hence allows only light to pass through a single plane.

A vast amount of software is available for objectively documenting the clinical features of digitized images. Once identified, the computer then extracts features of the lesion important to the physician, e.g. color, hue, texture, degree of asymmetry, degree of border irregularity, diameter, perimeter, length and area, etc.

Multispectral Imaging System[43,44]

Surface-spectral reflectance of an object is an inherent physical property of the object. Spectrophotometric intracutaneous analysis scope (SIAscope™) and Melafinder™ are two dermascopes using multispectral images as inputs for subsequent computer analysis. The SIAscope™ consists of a hand-held imaging probe covering a 12 mm diameter area that is placed in contact with the skin surface. High intensity LEDs illuminate the skin surface with eight consecutive discreet wavebands between 400 nm and 1000 nm, i.e. covering the visible spectrum and a small range of near infrared rays. These wavelength-dependent images provide information on the concentration, distribution and position of skin chromophores. The SIA algorithm determines the amount of collagen within the papillary dermis, using the infrared waveband, the epidermal and/or dermal melanin distribution, vessel distribution and topography of the dermal epidermal junction. This information is then displayed in different SIA graphs and corresponding images to assist the physician in diagnosis.

Ultrasound Imaging System[45-48]

This technique records the reflection of high frequency ultrasonic waves by the various components of the skin. Ultrasonic waves propagate through matter and their velocity is determined by the physicochemical properties of the tissue, among which the presence of water content is a major factor, i.e. a tissue free from water is non-echogenic. They cross skin structures and are reflected by the interfaces between different skin layers and some structural elements such as collagen bundles of the dermis. There are two basic types of ultrasonography with dermatologic applications. The most well established one is 20 MHz scanning, used to measure tumor thickness and /or skin thickness when treating inflammatory diseases such as scleroderma or psoriasis. Real-time sonography with 7.5–10 MHz probes has acquired an increasingly important role, since detecting subcutaneous tumors in a variety of clinical settings, including the preoperative stage and follow-up of melanoma surgery.

Ultrasound images are created due to the different acoustic properties of tissues. High-frequency sound impulses are transmitted into the skin and then reflected, refracted, or inflected when a tissue interface with different acoustic impedance is encountered. The intensity of the reflections at different depths in the skin is then plotted onto a display screen to give a one-dimensional graph, known as A-mode. The vertical cross-sectional image, which is the more familiar display of ultrasound data, is called B-mode scanning (brightness display). B-mode scanning uses the brightness level of multiple A-scans to build a 2D image. The current technology also allows 3D C-mode (computed) scanning of structures in skin *in vivo*. C-mode scans, still under development, may provide a better image than that from B-scans. The image of the echogenic structure of the skin can be recorded and the parameters can be measured with automated image processing.

Measuring skin thickness was the first application of this technique. Age, corticosteroids, diseases of connective tissue, skin allergy and irritation induce changes in skin thickness.[48,49] Comparison with histological data is fair and the use of ultrasound imaging for measuring the invasion depth of different types of tumor is often routinely performed before surgery.[50,51] Changes occurring within the skin as a result of aging have been also investigated. Ultrasound imaging showed a Sub-Epidermal Non- (or Low-) Echogenic Band (SENEB or SLEB) in the upper dermis of elderly women which was ascribed to UV-induced alterations in the collagen and elastin network of the upper dermis (Fig.10);[48] a low echogenicity means decreased heterogeneity of the medium, a hallmark of skin photoaging.

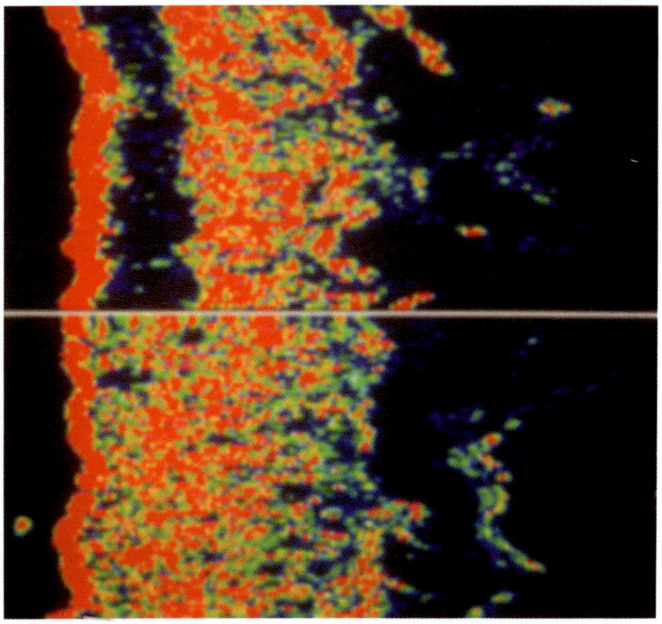

Figure 10: *In vivo* ultrasound image of sun-exposed skin (up) versus sun-protected skin (down): visualization of a Sub epidermal nonechogenic band in sun-exposed skin
©L'Oréal Research and Innovation

Optical Coherence Tomography[52-54]

Optical coherence tomography (OCT) is analogous to ultrasound B imaging, albeit using light instead of sound waves. It can be described as an intermediate imaging device between ultrasound and Confocal Scanning Laser Microscopy. The OCT technique is based upon the principle of Michelson interferometry. A pulse of near infrared, low coherence (super luminescent diode) light is split in such a way that half of the beam is sent to the specimen and half to a scanning reference mirror system. The light on the specimen is focused on the papillary skin layers, back scattering and recombining with the other reference beam of light reflected from the mirror system. An interference signal is only detected when the optical paths of both arms match with the coherence length of the light source. Measurement of the interference pattern allows the position within the tissue to be recorded where light is reflected. It is the reflectiveness of different components of tissues, such as cell membranes and melanin that provides contrast in the images. A 2D cross-sectional image is built up by lateral scanning across the tissue. Hence, much deeper layers of the skin can be imaged without much scattering as compared to ultrasound techniques. However, acquiring 2D OCT images is not sufficient to fully describe the 3D morphology of biological samples under study.

Optical coherence tomography images of healthy skin show some similarities with ultrasound images: a strong entrance signal corresponds to the amount of light reflected by the skin. Depending on the resolution level of the OCT device used, some other details of skin structure can be distinguished, e.g. the SC layer (two parallel lines) and the interface between the epidermis and the dermis

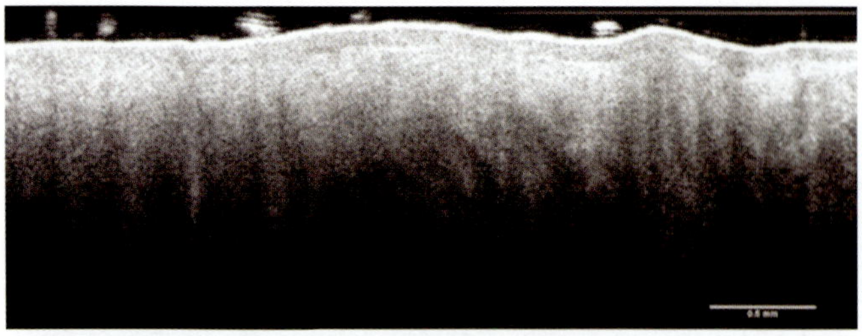

Figure 11: Optical coherent tomography (OCT) image of the crow-pad skin: Stratum corneum, epidermis and upper dermis may be distinguished
©L'Oréal Research and Innovation

owing to different gray levels (Fig. 11). Epidermis signal is less intense than that of the dermis one.[55] Due to a higher thickness, the SC and living epidermis are easily visible on the fingertips. In this area, sweat ducts can be recognized. The effects on skin of treatment by some drugs and cosmetics can be investigated using OCT imaging and have been reported. Other studies characterize irritant dermatitis, psoriasis, wound healing and skin tumors.[53] Effect of aging on the dermal-epidermal junction in women has been recently published.[52]

Magnetic Resonance Imaging

Developed in the early seventies, magnetic resonance imaging (MRI) is based on the interaction of an applied magnetic field with the spin of protons. The method is now routinely used in hospitals for clinical diagnosis. Magnetic resonance imaging is a highly flexible technique for making images of the whole human body. A Hydrogen (proton) nucleus behaves like a small magnet, implying that when the body is exposed to a strong external magnetic field, its own protons will align with the magnetic field. When properly excited, the protons (spin momentum) rotate around the direction of the applied magnetic field, producing a measurable signal in a nearby detector coil. The frequency of precession movement being proportional to the local magnetic field, making the field varying across the body, the signals arising from different locations are distinguished according to their frequency.

There are three basic components in a MRI system: (1) a large, static magnetic field (e.g. 3 Tesla for the human imagers at the Center; (2) radiofrequency (RF) coils that are used as a transmitter to excite the MR signal, and as a receiver to detect the MR signal; and (3) gradient coils that are pulsed on and off to produce linear gradients of the magnetic field for imaging. MRI techniques involve pulsing currents through the RF and gradient coils, explaining that this particular technique is often referred as a pulse sequence. By varying the pulse sequence, one can produce a huge range of images of different spatial and temporal resolutions and with a substantially high contrast between tissues in the image.

Magnetic resonance imaging displays good contrast in soft tissue. The increase in total proton density associated with changes in water structure alters free mobile protons in the epidermis, dermis, and subcutaneous tissue. These changes lead to increased contrast and brightness in MRI images (Fig. 12).

The major advantage of MRI is that it makes it possible to characterize the skin in a given region of interest by measuring the density of protons and T1 and T2 relaxation times. This was applied to skin aging studies.

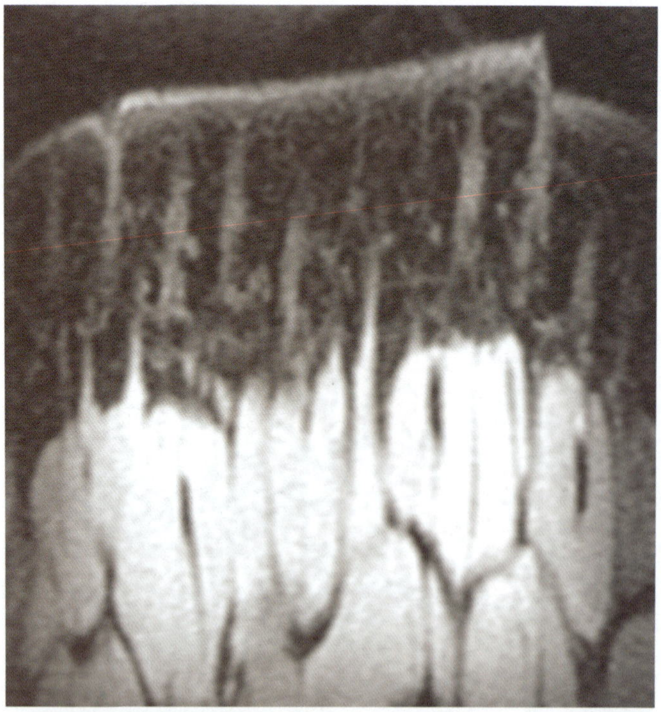

Figure 12: Magnetic resonance imaging of back skin: The epidermis with its pilosebaceous units can be distinguished. Some invasions of hypodermis into the dermis can also be noticed
©L'Oréal Research and Innovation

It was demonstrated that free water was higher in the epidermis than in the dermis irrespective of age and that free water was higher in the upper dermis of elderly (more than 70 years) as compared to fairly young (less than 40 years) adults.[56] Other published work deals with the measurement of the hydration gradient in the callus of the foot and the effect of a cosmetic treatment.[57] MRI was also used to study the precise location of hyaluronic acid in the upper dermis and its time-course following injection.[58]

Confocal Laser Microscopy[59,60]

The confocal laser microscope is a novel and interesting non-invasive tool for imaging skin lesions and subsurface skin lesions that are not visible to the naked eye or by dermatoscopy. It is based on the principle that when a diode laser beam crosses the skin, the reflected light is used to construct detailed images of optical sections through the tissue. A laser provides excitation light of high intensity. The laser light is reflected from a dichroic mirror. From there, it hits two mirrors which scan the laser light across the sample. Emitted light from the sample gets de-scanned by the dichroic mirror and is focused onto the pinhole after being measured by a detector (photomultiplier tube). As a limiting factor, any slight movement of the skin or body prevents the correct acquisition of images. The detector attached to a computer helps to build up the image one pixel at a time. The detection of backscattered light along with differences in the tissue refractive index helps in high resolution of cellular detail and contrast when examining thin sections, thus making staining unnecessary.

Nowadays, two different imaging modes are available for application in dermatology: (1) the reflectance mode; and (2) the fluorescence mode. In the first mode, contrast comes from changes in the refractive index of skin structural components. It is well established as a clinical diagnostic tool for the diagnosis of melanoma and non-melanoma skin cancers, and also for a wide range of other skin diseases. In the fluorescence mode, only fluorescent reemitted light (at a longer wavelength than that of the excitation light) is recorded. Contrast is achieved by utilizing the inherent refractive index properties of the various cellular microstructures. In vivo, reflectance mode is the most routinely used.

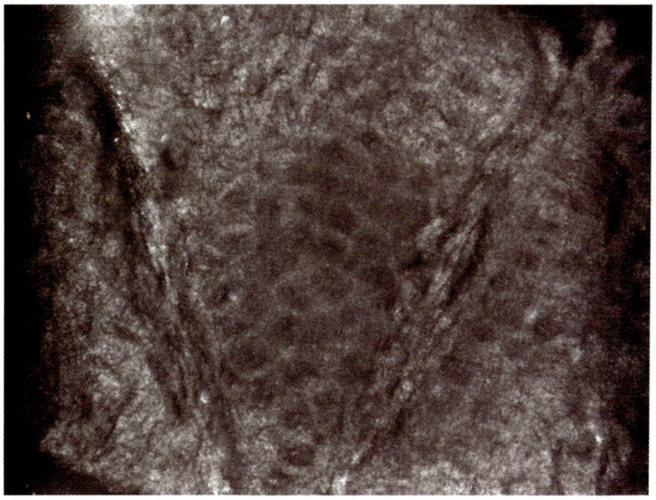

Figure 13: Confocal image of forearm skin (Horizontal section along the dermal epidermal junction)
©L'Oreal Research and Innovation

This type of measurement is quite accurate but is eventually possible on a very tiny surface area only. SC thickness as well as that of living epidermis can be measured with a very high accuracy.[47,61] Single cells can also be observed in their natural environment with quite good contrast, they can be counted and their diameter precisely measured. The dermal epidermal junction can also be easily studied due to the high reflectivity of melanin (Fig. 13). By counting the number of papillae in a given unit area, the inter-digitation between epidermis and dermis can be estimated. Data on the effects of repeated sun exposure, photoaging and aging have been reported.[62]

In clinical research, confocal microscopy seems to be a very promising technique for differentiating in vivo between equivocal lesions such as melanomas and other melanocytic lesions.[63] Other studies have been conducted for a better characterization of lentigines.[64]

Multiphoton Imaging of the Skin

Unlike confocal microscopy, when used in the fluorescent mode, multi- or two-photon microscopy (TM) produces fluorescence as a result of simultaneous absorption of two photons having the same energy. When a chromophore is excited, part of its energy is dissipated through the sample, while another part is emitted as a fluorescent photon with the energy lower than the total absorbed energy. Besides

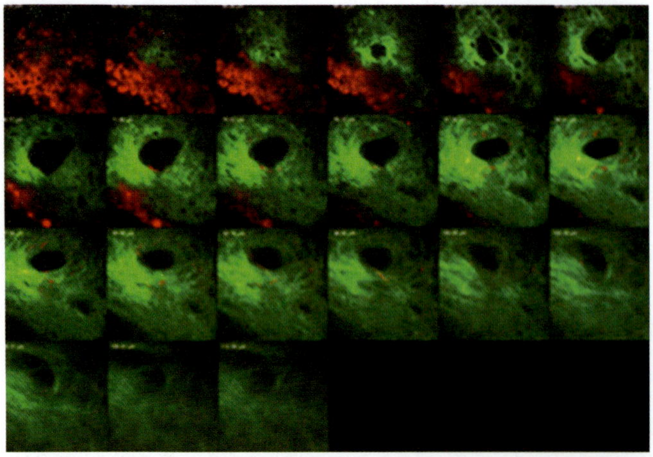

Figure 14: *In vivo* multiphoton images of forearm skin corresponding to 21 successive sections from upper down to mid-dermis. Elastic fibers are coded in red, collagen in green ©L'Oréal Research and Innovation

this two-photon auto-fluorescence (TPA) however, another type of deactivation of the chromophore takes place: some photons are emitted and their energy is the total amount of energy of the two incident photons. The latter emission type is called "second harmonic generation (SHM)". It is of particular relevance for looking at collagen which generates "second harmonic" photons at 410 nm corresponding to the simultaneous absorption of two photons with a wavelength of 820 nm.[65,66] The only way to produce simultaneous absorption of several photons by the same molecule is to use an ultrafast (femtosecond) laser in the infra-red range (tuning possibility 730–960 nm: MaiTai, Spectra Physics, Coherent, Chameleon). Such a laser can deliver a high power in a very short period (about 10–15 p-seconds). The total energy focused at a given point into the skin (the focal point) is minimized by modulating the laser impulse at 80 MHz. A commercially available TM device is DermalInspect (JenLab GmbH, Jena, Germany).

TM technique is quite recent. Masters et al. demonstrated the ability to quantify NADPH autofluorescence for assessing the metabolic states of human epidermal cells *in vivo*.[67] Other authors showed that TM enabled "optical biopsies" of inner epidermis and upper dermis to be recorded.[68] For instance, cells of the stratum granulosum, the stratum spinosum and the stratum basale could be differentiated according to the fluorescence level of their nuclei and their shape. An interesting application of TM is assessment both of the elastin and the collagen content on the same optical section (Fig. 14).[69,70] Elastin is evaluated from (TP) and collagen from (SH). Such studies demonstrate a progressive decrease in collagen and a relative increase in elastin with aging. The ratio of SHG to TPA could provide a quantified index of photoaging.[71]

TM was also used to study dermatological disorders such as psoriasis and skin cancer within pigmented area. Further studies in these fields, however, are needed before reaching any final conclusion. TM technique was used for screening the effects of drug *in situ*.[70] When a topical cream contains an active fluorescent ingredient, the penetration level of the ingredient into a given skin layer can be estimated.[71]

REFERENCES

1. Leveque JL, De Rigal J. Impedance method for studying skin moisturization. J Soc Cosmet Chem. 1983;34:419-25.
2. Fluhr JW, Gloor M, Lazzerini S. Comparative study of 5 instruments measuring stratum corneum hydration. Skin Res Tech. 1999;5:161-70.
3. Kazaka G, Courage W. Courage Kazaka Electronics, Köln, Germany, technical information concerning the digital measuring probes of Corneometer CM. 2004; 825.
4. Leveque,JL, Querleux B. Skin Chip©, a new tool for investigating the skin surface in vivo. Skin Res Technol. 2003;9:343-7.
5. Pierard GE. Leveque JL. What is Skin Chip? From silicon image sensor to skin chip. Dermatology. 2004;208:291-2
6. Batisse D, Giro, F, Leveque JL. Capacitance imaging of the skin surface. Skin Research Technol. 2006;12:99-104.
7. Thune P, Nilsen T, Hanstad IK, et al. The water barrier function of the skin in relation to the water content of stratum corneum, pH and skin lipids. The effect of alkaline soap and syndet on dry skin in elderly, non-atopic patients. Acta Derm Venereol. 1988;68:277-83.
8. Tagami H, Kobayashi H, Kikuchi K. A portable device using a closed chamber system for measuring Transepidermal water loss: comparison with the conventional method. Skin Res Technol. 2002;8:7-10.
9. Barel AO, Clarys P. Study of the stratum corneum barrier function by transepidermal water loss measurements: comparison between two commercial instruments Evaporimeter and Tewameter. Skin Pharmacol. 1995;8:186-90
10. Wa CV, Maibach HI. Mapping the human face: biophysical properties. Skin Res Technol. 2010;16:38–54.
11. Gloor M, Hirsch G, Willebrandt U. Use of infrared spectroscopy for the in vivo measurement of water content of the horny layer after application of dermatologic ointments. Arch Dermatol Res. 1981;271:305-13
12. Caspers PJ, Lucassen GW, Puppels GJ. Combined in vivo confocal Raman spectroscopy and confocal microscopy of human skin. Biophys J. 2003;85:572-80.
13. Chrit L, Hadjur C, Morel S, et al. In vivo chemical investigation of Human skin using confocal Raman fiber optic microprobe. J Biomed Optics. 2005;10:1-11.

14. Walling PL, Dabney JM. Moisturization in skin by near infrared spectroscopy. J Soc Cosmet Chem. 1989;40:151-71.
15. De Rigal J, Losch MJ, Bazin R, et al. Near-infrared spectroscopy: A new approach to the characterization of dry skin. J Soc Cosmet Chem. 1993;44:197-209
16. Charakida A, Charakida M, Chu AC. Double-blind, randomized, placebo-controlled study of a lotion containing triethyl citrate and ethyl linoleate in the treatment of acne vulgaris. Br J Dermatol. 2007;157:569–74.
17. Nouveau-Richard S, Zhu W, Li YH, et al. Oily skin: specific features in Chinese women. Skin Res Technol. 2007;13:43–8.
18. Kazak G, Courage W. Courage Kazaka Electronics, Köln, Germany, technical information concerning the Cutometer. 2004.
19. De Rigal J, Lévêque JL. In vivo measurement of the *stratum corneum* elasticity. Bioeng Skin. 1985;1:13–23.
20. Ohshima H, Kinoshita S, Oyobikawa M, et al. Use of Cutometer area parameters in evaluating age-related changes in the skin elasticity of the cheek. Skin Res Technol. 2013;19: e23–e242.
21. Griffiths CEM. The clinical identification and quantification of photodamage. Br J Dermatol. 1992;127:37-42.
22. Murray BC, Wickett RR. Correlation between dermal torque meter, cutometer and Dermal phase measurements of human skin. Skin Res Technol. 1997; 3;10106
23. Tosti A, Compagno G, Fazzini ML, et al. A ballistometer for the study of the plasto-elastic properties of skin. J Invest Dermatol. 1997;69:315–7.
24. Paye M, Mac-Mary S, Elkhyat A, et al. Use of Reviscometer for measuring cosmetic induced skin surface effects. Skin Res Technol. 2007;13 343-9
25. Reviscometer: Courage-Khazaka Electronics GmBH, Köln, Germany, 2008.
26. Grove GL, Grove MJ, Leyden JJ, et al. Optical profilometry: an objective method for quantification of facial wrinkle. J Am Acad Dermatol. 1989:21:631–7.
27. Leveque JL. EEMCO guidance for the assessment of skin topography. J Eur Acad Dermatol. 1999;12:103-14
28. Couturaud V, Zahouani H, Broucho G, et al. Measurement of skin topography imaging by defocalization laser device. Proceedings of the 20th IFSCC Congress. 1998
29. Lagarde JM, Rouvrais C, Black D, et al. Skin topography measurement by interference fringe projection: a technical validation. Skin Res Technol. 2001;7:112–21.
30. Corcuff P, de Rigal J, Leveque JL. Skin relief and aging. J Soc Cosm Chem. 1983;3:177190.
31. Griffiths CEM. The clinical identification and quantification of photodamage. Br J Dermatol. 1992;127:37-42.
32. Latreille J, Gardinier S, Ambroisine L, et al. Influence of skin colour on the detection of cutaneous erythema and tanning phenomena using reflectance spectrophotometry. Skin Res Technol. 2007;13:236-41.
33. Liu W, Lai W, Wang XM, et al. Skin phototyping in a Chinese female population: analysis of four hundred and four cases from four major cities of China. Photodermatol Photoimmunol Photomed. 2006;22:184-8.
34. Moncrieff M, Cotton S, Claridge E, et al. Spectrophotometric Intracutaneous Analysis: a new technique for imaging pigmented skin lesions. Br J Dermatol. 2002;146:448–57.
35. Petitjean A, Sainthillier JM, Macmary S, et al. Skin radiance how to quantify? Validation of an optical method. Skin Res Technol. 2007;13:28.
36. Matsubara A, Liang Z, Sato Y, et al. Analysis of human perception of facial skin radiance by means of image histogram parameters of surface&and subsurface reflections from the skin. Skin Res Technol. 2012;18:265-71.
37. Wilhelm P, Enzo B, Peter E, et al. Bio Engineering of Skin: Skin Imaging and Analysis. Dermatology: Basic science series. 2007; 423-43.
38. Anderson RR. Polarized light examination and photography of the skin. Arch Dermatol 1991;127:1000–5.
39. Muccini JA, Kollias N, Phillips SB, et al. Polarized light photography in the evaluation of photoaging. J Am Acad Dermatol. 1995;33:76--9
40. Guillard G, Lagarde J. Skin lesions segmentation and quantification from 3D body's models. Skin Res Technol. 2005;11:123–31.
41. Nischal KC, Khopkar U. Dermoscope. Indian J Dermatol Venereol Leprol. 2005;71:300-3.
42. Benvenuto-Andrade C, Dusza SW, Agero AC, et al. Differences between Polarized Light Dermoscopy and Immersion Contact Dermoscopy for the Evaluation of Skin Lesions. Arch Dermatol. 2007;143:329-38.
43. Moncrieff M, Cotton S, Claridge E, et al. Spectrophotometric Intracutaneous Analysis: a new technique for imaging pigmented skin lesions. Br J Dermatol. 2002;146:448–57.
44. Guillard G, Lagarde J. Skin lesions segmentation and quantification from 3D body's models. Skin Res Technol. 2005;11:123–31.
45. Mlosek RK, Ebowska RM, Lewandowski MI et al. Imaging of the skin and subcutaneous tissue using classical and high-frequency ultrasonographies in anti-cellulite therapy. Skin Res Technol. 2011;17:46–8.
46. Wortsman XC, Holm EA, Wulf HC. Real-time spatial compound ultrasound imaging of skin. Skin Res Technol. 2008;10:23–31.
47. Nouveau-Richard S, Monot M, Bastien P, et al. In vivo epidermal thickness measurement: ultrasound vs. confocal imaging. Skin Res Technol. 2004;10:13--40.
48. De Rigal J, Escoffier C, Querleux B, et al. Assessment of aging of the human skin by in vivo ultrasonic imaging. J Invest Dermatol. 1989;93:621-25
49. Richard S, Duteil L, Poli F, et al. Echographic assessment of corticosteroid-induced skin thinning, including echogenicity measurement. Skin Res Technol. 1996;2:18-22.
50. Matthes U, Hoxtermann S, Hoffman K, et al. Acoustic microscopy in dermatology: normal skin structure and tumours, In: Altmeyer P, el Gammal S, Hoffman K, (eds). Ultrasound in dermatology. Berlin, Germany: Springer-Verla,; 1992.
51. Vilana R, Puig S, Sanchez M, et al. Preoperative assessment of cutaneous melanoma thickness using 10-MHz sonography. AJR Am J Roentgenol. 2009;193:639-43.
52 Querleux B, Baldeweck T, Diridollou S, et al. Skin from various ethnic origins and aging: an in vivo cross-sectional multimodality imaging study. Skin Res Technol. 2009;15:306-13.
53. Welzel J. Optical coherence tomography in dermatology: a review. Skin Res Technol. 2001;7:1-9.
54. Pierce MC, Strasswimmer J, Park BH, et al. Advances in optical coherence tomography imaging for dermatology. J Invest Dermatol. 2004;123:458-63.
55. Weissman J, Hancewicz T, Kaplan P. Optical coherence tomography of skin for measurement of epidermal thickness by shapelet-based image analysis. Optics Express. 2004;12: 5760-9.
56. Richard S, Querleux B, Bittoun J, et al . Characterization of the skin in vivo by high resolution magnetic resonance imagin : water behavior and age related effects. J Invest Dermatol. 1993;100:705-9.

57. Querleux B, Richard S, Bittoun J, et al. In vivo hydration profile in skin layers by high-resolution magnetic resonance imaging. Skin Pharmacol. 1994;7:210-6.
58. Gensanne D, Josse AM, Schmidt AM, et al. In vivo visualization of hyaluronic acid injection by high-resolution T2 parametric magnetic resonance images. Skin Res Technol. 2007;13:385-9.
59. Rajadhyaksha M, González S, Zavislan JM, et al. In vivo confocal scanning laser microscopy of human skin II: advances in instrumentation and comparison with histology. J Invest Dermatol. 1999;113:293-303.
60. González S, Swindells K, Rajadhyaksha M, et al. Changing paradigms in dermatology: confocal microscopy in clinical and surgical dermatology. Clin Dermatol. 2003;21:359-69.
61. Sauerman K, Clemann S, Jaspers S. Age related changes of human skin investigated with histometric measurements by confocal laser scanning microscopy in vivo. Skin Res Technol. 2002;8:52-6.
62. Gamblicher T, Sauerman K, Altintas MA. Effects of repeated sunbed exposures on the human skin. In vivo measurements with Confocal Microscopy. Skin Res Technol. 2004;20:27-32.
63. Pellacani G, Guitera P, Longo C, et al. The impact of in vivo reflectance microscopy for the diagnostic accuracy of melanoma and equivocal melanocytic lesions. J Invest Dermatol. 2007;127:2759-65.
64. Nakajima A, Funasaka Y, Kawana S. Investigation by in vivo reflectance confocal microscopy: melanocytes at the edges of solar lentigines. Exp Dermatol. 2012;21:18-21.
65. Konig K, Riemann I. High resolution multiphoton tomography of human skin with subcellular spatial resolution and picosecond time resolution. J Biomed Opt. 2003;8:432-9.
66. Zipfel WR, Williams RM, Christie R, et al. Live tissue intrinsic microscopy using multiphoton excited native fluorescence and second harmonic generation. Proc Natl Acad Sci USA. 2003;100:7075-80.
67. Masters BR, So PT, Kim KH, et al. Multiphoton excitation microscopy, confocal microscopy, and spectroscopy of living cells and tissues; functional metabolic imaging of human skin in vivo. Methods Enzymol. 1999;307:513-36.
68. Lin SJ, Wu RJ, Tan HY, et al. Evaluating cutaneous photoaging by use of multiphoton fluorescence and second harmonic generation microscopy. Optics Letters. 2005;30:2275-7.
69. Decencière E, Tancrède-Bohin E, Dokladal P, et al. Automatic 3D segmentation of multiphoton images: A key step for the quantification of human skin. Skin Res Tech. 2013;19:115124.
70. El Madani AH, Tancrède-Bohin E, Bensussan A, et al. In vivo multiphoton imaging of human skin: assessment of topical corticosteroid-induced epidermis atrophy and depigmentation. J Biomed Opt. 2012;17:026009.
71. Konig K, Ehlers A, Stracke F,Iet al. In vivo drug screening in human skin using femtosecond laser multiphoton tomography. Skin Pharm Physiol. 2006;19:78-88.

Chapter 3

In Vitro Skin Models

José Cotovio, *L'Oréal Research and Innovation, Aulnay-sous-Bios, France*
Christian Pellevoisin, *Episkin Academy, Lyon, France*
Davinder Parsad, *Postgraduate Institute of Medical Education and Research, Chandigarh, India*

INTRODUCTION

As the main barrier to the environment, the skin protects the whole body from external aggressions, being of bacterial, chemical or physical origin. Additionally, some specific associated appendages (eccrine, apocrine glands) actively participate in regulating the body temperature through sweat release. Skin is also a highly developed sensory organ and as such, it is continuously involved in the perception of environment (cold, warm, rough, smooth, etc.). Through its close relation with brain, it plays an important part in human communications since expressing our feelings (smiling, etc.) or emotions (blushing, flushing, etc.).

Skin is the largest organ of the human body, representing a surface of 1.5–2 m^2 and weighing 3–4 kilograms (excluding the hypodermis) in adults. It is organized into layered structures and consists of an outermost epidermis, the upper part in contact with environment (first barrier) and an underlying dermis. The whole structure rests upon a subcutaneous adipose tissue (hypodermis) the thickness of which varies according to body area. Epidermis is a stratified epithelium, with a varying thickness from 0.05 millimeter on the eyelids to 1.5 millimeter on the soles of the feet. It continuously self-renew with a 3–4 week turnover time. It is mostly composed of keratinocytes which divide in the basal layer of the epidermis and further undergo a differentiation process while migrating towards the surface of the skin to ultimately form the stratum corneum (SC) layer. During differentiation, specific proteins and lipids are synthesized, playing an important role in the formation of this horny layer that ultimately constitutes the first line of skin.

Unraveling the complexity of Mother Nature by building simplified systems has always been a scientific challenge, attempting to learn by approaching its intricacy, mimicking its structure and mirroring its functions. Models are challenged to check how they could reproduce what is known or predict the unknown. Rebuilding skin, *in vitro*, obeys to such logic, in creating models of reconstructed skin structures. Characterizing and testing these models *vis à vis in vivo* reality generates new knowledge, in turn helps to build more complex models, under a virtuous cycle. Nowadays, we are far from integrating all the level of complexity of *in vivo* organs but existing models already have a large number of applications in the fields of medical, basic research or predictive evaluation of chemicals, drugs or cosmetics.

WHY DO WE NEED *IN VITRO* ENGINEERED SKIN?

Medical applications were the obvious initial drivers of reconstructing skin. However, it became soon evident that 3D reconstructed human skins could also be used in fundamental research and/or as tools for predicting the efficacy and safety of chemicals, drugs or cosmetics.

Research on artificial skin equivalents to treat burned patients was initiated as early as mid-1960s.[1] Generally speaking, damaged skin can self-rebuild unless a too severe damage has occurred. Indeed, a compromised skin barrier will likely result to severely increase transepidermal water loss. This raises an urgent need for the organism to recover its protective barrier to prevent both water loss and a subsequent possible infection. When the area of damaged skin is limited, autografts can be performed using skin samples taken from healthy parts of the body for covering the wounds. In case deep dermal and full-thickness wound/burnt area are larger than half the surface of the total body skin, these healthy skin areas are not large enough to cover the wound, and autologous (i.e. originating from the patient) epidermal sheets developed from *in vitro* culture technologies must be used.[2] Reconstructing human skin *in vitro* consists in associating cells with natural or synthetic polymers to reproduce certain physiological functions of epidermis and/or dermis. In 1979, first reconstructed epidermis with a functional horny layer was achieved.[3,4] Since, different models have been perfected to reconstruct *in vitro* either the structure of the epidermis alone or the whole full thickness dermoepidermal unit.

Beyond clinical uses of engineered skin, many non-clinical applications have been developed with 3D reconstructed skin models. Engineered skin has strong value for fundamental research for studying the biology and the physiology of human healthy skin and/or skin diseases. They allow different functions to be investigated, such as skin barrier, cell to cell and cell to extracellular matrix (ECM) interactions, wound healing, pigmentation control, mechanical properties or skin aging.[5-8]

The use of animal models for assessing the safety of chemicals, in humans has been increasingly questioned. The study by Olson et al. in 2000, gathering data from 12 pharmaceutical companies on 150 compounds, showed than skin and liver are the two organs that offer the poorest correlation for toxicity between animals and humans.[9] Over the past decades, a number of drugs have been withdrawn due to adverse effects observed at late stages of development or post-marketing because of a lack of predictability of conventional preclinical safety tests.[10,11] This underlines the need for *in vitro* models, which better mimic human skin, as 3D reconstructed skin models do. For both, toxicology and efficacy purposes, the added value of skin 3D models is not only scientific or economic but ethical too with regard to the 3R principle (Replacement, Reduction and Refinement of animal tests).[12] The first *in vitro* method ever accepted by regulators, as full replacement of animal, was the Episkin test assessing skin corrosivity, in 1998.[13]

The coming years will certainly confirm the increasing use of *in vitro* skin models, which allow better physiological interactions between different skin cells to take place, unlike standard 2D systems where they cannot efficiently occur. We are still far from integrating all the levels of complexity of *in vivo* organs' physiology and regulation but the latest technical and scientific discoveries open ways to better integrate models' complexity *in vivo* functional features and interactions. These issues will necessarily need appropriate and subtle specific developments of the materials used for building and supporting the tissues. For example, (1) scaffold allow skin cells to form structured epithelia (similar to the targeted *in vivo* functional biological system); (2) to communicate with each other; and (3) to mimic as close as possible the behavior of normal skin cells when exposed to agents of all kinds (biological, xenobiotics). Basic scaffoldings made of non-biodegradable material may lack any functioning vasculature or immune system, and as such cannot always be used as a complete substitute for *in vivo* animal or human studies. Nevertheless, they possess the significant advantage of accepting different cell types to assess their relevance to the skin biological phenomenon under investigation.

Large-scale production of standardized models used to evaluate product safety, to find new active substances and/or to achieve research studies, contributes to strengthen the relevance of these tools. Through supporting integrated decision-making process during research and development phases, 3D *in vitro* skin models contribute to reinforce many areas, some of which are described in this review.

PRINCIPLES OF SKIN ENGINEERING

Reconstructed Skin Adventure: Key Developments

The pioneers of tissue culture are the US biologist Ross Harisson in 1907 and the French Nobel Prize Winner Alexis Carrel with his works on tissues and organs culture.[14] Beyond medium and condition of culture, the limiting factor is access to a sufficient number of cells. Thanks to previous findings of Theodore Puck who demonstrated that a layer of lethally irradiated epithelial cells could be used as a source of mitogens allowing a second population of cells to proliferate,[15] keratinocytes were first reliably cultured at the laboratory scale about 35 years ago. The reconstructed skin adventure began

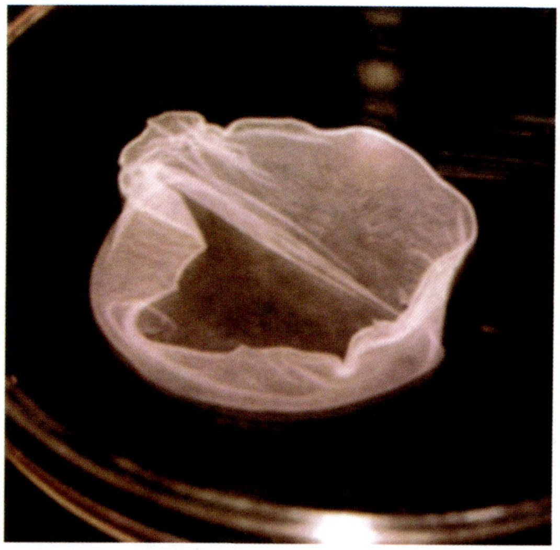

Figure 1: *In vitro* epithelium composed of keratinocytes cultured in immersed conditions. Epithelium sheets represent 2–3 layers of undifferentiated cells
©L'Oréal Research and Innovation

when James Rheinwald and Howard Green[16,17] at the Harvard Faculty of Medicine, cultivated keratinocytes in series on a base network of "nurse" fibroblasts (irradiated Swiss 3T3 mouse fibroblasts as the feeder layer) and succeeded in obtaining small sheets of epithelium two to three layers thick (cultured epithelial autographs) that were used to treat burnt persons.[18]

However, first epidermal substitutes composed of few layers of human keratinocytes did not present a functional horny layer and were far from resembling the *in vivo* tissue (Fig. 1). Indeed, several studies clearly highlighted the role of cell-cell and cell-ECM components interactions responsible for the cell-tissue behavior.[19,20] The first reconstructed epidermis model topped with a horny layer was perfected in 1979.[3] Mimicking the *in vivo* situation, the reconstructed epidermis equivalents consisted of seeded human keratinocytes (extracted from human skin biopsies) on the top of a cell-free dermal substitute for about 2 weeks at the air-liquid interface.[4] Simple dermal substitutes containing fibroblasts are also of importance for clinical use in case of severe burns and wounds.[21] Today, skin equivalents can be divided into three categories: (i) epidermal substitutes; (ii) dermal substitutes; and (iii) full thickness models containing both epidermal and dermal components.[16]

Main Steps in the Reconstruction of Epidermis

Over the last years, *in vitro* skin models have been perfected by adding different cell types, allowing various skin functions to being simulated. Whatever the *in vitro* skin model, reconstruction usually follows similar process key steps: keratinocytes are isolated from the epidermis of skin biopsies or from the external sheath of a hair follicle and further cultured as monolayers[4] in order to amplify the number of cells and to set up easy-to-use cell banks. In a second step, keratinocytes are "seeded" and allowed to

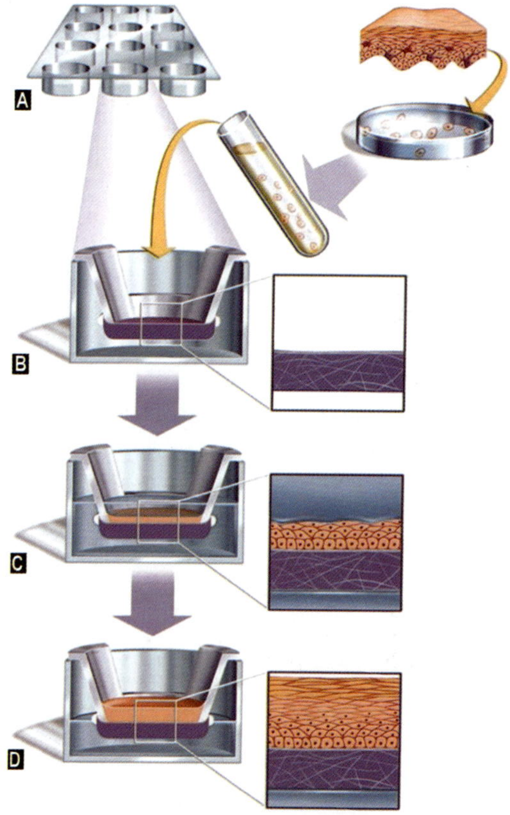

Figure 2: *In vitro* reconstruction main steps of the human epidermis model EpiskinTM. **A,** Extraction and amplification of keratinocytes in large amounts. **B,** Seeding keratinocytes on the top of a collagen matrix and incubation in immersed conditions at 37°C, 5% CO_2. **C,** Proliferation phase of keratinocytes in immersed conditions, incubation at 37°C, 5% CO_2. Cells first grow horizontally forming a simple epithelial sheet covering the collagen matrix support. Then some layers form, following a vertical migration of the cells. **D,** Air exposed period: cells brought into contact with the air. This step is mandatory for the stratification and full differentiation of the epidermal structure in 3D
©L'Oréal Research and Innovation

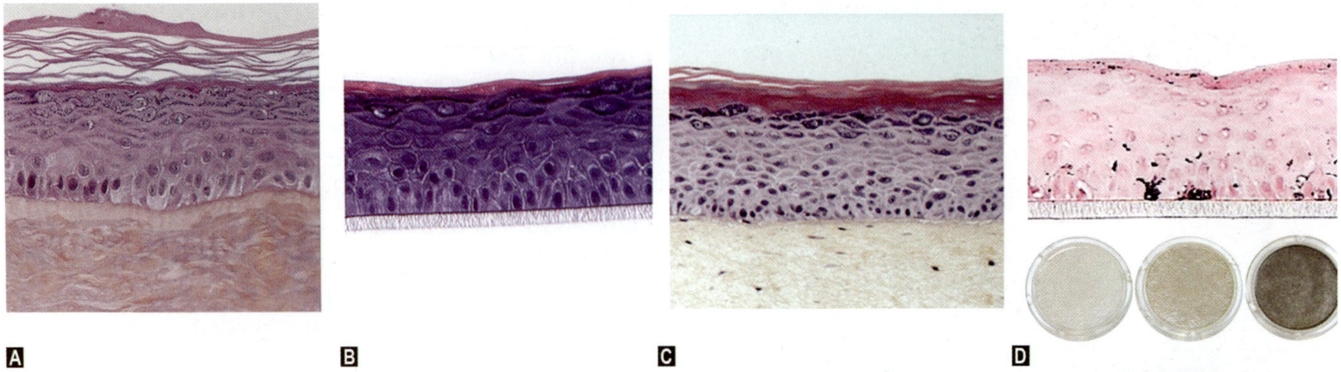

Figure 3: Examples of reconstructed epidermis and full thickness skin models. Optical microscope pictures showing vertical sections of the tissues (HE/HES staining, 60x magnification). **A,** Reconstructed epidermis EpiSkinTM model: Reconstructed human epidermis (RHE) using an a-cellular collagen matrix as support. **B,** Reconstructed epidermis SkinEthicTM RHE model : Reconstructed human epidermis using an artificial membrane as support. **C,** Full thickness skin model: Reconstructed skin with full differentiated epidermis and a fibroblast-populated collagen matrix as dermal support. **D,** Pigmented epidermis SkinEthicTM RHPE model: Reconstructed pigmented epidermis with melanocytes of different phototypes (No: no melanocytes, Ph.II: skin phototype II, Ph.IV: skin phototype IV) ©L'Oréal Research and Innovation

proliferate onto the surface of a support, which can be either a de-epidermized dermis (DED: dermis whose cells have been eliminated by successive freezing/thawing steps), or a biomaterial often based on collagen. This second step of the culture consists in obtaining a monolayer of keratinocytes by placing the cells and the dermal substitute immersed in the culture medium. During this step, other types of epidermal cells (e.g. melanocytes) may be added to keratinocytes depending on the model to be produced. In a third step, keratinocytes are brought into contact with the air (air exposed period) where they differentiate and stratify spontaneously to form all the layers of a fully differentiated epidermis including the horny layer which provides the reconstructed epidermis with its barrier function (Fig. 2).

Furthermore, it is possible to produce a dermal equivalent by mixing native collagen Type I and living fibroblasts according to the conditions that lead to the formation of a dermal tissue. Thus, an important additional step is taken when this living dermal compartment containing fibroblasts is used during the epidermal reconstruction process, ending up to a full thickness skin equivalent including the skin's two major cell types (keratinocytes and fibroblasts).[22]

Important developments in culture media composition and skin cells' knowledge allowed other important cells such as melanocytes and Langerhans cells (LC) to being included together with keratinocytes in the epidermis compartment and opened new fields of investigation.[23,24] See reconstructed tissue examples in Figure 3.

Several specific substrates have been used to create the dermal structure *in vitro* including DED,[4,25,26] collagen lattices,[27] collagen-glycosaminoglycan matrices,[28,29] chitosan cross-linked collagen-glycosaminoglycan matrices[30] and also biodegradable matrices.[31] Most of these reconstructs help in the development of new insights in processes linked to wound healing as critical improvement in the epidermal barrier function or the re-epithelialization sequences[32,33] and the dynamics of basement membrane formation.

In the future, new technologies could revolutionize the way to rebuild skin equivalents. Bio-printing is a newly opened area of research and engineering that involves printing devices to print in 3D tissues or organs. Cells, embedded in a gel, are printed or deposited onto a surface, layer by layer up to reproduce the desired tissue. Recently, an American team conducted a proof-of-concept study showing that this technology could be used to build a model of full thickness skin.[34]

Industrial Standardized Production of 3D Skin Models

Regular use of 3D skin models in anticipated and well-planned studies entail for users the availability of and easy access to standardized reproducible tissues. Some biotechnology companies like SkinEthic (www.Skinethic.com) are devoted to the development and production of robust models aiming at providing tools for efficacy and safety screenings of substances and/or finished cosmetic, pharmaceutical and industrial products. Specific cell culture process allows human tissues with well-characterized histology, functionality and ultra-structure features to be produced at a large scale. The latter mainly based upon reconstructed human epidermis (RHE), using a biological or non-biological support, possibly containing human melanocytes with different pigmented levels (phototype II to VI) (Table 1). Human corneal epithelium tissue using similar inserts is also part of the available industrial models (SkinEthic™ - HCE model).[35] Standardized large scale manufacturing processes are certified by ISO9001 standard. Reproducibility of batches and quality control are generally evaluated by histological scoring and response to a reference test-chemical. Such models are well designed for industrial application. They are produced in 6, 12, 24 or 96 well plates (Fig. 4). They are robust, easy to handle and can be used for high throughput screening (HTS) application.

Table 1: Examples of marketed reconstructed human epidermis models

SkinEthic™ RHE small (0.5 cm²) SkinEthic™ RHE large (4 cm²) SkinEthic™ RHPE large (0.5 cm²)	EpiSkin™ small (0.38 cm²) EpiSkin™ large (1 cm²)

Abbreviations: RHE, Reconstructed human epidermis

FUNCTIONAL HUMAN RECONSTRUCTED SKIN MODELS

Since it is not yet possible to reproduce an exact copy of the skin, the challenge then becomes to reproduce some physiological functions of this organ. Depending on the function studied, specific models are designed. The model is thus not "reality", but is based upon observations of reality. It is therefore necessary to characterize it and to identify its limits to avoid a biased simplistic representation, though, to the extreme, "The relevance of a model is not measured by its veracity but by its usefulness".[36] Understanding the biology of the skin require the design of such tools and implies constant improvement and adjustments of reconstructed skin models while focusing in depth on various aspects of skin properties and cells-cell as well as tissue interactions. Hopefully, each new model increases knowledge about skin physiology and contributes to enlarge functionality and fields of investigation.

In Vitro Barrier Function

In vivo, skin offers a remarkable barrier function that is mostly linked to the unique compositional and structural characteristics of its thin outermost layer (about 10–15 microns on the forearm), the SC.[37] The barrier property of the skin influences several mechanisms including drug delivery, absorption kinetics, biotransformation, and excretion. This explains the importance for *in vitro* skin tissues to exhibit an epidermal/dermal barrier function

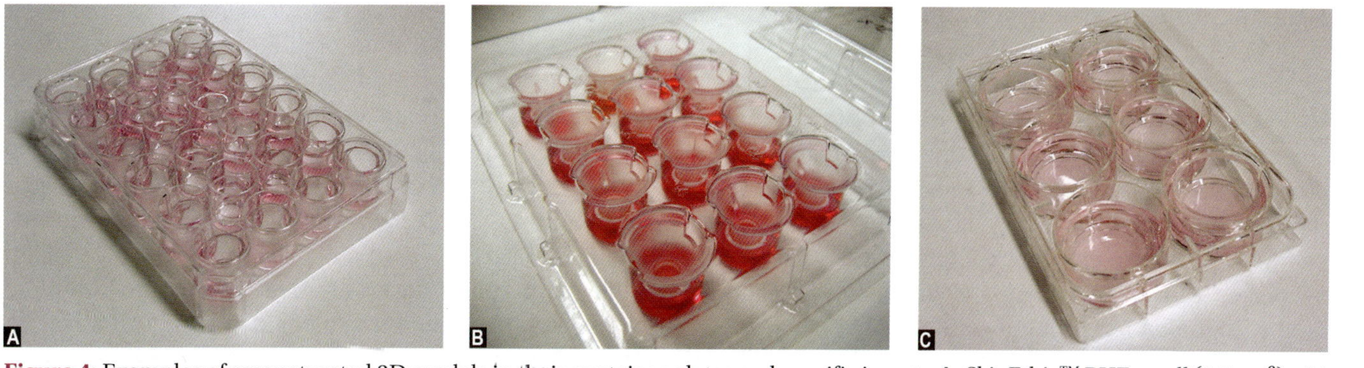

Figure 4: Examples of reconstructed 3D models in their container plates and specific inserts. **A,** SkinEthic™ RHE small (0.5 cm²) x 24 tissues. **B,** EpiSkin™ large (1 cm²) × 12 tissues. **C,** SkinEthic™ RHE large (4 cm²) × 6 tissues
©L'Oréal Research and Innovation

that mimics the behavior of the human skin in response to a given treatment or stress. Barrier function depends upon biological processes involved in epidermal homeostasis, such as proliferation, differentiation and lipogenesis. It is usually assumed that the barrier properties mostly rely on the composition and structure of SC hydrophobic intercellular domain that is filled with a well-defined lamellar lipid structures. Previous studies have shown that, under various culture conditions, the presence of a reconstructed and differentiated epidermis dramatically reduces the permeability of a DED, although the final skin equivalent still exhibits a higher permeability as compared to normal skin. Conditions that favor terminal differentiation of the keratinocytes, such as maintaining the cultures in delipidized serum clearly improved the barrier function.[38] Differences in SC lipid organization in reconstructed epidermis may be ascribed to variations in fatty acid content and profile, indicating that culture conditions are instrumental to generate *in vitro* epidermis with SC barrier properties close to native human tissue.[39] To date, engineered and standardized models which are close to native human skin in terms of morphology, lipid composition, calcium gradient and differentiation markers are commercially available[40-42] and currently involved in experimental procedures. Although permeation of these RHE exceeds that of human epidermis, the ranking of tested substances reflects the ranking observed through human epidermis.[43]

In Vitro Epidermal Compartment and Pigmentation

Variation in human skin color results, in a large part, from the total amount and quality (pheo/eumelanin ratio) of a natural pigment, the melanin. The latter is produced by the highly specialized cells, the melanocytes, located in the epidermal basal layer. Various functions are attributed to melanin, ranging from photoprotection (absorbing, scattering and reflecting light) to antioxidant properties (free radical scavenger). Dysregulations of melanocyte homeostasis and/or melanogenesis lead to various hyper- or hypo-pigmented disorders. Treatment of these disorders implies a better understanding of the pigmentatory function. Since the early 1990s, melanocytes were introduced in 3D skin models[23,44] and it became thereby possible to study more deeply the human pigmentatory function. Modeling the skin pigmentation unit opened the way to a better understanding of human melanogenesis modulation, such as the repressive influence of the dermal fibroblasts,[45] mechanisms of melanosome transfer[46] or autocrine and paracrine signaling networks between keratinocytes/melan-ocytes.[47,48] Caucasian skins are characterized by small melanosomes and light pigments, such as pheomelanins whereas dark skins are characterized by larger melanosomes, a higher amount of melanin and, mostly, that of the black pigments, eumelanins.[49] These various skin phototypes can be reproduced *in vitro*, not by changing the number of melanocytes, but by selecting melanocytes from donor of different ethnic origins.

Industrial pigmented tissues are commercially available (i.e. SkinEthic RHPE model, www.SkinEthic.com) thus enabling depigmentation/pro-pigmentation mechanisms to be investigated in standardized engineered tissues with selected phototypes.[35,50,51]

In Vitro Epidermal Compartment and Immunity

Langerhans cells are epidermal immunocompetent cells that play a key role in contact hypersensitivity.[52] The incorporation of LC in the epidermal compartment results in an "immunosensitive" 3D reconstructed tissue. Unlike keratinocytes, epidermal LC do not multiply *in vitro*, making essential to use precursors, such as CD34+ cells from blood (bone marrow derived).[53] A first culture step supports proliferation and differentiation of these precursors, particularly into dendritic cells.[54] When seeded with keratinocytes onto the dermal substrate, these dendritic cells continue their differentiation into LC during the epidermal reconstruction steps. They spontaneously become located at suprabasal level and express specific markers. These cells are functional since reacting to the application of allergens onto the surface of the reconstructed epidermis. As in normal skin, the activation of LC is expressed by the shortening of cell dendrites and, in certain cases, by a decrease in the number of LC in the epidermal compartment.

Incorporation of LC in the reconstructed epidermis EpiSkin (1 cm^2) revealed a dense network of LC located in the suprabasal layers visible by immunostaining. Exposure to the known sensitizer Nickel Sulfate or to solar light, affected LC behavior in a similar way as described *in vivo*, i.e. a reduction in the number of cells, dendritic morphological alteration, a decrease in langerin synthesis.[44] Such a model could open the prospect for studying the first stages of contact allergy reactions.

In Vitro Epidermal Compartment and Metabolism

Skin plays an important role in the detoxification and metabolism of xenobiotics in necessary contact with epidermis (i.e. drugs, cosmetics, etc.) or environmental substances and pollutants. The phase I metabolism of xenobiotics is catalyzed by cytochrome P450 and other oxidoreductases (esterases, epoxide hydrolases, alcohol and aldehyde dehydrogenases, etc.) which transform hydrophobic chemicals into more polar hydrophilic compounds. Phase 2 metabolism is catalyzed by transferases (UDP-glucuronosyl transferases, glutathione-S-transferases, sulfotransferases, etc.) that add conjugated groups to increase hydrophilicity and clearance, thus avoiding bioaccumulation and potential intracellular toxicity. Skin biotransformation of endogenous as well as exogenous compounds represents about 1/50th of the liver biotransformation capabilities Nevertheless, if activities of xenobiotic enzymes are relatively low per square centimeter of skin as compared to liver, such activities become more significant when considering that the skin is the biggest organ (surface area 1.5–2 m^2, 5–6% of the body weight for an adult). The low level of phase I enzymes as compared to liver made the skin a detoxification rather than an activation organ.

The xenobiotic metabolism of several reconstructed models, such as EpiSkin or SkinEthic RHE has been compared to that of human skin. Gene expression profiles of 61 phases I and II metabolizing enzymes in the reconstructed epidermis EpiSkinTM model, as well as in a reconstructed full thickness tissue, showed strong similarity to those in skin *in vivo*.[55] Study of protein expression profiles confirmed the similarity observed at the mRNA level between reconstructed models and whole skin.[56-58]

Recently, the enzymatic activities of xenobiotic enzymes was measured and compared between reconstructed epidermis and whole skin. Weak cytochrome P450-dependent mono-oxygenases (phase I enzymes) and high transferases (phase II enzymes) activities confirm that whole skin and skin models exhibit limited activation metabolism, and much greater detoxification capacities. These results demonstrate that skin models are similar to *in vivo* skin, in terms of metabolic functionality towards the investigated xenobiotics.[59, 60]

Skin is a well-recognized site of production and metabolism of steroids. Recent studies highlighted similar profiles of steroidogenic gene expression and activity between EpiSkin™ and human epidermis, suggesting the possible use of this *in vitro* tissue as a model for studying steroid metabolism related to cell differentiation.[61]

In Vitro Dermal Compartment

The availability of dermis equivalents has opened the way to specific research applications. Some of these scaffolds, such as collagen sponges or biopolymers not only enable fibroblasts to be introduced and to produce *in situ* ECM but also make it possible to reconstruct endothelial cells harboring dermis. Under specific *in vitro* conditions, endothelial cells can produce tubular structures mimicking the walls of blood capillaries.[62,63] From the availability of such models, promising approaches to angiogenesis and related proteolysis processes can be anticipated. Fibroblast population itself is composed of dynamic cells characterized by sub-population, which are functionally and morphologically heterogeneous, according to the body site.[64,65] Besides, fibroblasts originating from a single tissue (dermis) do not represent a homogeneous population but rather include specific subsets, i.e. fibroblasts from papillary superficial dermis and fibroblasts from the reticular deeper dermis.[66,67]

These two types of fibroblasts used in classical culture on plastic supports, exhibit very different morphologic and secretory properties. Furthermore, incorporating these different phenotypes in reconstructed skin allow a three-dimensional architecture with deep-related regional specificities to be reproduced,[68] raising the question of differential age-related changes in fibroblast subpopulations and resulting changes in skin structure and properties.

Stem Cells, the New Bricks for Skin Reconstruction?

Pluripotent stem cells persist in adult tissue. They ensure the survival and renewal of tissue throughout the life of the individual. They are capable of self-renewal and can give rise to cells with a limited proliferation capacity, i.e. the source of differentiated cells. Epidermal stem cells are located within the hair follicle[69] and the interfollicular epidermis[70] and have considerable potential for proliferating *in vitro*. At present, stem cells are difficult to isolate because they have only been partially characterized: they practically express no surface markers (amongst those known, up to now) except certain adherence proteins which hold them in place. A more precise "identity card" of epidermal stem cells is needed to allow us to select them more easily. Although these cells are already some way along a differentiation pathway (that of epidermal cells), they retain a considerable plasticity. Thus, under the influence of appropriate dermal signals, it is possible to orientate their differentiation towards hair follicles, sebaceous glands and sweat glands. However, the behavior of these cells is regulated by a natural mechanism, which limits the possible number of cell divisions. This "internal clock" is controlled by the progressive loss of DNA sequences located at the end of the chromosomes (telomeres). Studying this clock *in vitro* shows that the potential for cell division is reduced when cells are multiplied in culture, and one of the primary future objectives will be the decoding and mastering of the "mitotic clock" of these cells.[71-73]

IN VITRO SKIN MODELS FOR RESEARCH AND DEVELOPMENT

In vitro skin models improve the understanding of the skin in several ways. In itself, the process of "building" the model generates knowledge; it is necessary to (1) understand the mechanism one wishes to model; (2) identify the cellular participants; and (3) find the proper culturing conditions to promote their proliferation and differentiation, etc. It is often cross-disciplinary process that promotes exchanges and transfers of skills between different experts. In the same way, characterization of the model and comparison with human skin both increase the understanding of this organ. Knowledge is still generated when the model does not respond as expected. Successfully incorporating melanocytes, LC or stem cells into an epidermis necessitates a high understanding of these cell types and of their interactions. Verifying their presence and their functionality leads to greater knowledge of the regulating mechanisms that govern them.

Once constructed and characterized, the model is an exceptional tool for the researcher. The availability, reproducibility, and access to numerous parameters (proteomic and genomic analyses, assays, morphology, etc.) pave the way for innumerable fields of experimentation. The contributions of reconstructed skin are significant in many lines of research, for example: UV sensitivity, specific ethnic characteristics, skin sensitization and allergy, SC lipids, chronological aging. The following paragraphs illustrate, through examples, some of the contributions of reconstructed skin to the understanding of the skin.

Studying Skin Aging

Chronological aging is a complex biological phenomenon that affects all organs. At the skin level, it is accompanied by characteristic clinical signs: wrinkles, slackening of tissues and pigmentation marks. Studies have shown changes in all the layers of the skin: decline in renewal of the epidermis, thinning of the epidermal layers, flattening and delamination of the dermal epidermal junction (DEJ). The dermis is also affected by a decrease in ECM glycosaminoglycans (GAGs), in the number of fibroblasts and their activity and a degradation of the ECM. Actinic aging induced by exposure to ultraviolet (UV) increases and accelerates these changes and is accompanied by specific signs, such as solar elastosis.

Reconstructed skins are tools of choice for understanding the biological mechanisms that accompany and induce the appearance of the clinical signs related to aging.

Two main mechanisms are involved in dermis alterations during skin aging:[74] atrophy and changes in architectural organization. Two regions are distinguished in the dermis: the papillary dermis, a region lying beneath the epidermis, and the reticular dermis. The influence of the origin, papillary or reticular, as well as the age of the fibroblasts (donors from 19 years to 74 years of age) on the morphogenesis of epidermis was evaluated in reconstructed skin models. It was shown that dermal equivalents containing papillary fibroblasts were more potent to promote morphogenesis of a correctly stratified and differentiated epidermis than those containing reticular fibroblasts. These differences decline with increasing donors' age (Fig. 5).[67] Matrix metalloproteinase (MMP)1 and VEGF secretion levels were increased in the presence of papillary fibroblasts, whereas MMP3

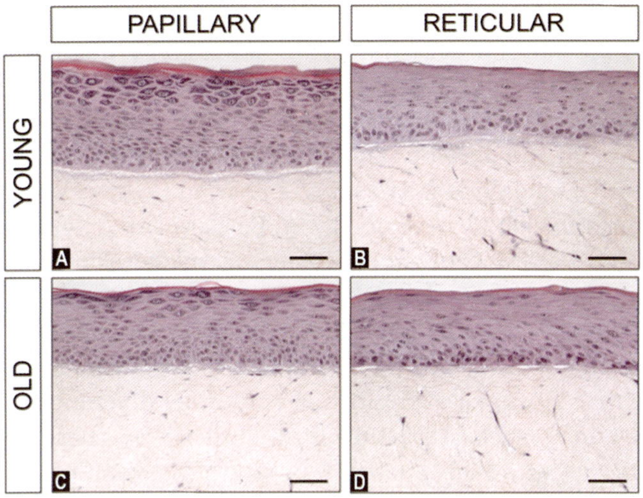

Figure 5: Age-related impact of Fp and Fr on the epidermal compartment in 3D Reconstructed skin. Keratinocytes from the same batch were seeded onto dermal equivalents containing papillary fibroblasts or reticular fibroblasts from young or old donors. Typical histological sections of reconstructed skin samples made with collagen contracted lattices containing: **A,** young papillary fibroblasts. **B,** Young reticular fibroblasts. **C,** Old papillary fibroblasts. **D,** Old reticular fibroblasts. Histology shows that only reconstructed skin with papillary fibroblasts from young donors induces morphogenesis of a well-stratified and well-differentiated epidermis (A)
©L'Oréal Research and Innovation

and KGF levels were higher in the presence of reticular fibroblasts.[75] These models revealed that papillary and reticular fibroblasts exert distinct functions and activities in skin. These functional differences may have strong implications in wound healing and skin aging processes.

During chronological skin aging, the most visible changes occur in the superficial dermis: the DEJ tends to flatten and delaminate, the number of fibroblasts decreases as well as their capacity to synthesize some important proteins, such as collagen (skin cohesion), elastin (skin elastic properties) and proteoglycans (dermis hydration) and reticulation (cross-linking) of macromolecules occurs by glycation. Glycation (i.e. sugars reacting with the free amine of lysine and arginine in proteins) is a slow process with formation of cross-linking bonds bounds between collagen fibers, making the collagen network more rigid. A dermal equivalent made of collagen fibers preglycated by ribose (this sugar cross-links the collagen fibers) was developed, providing new insights into the role played by glycation end-products (AGEs) in the skin. These works highlight the influence of collagen glycation not only at a dermal level but also on the quality of epidermis through fibroblast regulation.[76,77]

Human skin is the only organ directly exposed to solarsun UV rays, a well-recognized environmental damaging factor responsible for photoaging.[78,79] Acute overexposure of human skin to UV's causes sunburn, altered pigmentation, inflammation, immune suppression, and dermal connective tissue damage. Chronic UV exposure can induce a disruption of normal architecture of the skin and ultimately cause premature photoaging. It may also cause skin cancer in worse cases. For a long time, UVB rays were held to be the only UV rays detrimental to the skin since mainly responsible for sunburn and direct DNA damage to epidermal cells. Biologists observed that UVA rays, which penetrate deeper into the skin, are also harmful since they directly alter the dermal compartment. Through an oxidative stress process (generation of reactive oxygen free radicals), they damage the fibroblasts and promote the synthesis of proteins responsible for collagen breakdown. Using models of full-thickness reconstructed skin containing both the epidermis and the dermis; it was shown that keratinocytes participate indirectly in the photoaging process. Under the influence of UVB, they release soluble factors which cause dermal fibroblasts to synthesize proteolytic enzymes MMP that degrade collagen and other ECM proteins of the dermal connective tissue.[80] Identifying early biological events that occur post UV exposure is therefore essential for studies on photoprotection. Using full-thickness skin models, the effects of UV's (UVB and UVA) have been investigated. UVB-induced damages that essentially occur at epidermal level, with the formation of sunburn (apoptotic) cells and DNA lesions, whereas UVA-induced damages are mostly located within the dermal compartment.[81,82] The effects of cumulative exposure to each type of UV radiation and their possible synergy can be studied using full thickness skin models and combining fine adjustments of simulated exposure and specific treatments. Likewise, significant advances in the knowledge of chronological aging/photoaging are anticipated from the use of "aging" skin models/UV-exposed skin models, thus providing new strategies in anti-aging research.

Studying Wound Healing

Re-epithelialization of damaged skin relies on the migration of epidermal cells (keratinocytes) into the wound, leading to the reconstruction of an organized, stratified and squamous epithelium that will permanently cover the wound defect and restore main functions. Regeneration of a functional epithelium depends on several important tissue structures, such as the quality of DEJ that anchors the epidermis to the dermis and the terminal differentiation of keratinocytes forming the highly protective cornified envelope.[83,84] These complex processes require continuous communication between cells through soluble factors (i.e. cytokine release), cell-to-cell contacts and cell-to-matrix interactions. One of the major applications of engineered skin substitutes for wound healing is to promote *in vivo* healing of cutaneous wounds and dermal reconstruction. A variety of scaffolds have been fabricated based on materials ranging from natural skin components to synthetic substrates.[85] Nevertheless, the pattern of wound healing has been debated for a long time and yet remains unclear. Thus the chronology of events must be studied with the full spectrum of changes that can develop spatially.[86] Using reconstructed full thickness skin as wound healing model with functional living dermis and epidermis, it has been shown that spatial distribution of keratinocyte re-epithelialization relies on complementary mechanisms from passive cell displacement to cells "crawling" at the tip of progressing neoepidermis.[86] More complex models including endothelial cells and capillary-like tube formation mimicking the microvasculature of skin were used to characterize angiogenesis that occurs in response to injury and during wound healing. Recovery phenomena can be quantified using fluorescence-based, digital imaging microscopy, biochemical, and molecular approaches.[87] These models can bring new insights and new prospect to long-standing questions regarding wound recovery process in acute and chronic wounds.

Studying Specific Skin Diseases

Major consequences of exposure to UVs are skin photoaging and cancer development. Some dramatic effects of UV radiation are demonstrated in patients affected by the rare genetic disease xeroderma pigmentosum (XP),[88] characterized by a severe deficiency in the nucleotide excision repair of UV-induced DNA lesions. While normal cells do repair the lesions (mutations) induced by UV's with a specific repair enzyme, XP cells cannot. These patients show exacerbated sensitivity to the sun and develop skin cancers on exposed areas very early in childhood. Sarasin A et al. from Gustave Roussy Institute, jointly developed with Bernerd and Asselineau from L'Oréal Laboratories, a reconstructed skin model using keratinocytes and fibroblasts from XP patients. Thus, XP skin model comprising an epidermis and a dermal equivalent was successfully reconstructed *in vitro*. Abnormal expression of epidermal differentiation products, such as keratin K10 and loricrin, was observed as well as a high proliferation rate of XP keratinocytes as compared to normal ones. Furthermore and most strikingly, reconstructed XP skin showed numerous proliferative epidermal invasions within dermal equivalent. After UVB-induced DNA damage, long-lasting DNA damage was observed in all layers when skin was reconstructed from XP cells. In contrast, they were repaired within 4 days in reconstructed skin issued from normal cells.[89] Biologists are undertaking genetic correction trials by introducing the normal repair gene into XP keratinocytes. They are investigating whether skin reconstructed with genetically corrected cells behaves like normal skin as far as repair of DNA lesions induced by ultraviolet radiation is concerned.[90,91] This approach holds great hope for a long-term treatment of XP patients.

Melanoma is the most aggressive and deadly form of skin cancer. Metastasis of melanoma is a complex multistage process and the use of 3D reconstructed skin helped to understand the first stages of melanocytic transformation and invasion. Correct functioning of the epidermis, is regulated by the equilibrium between cell proliferation, differentiation and apoptosis. In normal skin, melanocyte behavior is mainly under the control of keratinocytes, which promote the expression of adhesion molecules, such as E-cadherin. In malignant melanocytes, the down-regulation of E-cadherin expression is associated with melanoma invasion and metastasis potential. This has been confirmed in 3D models of skin reconstructed with malignant melanocytes which have lost their invasive properties when they have been forced to express E-cadherin (transduction of E-cadherin-negative melanoma cells with full-length E-cadherin cDNA).[92] When melanocytes no longer express E-cadherin, but N-cadherin instead, they escape from the control of keratinocytes and start to communicate with the fibroblasts. Consequently, melanocytes migrate into the dermis rather than remaining in the epidermis. This altered dialogue between cells plays a role in the process of cancer development.[93,94]

Studying Epidermal Resident Stem Cells

In the medical field, use of stem cells should revolutionize applications of tissue engineering.[95] Stem cells are quiescent and undifferentiated cells. They rarely divide, and produce two types of cells by asymmetric divisions: cells identical to themselves, to constitute a permanent reservoir of their kind, and progenitor cells, which are programmed to differentiate after transient amplification into a specialized type of cells, such as red blood cells, liver hepatocytes or epidermal keratinocytes. It is possible to select keratinocyte populations enriched or depleted in stem cells from skin samples on the basis of the specific properties of these cells (Fig. 6).[96] First, they have a high capacity to adhere to collagen (related to the presence of molecules of α6β4 integrins strongly expressed at their surface) and this property is used to select a population called Adh+++ (accounting for 10% of the keratinocytes). Secondly, they have low or no expression of the epidermal growth factor receptor (EGF-R). This criterion allows a subpopulation called EGF-Rlow (2% of the starting population) to be selected by flow cytometry. An Adh+++ EGF-Rlow cell is capable of producing over 100 billion keratinocytes. An Adh+++ EGF-Rhigh cell strongly expressing the EGF receptor produces only 100 to 1000.

Keratinocyte population depleted in stem cells generates only a weakly stratified, poorly differentiated epidermis. Conversely, a population enriched in stem cells is capable of reconstructing a stratified and almost perfectly differentiated epidermis.

By varying only a single parameter, the enrichment in keratinocytic stem cells, it is possible to mimic the morphological signs of epidermal aging. Even though, as shown in a previous work, the amount of stem cells varies little in the course of aging, these models open up new approaches for studying the mechanisms of aging and loss of stem cell functionality. The concept of a stem cell "niche", inseparable from the function of the stem cells, still remains poorly understood. Such models with variable organogenic potential make it possible to study the nature of the signals and interactions that allow a stem cell to be and remain a stem cell (Fig. 7).

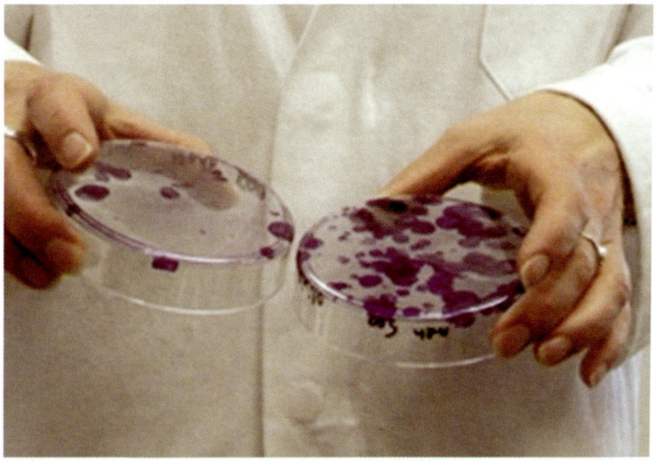

Figure 6: The colony forming efficiency. This culture test consists in seeding keratinocytes at low density (3,000 cells per dish), so as to obtain well-individualized colonies of clones, easily countable and easy to distinguish from a qualitative point of view. Example of keratinocyte populations depleted in stem cells (on the left) and enriched in stem cells (on the right)
©L'Oréal Research and Innovation

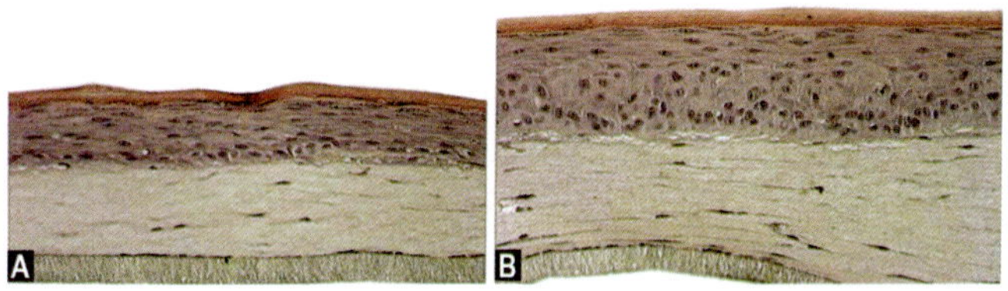

Figure 7: Histological sections of reconstructed skins with variable organogenic potential. **A,** Reconstructed skin with reduced number of functional regenerative cells. **B,** Reconstructed skin enriched in functional regenerative cells
©L'Oréal Research and Innovation

Clinical Applications

The most remarkable use of reconstructed epidermis aims at treating aims at treating major burns. Without epithelial coverage, defense lacks against contamination of the exposed underlying tissue or loss of fluid. The first clinical trials of grafts of autologous epithelia, obtained in culture, date back to 1979. Since then, biotechnology companies, such as Genzyme Biosurgery have been producing cultured epithelia for grafting purposes (www.genzyme.com). Cultured epithelial autografts (Epicel) have been available since the late 1980s. The hospital specialized structures send the laboratory a few square centimeters of the patient's skin (intact areas) and after two to three weeks of culture, more than a square meter of epidermis is produced and may be applied to the patient. This indicates that the keratinocytes have multiplied by about 10,000 times. The quality of the cell culture system and, in particular, maintaining the keratinocyte strains, which keep the capacity to regenerate the epidermis throughout life, is essential to ensure that the graft takes and that the epidermis lasts.

Other clinical areas of application for reconstructed skin involve the treatment of chronic wounds (e.g. leg ulcers in diabetic subjects or varicose ulcers). Two types of product can be used: patient cells (autologous) or cells from another person (allogeneic) due to the inability of epidermal keratinocytes and fibroblasts to stimulate a T-cell response. The US Company Organogenesis (www.organogenesis.com) and another one in Shanxi (PR China) produce allogeneic skin equivalents at an industrial scale for treating leg ulcers and burns. This artificial skin consists of both a dermal compartment and an epidermal compartment. Applied to the wound, it acts as a biological dressing. It releases growth factors and stimulates the patient's own cells. The latter also begin to secrete growth factors which promote healing and stimulate multiplication of the cells around the edge of the wound and their migration close to the ulcer. From a tissue-engineering point of view, such products have a capability of responding to the microenvironment and thus behave in a "smart" way to induce angiogenesis and granulation-tissue formation to regenerate the wound.

The manufacturing of cultured epidermis from epilated hair is another useful way of obtaining reconstructed skin.[97] The keratinocytes located along the external sheath of the hair have a high capacity to multiply, irrespective of the age of the patient. After several weeks of culture, it is possible to obtain small areas of epidermal tissue which are grafted onto the wound and help to close the ulcer. These models of reconstructed skin are also used to treat acute wounds which sometimes occur after a surgical procedure to remove an area of cancerous skin or a tattoo.

To date, tissue therapy with reconstructed skin has saved the life of thousands of major burnt victims and has provided new ways of treating ulcers. Nevertheless, reconstruction generally is neither perfect nor complete. Accordingly, biologists are continuously studying new substrates (for example fibrin films) which can assist the culture and transplantation of epithelia, promote reorganization and revascularization of the dermis and decrease scar formation.

IN VITRO SKIN MODELS FOR PREDICTIVE EVALUATION OF COMPOUNDS AND FINISHED PRODUCTS

The ability to reproduce several functions of human skin *in vitro* opens a large field for industrial applications. Thanks to *in vitro* skin models it is now possible to predict, early in their development phase, the effects, positive or negative, of new compounds, drugs, chemicals, cosmetics, medical devices, etc.

The development of new cosmetics requires a precise assessment of their safety and activity. A number of *in vitro* methods have been developed and proposed for this purpose. Methods using reconstructed epidermis or full thickness skin models have been introduced and are today commonly used to assess both efficacy and safety of cosmetic ingredients and formulations. These 3D skin models offer many advantages:

- Architecture close to that of native skin
- Presence of a SC, that forms a barrier to exogenous substances although less efficient than that of skin *in vivo*
- They can be used to measure a large variety of parameters related to the efficacy or safety of substances
- The air exposed surface allows ingredients/products with various physicochemical properties to be topically applied thus mimicking *in vivo* use.

Compared to classical *in vitro* 2D cell cultures, 3D models reproduce the complexity and richness of *in vivo* cell-cell and cell-ECM interactions. Reproducing this microenvironment is important since cellular interactions regulate several mechanisms, such as viability, proliferation, differentiation, morphology, protein synthesis and genome expression.[98] It has been shown that the gene expression profiles of keratinocytes from *in vitro* 3D reconstructed skin is much closer to *in vivo* human skin than keratinocytes cultivated in 2D.[99] In 2D models, cells are immersed in an aqueous culture medium which limits the testing to hydrosoluble substances. The use of *in vitro* skin models overcome this limitation and makes possible to apply substances, whatever their physicochemical forms (liquid, powder, gel) directly to the SC. The way the products tested are applied and the resulting exposure of the cells (barrier function, gradient of concentration) are closer to the *in vivo* conditions, as compared to 2D protocols.

Over the last 20 years, substantial work and investments have been devoted to the development of both *in vitro* and *ex vivo* methods. Thus, several validation studies based on test methods using organotypic models, reconstructed human tissues, simple cell assays, physicochemical assays or combination of tests were conducted. However, despite huge progress in the models used, numerous questions have been raised regarding mechanisms of action, classification, scope of applications and, finally, the need to identify testing strategies able to strengthen final predictions. *In vitro* reconstructed skin models, such as EpiSkin™, SkinEthic RHE and full thickness tissues are widely used today in both safety and efficacy pre-screening tests.[100] Their growing interest was followed in the last decade by several validations and acceptance for regulatory purposes.

PREDICTIVE TOXICOLOGY AND ALTERNATIVE METHODS

To date, any novel substance used in the composition of consumer products should undergo preliminary comprehensive toxicological evaluation process. However, the use of animal tests is strongly questioned and rightly criticized for both ethical and scientific reasons (methods with more or less subjective scoring, low inter-laboratory reproducibility, known differences in sensitivity with humans).[101,102] In Europe, the 7th amendment (2003/15/CE)[103] to the Cosmetics Directive, (76/768/EEC), introduced a ban on the use of animal tests to evaluate the human safety of cosmetic products and their ingredients. Since 2009, this ban covered "acute" toxicological end-points including those linked to skin and eye adverse effects. In March 2013, it was extended to other tests requiring repeated applications, e.g. repeat dose toxicity, sensitization, reproductive toxicity, carcinogenicity as well as toxicokinetics. This total ban of animal testing concerns not only products developed in Europe but any cosmetics intended to be marketed in Europe. Following the European model, Israel banned in 2013 the importation of cosmetics tested on animals. This regulation completed a 2007 ban of animal testing on domestic cosmetics. In June 2013, India became the first country in South Asia to decide a ban of animal testing for domestic manufacturing cosmetics. In May 2014, this ban was extended to all imported cosmetics. To fully enter in force, the Bureau of Indian Standards (BIS) is going to set down standards to allow the Drugs Controller General of India (DCGI) to make relevant amendments in acts and laws. Position of China about animal testing is also evolving rapidly. A new policy passed in December 2013 authorizes from June 2014 certain categories of cosmetics (such as soap, shampoo and some skin products) locally developed to be marketed without the need of animal test. Recently, in January 2014, the state of São Paulo in Brazil released a bill prohibiting cosmetics testing on animals.

The movement initiated in Europe with the 7th amendment to the cosmetics Directive progressively spreads out worldwide. This lead to a shift from a toxicology based on observation of effects into animals to a mechanistic approach based upon *in vitro* and *in silico* tests to predict potential adverse effects in human. The Cosmetic industry is at the forefront of this new paradigm in toxicology, but this will undoubtedly and increasingly concerns other industries, such as chemicals, medical devices or drug development.

Validated Versus Valid Methods

The diversity of existing *in vitro* models including reconstructed epidermis and skin tissues, together with their variety, represents a potential strong driver for the application of adapted and integrated *in vitro* methods. Reconstructed human skin presents several advantages that make it an alternative method of choice for evaluating some regulatory aspects of safety. It is a fully *in vitro* method based on biological systems close to the target organ of the products. The tests are reproducible, standardized and easily accessible. The evaluation parameters are simple and related to the *in vivo* or clinical damage. In addition, cutaneous engineering

Table 2: List of centers for validation of alternative methods in the world

Name	Acronym and website	Created
European Union Reference Laboratory for alternatives to animal testing	EURL ECVAM (formerly ECVAM) http://ihcp.jrc.ec.europa.eu/our_labs/eurl-ecvam	1991
Interagency Coordinating Committee on the Validation of Alternative Methods	ICCVAM http://ntp.niehs.nih.gov/go/iccvam	1994
Japanese Center for the Validation of Alternative Methods	JacVAM http://www.jacvam.jp/	2005
Korean Center for the Validation of Alternative	KocVAM http://www.nifds.go.kr/en/inter/kocvam.jsp	2009
Brazilian Centre for the Validation of Alternative Methods	BraCVAM	2011

allows finished products or ingredients to be evaluated under conditions very close to the final conditions of use. To date, several methods have been developed based upon *in vitro* skin to assess different toxicological end-points (skin penetration, skin corrosion/irritation, phototoxicity, genotoxicity).[104] However, an *in vitro* alternative method must be validated before being recognized by the concerned regulatory bodies. Validation is the process whereby the reliability and relevance of a particular approach, method, procedure or assessment is established for a defined purpose.[105] In Europe, the European Center for Validation of Alternative Methods (EURL-ECVAM) is devoted to the validation of alternative methods. It maintains the Tracking System on Alternative Methods (TSAR), a tool aimed at providing view on the status of alternative methods as they progress from purely scientific protocols submitted for prevalidation to being actively used within a regulatory context. Since the creation of ECVAM in 1991, four regional organizations have been created on the same principle in different countries (Table 2).

Today, two alternative methods based on *in vitro* skin models have been validated as full replacement methods to animal. These methods have been integrated in the test guidelines of the Organization for Economic Co-operation and Development (OECD): TG 431 for *in vitro* skin corrosion and TG 439 for *in vitro* skin irritation.

In the Field of Skin Corrosion and Irritation

Skin corrosion or dermal corrosion tests assess the potential of a substance to cause irreversible damage to the skin, namely visible necrosis through the epidermis and into the dermis, following the application of a test substance for the duration period of 3 minutes up to 4 hours. The historical Draize test developed in the 1940s causes severe discomfort and pain to animal and was part of the banned animal tests for 2013 deadline.[106] Many attempts have been made to replace the *in vivo* Draize rabbit skin corrosion test. Up to now, 6 methods have been validated between 1999 and 2006 and officially quoted in EU statements from the ECVAM advisory committee (ESAC). Amongst these, two validated methods were not based on reconstructed tissues: the Corrositex (artificial biobarrier), a corrosion test peer-reviewed by ICCVAM (report 1999), quoted in the ESAC 2000 statement and in the OECD guideline TG435; the Rat Skin Transepidermal Electrical Resistance—TER, validated by ECVAM, quoted in the ESAC 1998 statement and in the OECD guideline TG430.

Four validated test methods using *in vitro* reconstructed epidermis were validated by ECVAM and subsequently endorsed by ESAC: the EpiSkin™ model,[107] the EpiDerm™ model,[107] the SkinEthic™ RHE model[108] and the EST-1000 model.[109] All these *in vitro* methods based upon reconstructed epidermis were implemented in the EU Methods for testing dangerous substances and included in the OECD test guideline 431 (dedicated to human *in vitro* skin model tests methods). The Test Guideline 431 defines some general and functional rules and conditions needed to being evaluated before using the models for routine purposes. The last revision of TG 431 released in July 2013, includes a technical update on performance standards and the possibility to use some of the methods for the sub-categorization among corrosive chemicals.[110] From the four methods validated for distinguishing between corrosive and non-corrosive, only the EpiskinTM model can be used also for the sub-categorization of corrosive substances into two classes, 1A and 1B-1C, in accordance with the UN GHS.[111]

Skin irritation or dermal irritation is defined as reversible damage of the skin following the application of a test substance for up to 4 hours. Evaluation of the irritancy potential to human skin of any chemical or product used in the pharmaceutical or cosmetics industry is a requirement. The assessment of acute skin irritation has been usually performed on rabbit skin (Draize rabbit skin irritation test).[112] According to the test guideline 404[113] and involved determination of clinical signs, such as erythema and edema after single application to skin. Regarding potential misclassification[114] and ethical considerations, animal data could be very questionable and are subjected to regulatory issues.[115] Consequently, alternatives to these animal test procedures have been developed in different fields.[116,117] EpiSkin™ and EpiDerm™ test methods were evaluated for their ability to predict skin irritation[118] throughout an ECVAM formal validation study. On the basis of this study, ESAC (2007)[119] concluded that the EpiSkin™ Skin Irritation Test (SIT) showed evidence of being a reliable and relevant stand-alone test for predicting skin irritation as a replacement for the Draize Skin Irritation Test. The test method is able to distinguish between skin irritant and no-label test substances. In 2008, ESAC endorsed two additional skin models test methods for skin irritation testing: the EpiDerm skin irritation test method and the SkinEthic™ RHE skin irritation test method. Both showed results similar to the Validated Reference Method (VRM) EpiSkin™ test method, and are considered as valid replacement methods. Validated models, EpiSkin™,[119] EpiDerm™,[119] SkinEthic™ RHE[119] and LabCyte EPI-MODEL24 are included in the last version of the test guideline TG439 (July 2013). The VRM (EpiSkin™) protocol was based on a short treatment time (15 min) followed by an extended 42 hour post-treatment incubation period. The prediction model mainly based on the formally validated viability measurement (MTT test) combined with the useful adjunct IL-1α and appropriate cut-off values (prediction model) allowed 2 chemical classes to be drawn up in accordance with the EU new Classification Labeling and Packaging (CLP): Irritants (=Globally Harmonized System class 2) and non-classified substances. Applied to a set of 184 substances, including references and industrial chemicals covering diverse physical-chemical categories, the performances of the EpiSkin™ test-method were well balanced with 85% sensitivity, 86% specificity and 86% accuracy.[120]

These validated tools are part of the necessary and useful battery of alternative methods allowing industrial non-animal testing strategies to be used. Assessing performance of test methods on a large number of chemicals and products relevant to industrial needs, will help to concretely determine and adjust applicability domains (industry specific) while identifying the remaining gaps.

In the Field of Skin Phototoxicity

Photoirritation is an adverse acute, inflammatory and non-immunologically mediated skin reaction that occurs after a single contact with a photoreactive chemical, under sun exposure. Since 2000, the *in vitro* 3T3 NRU phototoxicity test is the only *in vitro* test validated for evaluating the acute phototoxicity of a chemical. However, this monolayer culture of fibroblasts is a simple basic system lacking connections and interactions between different cell types and ECM.[121] To overcome these limitations, an *in vitro* EpiSkin™ phototoxicity assay (EPA) was developed. EPA performance (on 17 reference chemicals), showed a very good overall accuracy of 94%.[122] Interestingly, the EPA takes into account the influence of the administration route (topical treatment versus a systemic-like administration) in the prediction of phototoxic potency.

Similar protocols based on viability assessment were applied to different skin and epidermis reconstructed models.[123,124] The promising performance of EPA showed that the EpiSkin™ model is an interesting tool which is able to integrate decision-making processes to address the question of phototoxicity linked to the administration route. Using the industrial epidermis SkinEthic™ RHE model showed that exposure to solar simulated radiation (SSR) induced phototoxic features, such as the formation of sunburn cells and DNA damages (fragmentation) with the activation of caspase-3 protease in keratinocyte basal layers, which opens possibilities for evaluating the photoprotective capacity of cosmetic formulations.[125]

In the Field of Genotoxicity

Genotoxicity refers to processes which alter the structure, information content or segregation of DNA and which are not necessarily associated with mutagenicity. Thus, tests for genotoxicity include tests that assess induced damages to DNA (but not direct evidence of mutation). Genotoxicity and mutagenicity evaluations are important and early steps in the safety assessment of chemicals for industrial development and regulatory purposes. Although many *in vitro* tests are routinely used and accepted by regulatory agencies, their accuracy to predict the mutagenic/genotoxic potential in humans is frequently questioned.[126] In 2007, a workshop of experts underlined the fact that genotoxicity tests in 2D culture of mammalian cells *in vitro* produced a remarkably high and unacceptable occurrence of irrelevant positive results. The only way to confirm such results would imply an *in vivo* rodent carcinogenicity test. Among the proposals made to overcome this limitation, the experts concluded that the use of 3D *in vitro* skin models was a promising way. They indeed present clear advantages (organ structure, functionality, standardized production, availability, etc) as *in vitro* screening tools for genotoxicity. Specific protocols to perform the comet assay (genotoxicity test) on EpiSkin™ were developed both with UV exposure and/or reference chemicals (Lomefloxacin, 4-nitroquinoline-N-oxide) as stress agents. Pretreatment with the sunscreen Mexoryl SX® was able to clearly reduce the extent of UV-induced DNA damages assessed by the comet signal. A second approach was developed, taking advantage of the barrier function and metabolic capacities of the EpiSkin™ model, to drive the response to a topically applied test chemical and its possible metabolites. A specific co-culture system using a target lymphoma cell line (L5178Y) underneath the epidermis was performed for the evaluation of micronucleus induction after topical application of the test-substance. This approach aims at improving the relevance of exposure conditions for testing further products to be applied onto the skin.[127] This could improve the predictive value of a genotoxicity assessment as compared to those afforded by existing *in vitro* tests and, therefore, could be used as follow-up tests in case of positive results from the standard *in vitro* genotoxicity testing battery. Another approach under validation is to conduct the micronucleus test and the comet assay directly on 3D human reconstructed skin models.[128] Validation studies of the micronucleus test using the human reconstructed skin models are coordinated and funded by Cosmetics Europe and, in the case of the 3D Skin Comet assay, by a joint effort between Cosmetics Europe and a German Consortium funded by BMBF.[129]

In the Field of Skin Penetration and Metabolism

Assessment of systemic risks after dermal exposure requires reliable models and protocols. To better evaluate and understand the needs for safety evaluation and the role of the tissue compartments, studies using infinite-doses versus finite-doses were conducted according to a validation-like format with several manufactured and "in house" reconstructed human skin models.[130] The authors demonstrated the suitable *in vivo*/*in vitro* correlation as regards test-chemicals' ranking with EpiSkin™, EpiDerm and SkinEthic™ RHE, even though permeation of *in vitro* models still generally exceeds that of human excised skin. Studies using the EpiSkin™ model have demonstrated that percutaneous assays could be easily performed without specific or complex device, such as Franz cell.[131] This system simplifies the development of screening tests for evaluation of skin penetration of compounds with a high reliability and a high throughput. The permeation of essential oils was evaluated using SkinEthic™ RHE to establish the kinetics of release of active principles from cosmetic formulations. Diffusion and quantification of selected terpenes proved the method sensitive, simple and reproducible, thus providing a convenient model for safety/quality assessment of formulations.[132] Similarly, EpiSkin™ tissues were used to evaluate the absorption of vitamins C and E from topical micro-emulsions, allowing the best formulation able to enhance deposition of the tested vitamins in the tissue to be identified.[133]

Investigating the biotransformation of oxygen-sensitive aromatic diamines (AD) (used in oxidative oxidative hair coloring) during penetration through process following topical application onto the EpiSkin™ model, it was interestingly shown that the reconstructed epidermis had a clear capacity to activate N-acetylation, glucuronidation and sulfation enzymes, i.e. to metabolize and detoxify these AD derivatives. The data supports the growing evidence that ADs are transformed in human skin and suggests that current practices of safety assessment of ADs should take these essential findings into account.[134] The latter results evidenced the role of the barrier function together with the expression of metabolic capacities in 3D models (i.e. standardized SkinEthic™ RHE and EpiSkin™ epidermis) and thus support their use as simple and cost effective tools suited to efficacy/safety studies, overcoming availability problems usually encountered with human skin explants, but with the sound care when extrapolating results to clinical levels.[130]

Recently, the use of noninvasive imaging technology, such as confocal Raman spectroscopy or two photon imaging, provided new insights to study the permeation process and development of local toxicity.[135,136]

PREDICTIVE METHODS IN EFFICACY

In the area of efficacy, reconstructed skins allow active, new agents not only to be identified and their efficacy measured but also their activity characterized and their way of action deciphered. Extrapolating their results to real human skin is an important line of research.

In the Field of Skin Aging

Skin aging induces dramatic changes in the extracellular dermal matrix (ECM) as well as in the DEJ. Reversing or slowing down these phenomena could reduce these visible signs of aging. It was shown that topical application of a C-xylopyranoside derivative (C-beta-D-sylopyranoside-2-hydroxy-propane) to a reconstructed full thickness skin induced neo-synthesis of some matrix proteins, such as GAG and heparan sulfate proteoglycans. It additionally led to an improvement in the DEJ morphogenesis together with an increased collagen VII expression, all data thus suggesting beneficial effects on aged skin.[137] GAGs are major components of dermal ECM and participate in tissue cohesiveness and hydration. Through their ability to bind to and modulate the activity of a number of growth factors, GAGs are also involved in cell adhesion and migration, as well as skin organogenesis and wound healing. The structure and integrity of GAGs is therefore essential for skin homeostasis and regeneration. Some works suggest that age-related alteration of the dermal connective tissue may involve a remodeling of GAG expression and structure.[138,139] Further studies with *in vitro* skin models confirmed that C-xyloside strongly enhanced synthesis of GAG chains, but also induced significant changes in their size and structure. C-xyloside primed GAGs were exclusively chondroitin/dermatan sulfate with reduced chain size, increased O-sulfation, and changes in iduronate content and distribution.[140] This gives new insights into the effect of C-xyloside on GAG structure and activities, which opens up prospects and applications of such compound in skin repair/regeneration.

Differentiation/proliferation balance in keratinocytes strongly influences skin homeostasis. Topical application of the anti-aging reference retinol to *in vitro* skin model was shown to modulate differentiation. A combination of retinol and adenosine applied to the 3D skin model showed the ability of adenosine to potentiate retinol effects in accordance with results from a clinical application of a skin care product containing these agents.[141] A derivative of Jasmonic acid, a signal molecule synthesized by plants under stress, was studied on EpiSkin models to evaluate its effect on their regenerative potential. Morphological studies, immunohistochemical measurements and transcriptomic analyses were conducted. Preliminary results on the thickness and proliferation markers (Ki67 markers) showed an increase in the regenerative potential of the *in vitro* skin treated as compared to control. Transcriptomic and immunohistochemical studies showed that this activity was mediated by a stimulation of hyaluronasome, a complex of proteins involved in the synthesis (hyaluronate synthetase HAS3 and HAS2), maturation (hyaluronidase) and fixation of hyaluronic acid on specific receptors (CD44). However, this increase in the epidermal hyaluronic content and keratinocyte proliferation does not disrupt normal differentiation of the epidermis, unlike retinol, which tends to inhibit this process.[142] Further tests using a full thickness model showed an increased synthesis of collagens IV and VII and laminin 5, essential components of the DEJ. Further clinical studies have confirmed, *in vivo*, the efficiency of the Jasmonic derivative and its antiaging potential.[143]

In the Field of Photoprotection

Besides beneficial effects of sunlight, excessive or repeated exposure is known to induce oxidative stress resulting from reactive oxygen species (ROS) production in skin, a major contributor to the deleterious effects following UVA exposure. Among the mechanisms known to be involved, iron plays a central role[144] and can act as a catalyst of uncontrolled oxidation reactions with cell components.[145] Applying iron chelators to the EpiSkin™ model *in vitro* potentially offers an effective way to protect skin against UVA insults,[146] but found hard to being achieved without disturbing iron homeostasis. Recently, a novel compound (Sideroxyl) developed to avoid these potentially harmful side effects was evaluated in reconstructed human skin model. Designed to acquire its strong chelating capacity only during oxidative stress following an intramolecular hydroxylation process, this ingredient demonstrated protective efficiency against UVA deleterious effects at molecular, cellular and tissue levels. The use of *in vitro* reconstructed tissue allowed several endpoints to be measured including carbonyl increase, intracellular ROS, DNA damage (comet assay) and MMP-1 synthesis and release, altogether suggesting that such an ingredient may prevent UVA-induced damage in human skin in complement to sunscreens, especially in the long wavelength UVA range (370–400 nm).[147]

The structure of the 3D models and the presence of an air-exposed SC make them tools of choice for the topical application of finished products. Application of a product containing Mexoryl SX® sunscreen before solar simulated sunlight exposure (conditions mimicking *in vivo* use) revealed the ability of the sunscreen to inhibit almost completely the UV-induced pigmentation.[148] The *in vitro* evaluation of sunscreens after topical application allows their protective effects against UV to be investigated and proper selection of UV absorbers to be carried out and tested based upon their absorption spectrum.[72,73] Recent definition of a standard "daily ultraviolet radiation" (DUVR) allowed non-zenithal sun exposure conditions to be reproduced on *in vitro* models. Two commercial sunscreen products with similar sun protection factor (SPF) but different absorption profiles over the UVA range, were evaluated on reconstructed human skin. Using vimentin immunostaining for dermal fibroblasts, and MMP1 secretion, it was shown that sun-screening profile of the product should be well balanced with a sufficient level of UVA absorption,[149] to ensure an efficient daily photo protection from DUVR.

In the Field of Modulation of Pigmentation

N-acetyl glucosamine (NAG) is an amino sugar precursor in human skin of the high molecular weight water-binding polymer hyaluronic acid. It has been shown effective in reducing the appearance of hyperpigmented spots.[150] Through inhibiting the glycosylation of Tyrosinase, a key enzyme in the production of melanin.[151] To identify additional mechanisms by which NAG might affect melanin production, a transcriptomic study of the effect of NAG was conducted onto the SkinEthic model of reconstructed human pigmented epidermis (RHPE). The results showed several expression changes (up-regulation and down-regulation), some of them being related to synthesis and regulation of intracellular cytoskeletal proteins involved in melanosomes transport within the cells.[152] Thus, several mechanisms may be operative in the observed effects of NAG onto pigmentation. Produced in an industrial scale, these *in vitro* pigmented skin models are able to reproduce different skin phototypes. They are powerful tools to screen the pro- or depigmentating efficacy of new compounds.[153,154] Such model has been also used to develop RNA silencing (siRNA) strategies to modulate skin pigmentation. After selecting a potent siRNA compounds that which targets the tyrosinase gene, its efficacy was assessed during reconstruction of a RHPE model. Melanocytes derived from the dark-dark-pigmented phototype VI skin were used for the reconstruction of a phenotypically silenced epidermis. A visible and long-term pigmentation interference effect (lasting more than 30 days) was observed in the SkinEthic RHPE model.[155] This knock down of tyrosinase expression was indeed transient since reconstructed epidermis started recovering pigmentation at day 39 and thus did not irreversibly affect melanocyte differentiation. The pigmented reconstructed epidermis therefore becomes a precious tool for studying the effect of various topical applications and vectors as well as selecting, evaluating and designing new dermatological interventions, tools and targets.

CONCLUSION

This chapter gives an overview of several medical, industrial and research applications of skin engineering. Since the first reconstructed epidermis in the 1980s, a lot of advances have been realized. With the emergence of new tools, such as bioprinting, organ on a chip, stems cells and transduced cells we can predict an acceleration and a revolution for the coming years of the reconstructed skin models and of their applications.

REFERENCES

1. Hall CW, Liotta D, De Bakey ME. Artificial skin. Trans Am Soc Artif Intern Organs. 1966;12:340-5.
2. Herndon DN, Gore D, Cole M, et al. Determinants of mortality in pediatric patients with greater than 70% full-thickness total body surface area thermal injury treated by early total excision and grafting. J Trauma. 1987;27:208-12.
3. Pruniéras M. Epidermal cell cultures as models for living epidermis. J Invest Dermatol. 1979;73:135-7.
4. Pruniéras M, Régnier M, Woodley D. Methods for cultivation of keratinocytes with an air-liquid interface. J Invest Dermatol. 1983;81:28-33.
5. Ferraris C. La peau reconstruite. Pour la Science. 2005;333:70-5.
6. MacNeil S. Progress and opportunities for tissue-engineered skin. Nature. 2007;45:874-80.
7. Carlson MW, Alt-Holland A, Egles C, et al. Three-dimensional tissue models of normal and diseased skin. Curr Protocols Cell Biol. 2008;41:1-17.
8. Groeber F, Holeiter M, Hampel M, et al. Skin tissue engineering — In vivo and in vitro applications. Adv Drug Deliv Rev. 2011;128:352-66.
9. Olson H, Betton G, Robinson D, et al. Concordance of the Toxicity of Pharmaceuticals in Humans and in Animals. Regul Toxicol Pharmacol. 2000;32:56-67.
10. Li AP. Accurate prediction of human drug toxicity: a major challenge in drug development. Chem Biol Interact. 2004;150:3-7.
11. Ledford H. Translational research: 4 ways to fix the clinical trial. Nature. 2011;477:526-8.
12. Russell WMS, Burch Rl. The principles of humane experimental technique. London: Methuen; 1959.
13. ECVAM. Statement on the scientific validity of the EpiskinTM test (an in vitro test for skin corrosivity). ESAC Statement. 1998.
14. Carrel A, Burrows MT. Cultivation of adult tissues and organs outside the body. JAMA. 1910;55:1379-81.
15. Puck TT, Marcus PI. Clonal growth of mammalian cells in vitro; growth characteristics of colonies from single HeLa cells with and without a feeder layer. J Exp Med. 1956;103:273-83.
16. Rheinwald JG, Green H. Serial cultivation of strains of human epidermal keratinocytes: the formation of keratinizing colonies from single cells. Cell. 1975;6:331-43.
17. Green H, Kehinde O, Thomas J. Growth of cultured human epidermal cells into multiple epithelia suitable for grafting. Proceedings of the National Academy of Science of the US. 1979;76:5665-8.
18. O'Connor NE, Mulliken JB, Banks-Schlegel S, et al. Grafting of burns with cultured epithelium prepared from autologous epidermal cells. Lancet. 1981;1:75-8.
19. Bissell MJ, Hall HG, Parry G. How does the extracellular matrix direct gene expression? J Theoret Bio. 1982;99:31-68.
20. Lin CQ, Bissell MJ. Multi-faceted regulation of cell differentiation by extracellular matrix. FASEB J. 1993;7:737–43.
21. Boyce ST, Warden GD. Principles and practices for treatment of cutaneous wounds with cultured skin substitutes. Am J Surg. 2002;183:445-56.
22. Asselineau D, Bernard BA, Bailly C, et al. Epidermal morphogenesis and induction of 67kD keratin polypeptide by culture at the liquid-air interface. Exp Cell Res. 1985;159:536-9
23. Haake AR, Scott GA. Physiologic distribution and differentiation of melanocytes in human fetal and neonatal skin equivalents. J Invest Dermatol. 1991;96:71-7.
24. Facy V, Flouret V, Regnier M, et al. Langerhans cells integrated into human reconstructed epidermis respond to known sensitizers and ultraviolet exposure. J Invest Dermatol. 2004;122:552-3.
25. Régnier M, Schweizer J, Michel S, et al. Expression of high molecular weight (67K) keratin in human keratinocytes cultured on dead de-epidermized dermis. Experimental Cell Res. 1986;165:63-72.
26. Ponec M, Weerheim A, Kempenaar J, et al. Lipid composition of cultured keratinocytes in relation to their differentiation. J Lipid Res. 1988;29:949-62.
27. Bell E, Ehrlich HP, Sher S, et al. Development and use of a living skin equivalent. J Plast Rec Surg. 1981;67:386.
28. Boyce ST, Christianson D, Hansbrough J. Structure of a collagen-GAG skin substitute optimized for cultured human epidermal keratinocytes. J Biomat Res. 1988;22:939-57.
29. Black AF, Bouez C, Perrier E, et al. Optimization and characterization of an engineered human skin equivalent. Tissue Engineering. 2005;11:723-33.
30. Shahabeddin L, Berthod F, Damour O, et al. Characteri-zationof skin reconstructed on a chitosan-cross-linked collagengly-cosaminoglycan matrix. Skin Pharmacol. 1990;3:107-14.
31 El Ghalbzouri A, Lamme EN, van Blitterswijk C, et al. The use of PEGT/PBT as a dermal scaffold for skin tissue engineering. Biomaterials. 2004;25:2987-96..
32. Boyce ST, Supp AP, Swope VB, et al.Vitamin C regulates keratinocyte viability, epidermal barrier, and basement membrane formation in vitro, and reduces wound contraction after grafting of cultured skin substitutes. J Invest Dermatol. 2002;118:565-72.
33. Harrison CA, Heaton MJ, Layton CM, et al. Use of an in vitro model of tissue-engineered human skin to study keratinocyte attachment and migration in the process of reepithelialization. Wound Rep Reg. 2006;14:203-9.
34. Lee V, Singh G, Trasatti JP, et al. Design and Fabrication of Human Skin by Three-Dimensional Bioprinting. Tissue Eng Part C Methods. 2014;20:473-84.
35. De Brugerolle A. SkinEthic Laboratories, a company devoted to develop and produce in vitro alternative methods to animal use. ALTEX. 2007;24:167-71.
36. Obin JP, De Vecchi G, Carmona-Magnaldi N. Faire construire des savoirs.Paris: Hachette Education;2008.
37. Madison KC. Barrier Function of the Skin: "La Raison d'Être" of the Epidermis. J Invest Dermatol. 2003;121:231-41.
38. Régnier M, Caron D, Reichert U, et al. Reconstructed human epidermis: a model to study in vitro the barrier function of the skin. Skin Pharmacol. 1992;5:49-56.
39. Ponec M, Gibbs S, Pilgram G, et al. Barrier function in reconstructed epidermis and its resemblance to native human skin. Skin Pharmacol App Skin Physio. 2001;14:63-71.
40. Boelsma E, Gibbs S, Faller C. Characterization and comparison of reconstructed skin models: morphological and immunological evaluation. Acta Dermatol Venerol. 2000;80:82-8.
41. Ponec M, Boelsma E, Weerheim A, et al. Lipid and ultra structural characterization of human reconstructed skin models. Int J Pharm. 2000;203:211-21.
42. Barbotteau Y, GontierE, Barberet P, et al. Reconstructed human epidermis: A model to study the barrier function. Nucl Instr Meth Phys Res. 2005;B231:286-91.
43. Schäfer-Korting M, Bock U, Diembeck W, et al. The Use of Reconstructed Human Epidermis for Skin Absorption Testing: Results of the Validation Study. Altern Lab Anim. 2008;36:161-87.
44. Régnier M, Schmidt R. Reconstruction of an epidermal melanin unit

by co-cultures of normal human keratinocytes (NHK) and normal human melanocytes (NHM). J Invest Dermatol. 1994;102:596.

45. Hedley SJ, Layton C, Heaton M, et al. Fibroblasts play a regulatory role in the control of pigmentation in reconstructed human skin from skin types I and II. Pigment Cell Res. 2002;15:49-56.
46. Topol BM, Haimes HB, Dubertret L, et al. Transfer of melanosomes in a skin equivalent model in vitro. J Invest Dermatol. 1986;87:642-7.
47. Valyi-Nagy IT, Murphy GF, Mancianti ML, et al. Phenotypes and interactions of human melanocytes and keratinocytes in an epidermal reconstructed model. Lab Investig. 1990;62:314-24.
48. Duval C, Chagnoleau C, Pouradier F, et al. Human Skin Model Containing Melanocytes: Essential Role of Keratinocyte Growth Factor for Constitutive Pigmentation—Functional Response to α-Melanocyte Stimulating Hormone and Forskolin. Tissue Eng Part C Methods. 2012;18:947-57.
49. Alaluf S, Atkins D, Barrett K, et al. Ethnic variation in melanin content and composition in photoexposed and photoprotected human skin. Pigment Cell Research. 2002;15:112-8.
50. Sahuc F, De Wever B, Rosdy M. Human pigmented epidermis reconstructed in chemically defined medium used for the evaluation of modulation of pigmentation. 12th Annual Meeting of the European Society of Pigmented Cell Research. Paris September 2004.
51. Sahuc F. Reconstructed Human Pigmented Epidermis (RHPE): An *in vitro* Model for the Evaluation of Melanogenesis. SÖFW-Journal. 2009;135:31-5.
52. Kimber I, Basketter DA, Gerberick GF, et al. Allergic contact dermatitis. Int Immunopharmacol. 2002;2:201-11.
53. Katz SI, Tamaki K, Sachs DH. Epidermal Langerhans cells are derived from cells originating from bone marrow. Nature. 1979;282:324-6.
54. Régnier M, Staquet MJ, Schmitt D, et al. Integration of Langerhans cells into a pigmented reconstructed human epidermis. J Invest Dermatol. 1997;109:510-2.
55. Luu-The V, Duche D, Ferraris C, et al. Expression profiles of phase 1 and phase 2 metabolizing enzymes in human skin and the reconstructed skin models EpiSkin and full thickness model from EpiSkin. J Steroid Biochem Mol Biol. 2009;116:178-86.
56. van Eijl S, Zhu Z, Cupitt J, et al. Elucidation of Xenobiotic Metabolism Pathways in Human Skin and Human Skin Models by Proteomic Profiling. 2012;7:e41721.
57. Pham MA, Magdalou J, Siest G, et al. Reconstituted epidermis : a novel model for the study of drug metabolism in human epidermis. J Invest Dermatol. 1990;94:749-52.
58. Vecchini F, Bernard BA, Magdalou J, et al. Constitutive and inducible expression of drug metabolizing enzymes in cultured human keratinocytes. Br J Dermatol. 1994;132:14-21.
59. Eilstein J, Léreaux G, Budimir N, et al. Comparison of xenobiotic metabolizing enzyme activities in ex vivo human skin and reconstructed human skin models from SkinEthic. Arch Toxicol. 2014;22.
60. Hewitt NJ, Edwards RJ, Fritsche E, et al. Use of human in vitro skin models for accurate and ethical risk assessment: metabolic considerations. Toxicol Sci. 2013;133:209-17.
61. Luu-The V, Ferraris C, Duche D, et al. Steroid metabolism and profile of steroidogenic gene expression in Episkin: high similarity with human epidermis. J Steroid Biochem Mol Biol. 2007;107:30-6.
62. Black AF, Berthod F, L'Heureux N, et al. In vitro reconstruction of a human capillary-like network in a tissue-engineered skin equivalent. FASEB J. 1998;12:1331-40.
63. Boenhke K, Mirancea N, Pavesio A, et al. Effects of fibroblasts and microenvironment on epidermal regeneration and tissue function in long term skin equivalents. Eur J Cell Biol. 2007;86:731-46.
64. Castor CW, Prince RK, Dorstewitz EL. Characteristics of human fibroblasts cultivated in vitro from different anatomical sites. Lab Investig. 1962;11:703-13.
65. Rinn JL, Bondre C, Gladstone HB, et al. Anatomic demarcation by positional variation in fibroblast gene expression programs. PlOS Genetics. 2006;2:1084-96.
66. Sorrell JM, Caplan AI. Fibroblast heterogeneity: more than skin deep. J Cell Sci. 2004;117:667-75.
67. Mine S, Fortunel NO, Pageon H, et al. Aging alters functionally human dermal papillary fibroblasts: A new view of skin morphogenesis and aging. PloS ONE. 2008;3:e4066.
68. Asselineau D, Pageon H, Mine S. Fibroblast subpopulations: a developmental approach of skin physiology and aging. J Société Biol. 2008; 202:7-14.
69. Commo S, Gaillard O, Bernard BA. The human hair follicle contains two distinct K19 positive compartments in the outer root sheath: a unifying hypothesis for stem cell reservoir? Differentiation. 2000;66:157-64.
70. Mascré G, Dekoninck S, Drogat B, et al. Distinct contribution of stem and progenitor cells to epidermal maintenance. Nature. 2012;489:257-62.
71. Grégoire S, Patouillet C, Noé C, et al. Improvement of the experimental setup for skin absorption screening studies with reconstructed skin Episkin. Skin Pharmacol Physiol. 2008;21:89-97.
72. Murthy V. Telomerase activity in human umbilical cord cell populations containing hematopoietic stem cells. 2002. http://www.wpi.edu/Pubs/ETD/Available/etd-0430102-105910/unrestricted/Murthy.pdf [2010-10].
73. Deshayes N, Rathman-Josserand M. Origines et sélection de progéniteurs et cellules souches épidermiques: Un défi pour l'ingéniérie tissulaire. J Société Biol. 2008; 202:43-54.
74. Lapierre CM. The aging dermis: the main cause for the appearance of "old" skin. Br J Dermatol. 1990;122:5-11.
75. Pageon H, Zucchi H, Asselineau D. Distinct and complementary roles of papillary and reticular fibroblasts in skin morphogenesis and homeostasis. Eur J Dermatol. 2012;22:324-32.
76. Pageon H, Bakala H, Monnier VM, et al. Collagen glycation triggers the formation of aged skin in vitro. Eur J Dermatol. 2007;17:12-20.
77. Pageon H, Zucchi H, Rousset F, et al. Skin aging by glycation: lessons from the reconstructed skin model. Clin Chem Lab Med. 2014;52:169-74.
78. Leyden J. What is photoaged skin? Eur J Dermatol. 2001;11:165-7.
79. Helfrich YR, Sachs DL, Voorhees JJ. Overview of skin aging and photoaging. Dermatol Nur. 2008;20:177-83.
80. Quan T, Qin Z, Xia W, et al. Matrix-degrading metalloproteinases in photoaging. J Invest Dermatol Symp Proc. 2009;14:20-4.
81. Bernerd F, Vioux C, Asselineau D. Evaluation of the protective effect of sunscreens on in vitro reconstructed human skin exposed to UVB or UVA irradiation. Photochem Photobiol. 2000;71:314-20.
82. Bernerd F, Asselineau D. An organotypic model of skin to study photodamage and photoprotection *in vitro*. J Am Acad Dermato. 2008;58:155-9.
83. Démarchez M, Sengel P, Pruniéras M. Wound healing of human skin transplanted onto the nude mouse. I An immunohistological study of the reepithelialization process. Dev Biol. 1986;113:90-6.
84. Démarchez M, Desbas C, Pruniéras M. Wound healing of human skin transplanted onto the nude mouse. II. An immunohistological and ultrastructural study of the epidermal basement membrane zone reconstruction and connective tissue reorganization. Dev Biol. 1987;121:119-29.
85. Zhong SP, Zhang YZ, Lim CT. Tissue scaffolds for skin wound healing and dermal reconstruction. Wiley interdisciplinary reviews: nanomedicine and nanobiotechnology. 2010;2:510-35.

86. Laplante A, Germain L, Auger FA, et al. Mechanisms of wound reepithelialization: hints from a tissue-engineered reconstructed skin to long-standing questions. FASEB J. 2001;15:2377-89.
87. Herman IM, Leung A. Creation of human skin equivalents for the in vitro study of angiogenesis in wound healing. Meth Mol Bio. 2009;467:241-8.
88. Ford JM, Hanawalt PC. Role of DNA excision repair gene defects in the etiology of cancer. Curr Top Microbiol Immunol. 1997;221:47-70.
89. Bernerd F, Asselineau D, Vioux C, et al. Clues to epidermal cancer proneness revealed by reconstruction of DNA repair-deficient xeroderma pigmentosum skin *in vitro*. Proc Natl Acad Sci USA. 2001;98:7817-22.
90. Warrick E, Garcia M, Chagnoleau C, et al. Preclinical corrective gene transfer in xeroderma pigmentosum human skin stem cells. Mol Ther. 2012;20:798-807.
91. Rouanet S, Warrick E, Gache Y, et al. Genetic Correction of Stem Cells in the Treatment of Inherited Diseases and Focus on Xeroderma Pigmentosum. Int J Mol Sci. 2013;14:20019-36.
92. Hsu MY, Meier FE, Nesbit M, et al. E-Cadherin Expression in Melanoma Cells Restores Keratinocyte-Mediated Growth Control and Down-Regulates Expression of Invasion-Related Adhesion Receptors. Am J Pathol. 2000;156:1515-25.
93. Sanzo M, Colucci R, Arunachalam M, et al. Stress as a possible mechanism in melanoma progression. Dermatol Res Pract. 2010;2010:483493.
94. Bonitsis N, Batistatou A, Karantima S, et al. The role of Cadeherin/Catenin complex in malignant melanoma. Exp Oncol. 2006;28:187-93.
95. Rathman-Josserand M, Deshayes N. Origins and selection of epidermal progenitors and stem cells: a challenge for tissue engineering. Journal de la Société de Biologie. 2008;202:43-54.
96. Fortunel NO, Hatzfeld JA, Rosemary PA, et al. Long-term expansion of human functional epidermal precursor cells: promotion of extensive amplification by low TGF-beta1 concentrations. J Cell Sci. 2003;116:4043-52.
97. Lenoir MC, Bernard BA, Ferracin J, et al. Growth and differentiation of human keratinocytes on the eye lens capsule. Res Arch Dermatol. 1985;278:120-5.
98. Aplin AE, Howe A, Alahari SK, et al.Signal transduction and signal modulation by cell adhesion receptors: the role of integrins, cadherins, immunoglobulin-cell adhesion molecules, and selectins. Pharmacol Rev. 1998;50:97-263.
99. Bernard FX, Pedretti N, Rosdy M, et al. Comparison of gene expression profiles in human keratinocyte mono-layer cultures, reconstituted epidermis and normal human skin; transcriptional effects of retinoid treatments in reconstituted human epidermis. Exp Dermatol. 2002;11:59-74.
100. Roguet R. The use of standardized human skin models for cutaneous pharmacotoxicology studies. Appl Skin Physiol Skin Pharmacol. 2002;15:1-3.
101. Christian MS, Diener RM. Soaps and detergents, alternatives to animal eye irritation tests. J Am Coll Toxicol. 1996;15:1-44.
102. York M, Steiling W. A critical review of the assessment of eye irritation potential using the Draize rabbit eye test. J Appl Toxicol. 1998;18:233-40.
103. Directive 2003/15/EC of the European Parliament and of the Council of 27 February 2003 amending Council Directive 76/768/EEC on the approximation of the laws of the Member States relating to cosmetic products (Text with EEA relevance). [online] Available from http://eur-lex.europa.eu/homepage.html [Accessed July 2014]
104. EURL ECVAM progress report on the development, validation and regulatory acceptance of alternative methods (2010-2013). ECVAM, EURL. [online] Available from http://ihcp.jrc.ec.europa.eu/our_labs/eurl-ecvam/eurl-ecvam-releases-2013-progress-report-development-validation-regulatory-acceptance-alternative-methods/at_multi_download/file?name=EURL_ECVAM_progress_report_cosmetics_2013.pdf. [Accessed July 2014].
105. GUIDANCE DOCUMENT ON THE VALIDATION AND INTERNATIONAL ACCEPTANCE OF NEW. OECD. [online] Available from http://www.oecd.org [Accessed July 2014]
106. Manual of decisions for implementation of the 6th and 7th Amendments to directive 67/548/EEC on dangerous substances. Updated version July 2004 (EUR 20519). Ispra, Italy. European Chemicals Bureau; European Commission JRC. EC. 2004.
107. Statement on the validity of in vitro tests for skin corrosion. ESAC. http://ecvam.jrc.it, 1998. [online] Available from https://eurl-ecvam.jrc.ec.europa.eu/[Accessed July 2014]
108. Statement on the validity of in vitro tests for skin corrosion. ESAC. 2006 [online] Available from https://eurl-ecvam.jrc.ec.europa.eu/ [Accessed July 2014]
109. Statement on the validity of in vitro tests for skin corrosion. ESAC. 2009 [online] Available from https://eurl-ecvam.jrc.ec.europa.eu/ [Accessed July 2014]
110. Test No. 431: *In Vitro* Skin Corrosion: Reconstructed Human Epidermis (RHE) Test Method. OECD (2013). [online] Available from: http://www.oecd-ilibrary.org/environment/test-no-431-in-vitro-skin-corrosion-reconstructed-human-epidermis-rhe-test-method_9789264203822-en;jsessionid=1040k85dsvq07.x-oecd-live-01. OECD Guidelines for the Testing of Chemicals, Section 4, OECD Publishing. [Accessed July 2014].
111. United Nations Globally Harmonized System of Classification and Labelling of Chemicals (GHS), Third revised edition. UN. UN New York and Geneva, p. 2009. [online] Available from: http://www.unece.org/fileadmin/DAM/trans/danger/publi/ghs/ghs_rev04/English/ST-SG-AC10-30-Rev4e.pdf. [Accessed July 2014].
112. Draize JH, Woodward G, Calvery HO. Methods for the study of irritation and toxicity of substances applied directly to the skin and mucous membranes. J Pharmacol Exp Therap. 1944;377-90.
113. OECD Guidelines for the Testing of Chemicals No. 404: Acute Dermal Irritation/Corrosion (2002). OECD. [online] Available from: http://www.oecd-ilibrary.org/environment/test-no-404-acute-dermal-irritation-corrosion_9789264070622-en. [Accessed July 2014].
114. York M, Griffiths HA, Whittle E, et al. Evaluation of human patch test for the identification and classification of skin irritation potential. Contact Dermatitis. 1996;34:204-12.
115. EU. Directive 2003/15/EC of the European Parliament and the council of 27 February 2003 amending council Directive 76/768/EEC on the approximation of the laws of the member states relating to cosmetic products. Off J Eur Union.2003;66:26-35.
116. Botham PA, Earl LK, Fentem JH, et al. Alternative methods for skin irritation: the current status. ECVAM skin irritation task force report. ALTA. 1998;26:195-211.
117. Cotovio J, Grandidier MH, Portes P, et al. The *in vitro* acute skin irritation of chemicals: optimisation of the EpiSkinSM prediction model within the framework of the ECVAM Validation Process. ATLA. 2005;33:329-49.
118. Spielmann H, Hoffmann S, Liebsch M, et al. The ECVAM International Validation on in vitro tests for acute skin irritation: report on the validity of the EpiSkin and EpiDerm assays and on the Skin integrity function test. Altern Lab Anim. 2007;35:559-601.
119. Statement on the validity of *in vitro* tests for skin irritation. ESAC. [online] Available from http://ihcp.jrc.ec.europa.eu/our_labs/eurl-ecvam. [Accessed July 2014].
120. Cotovio J, Grandidier MH, Lelièvre D, et al. *In vitro* acute skin irritancy of chemicals using the validated EPISKIN model in a tiered

strategy -results and performances with 184 cosmetic ingredients. AATEX Proc. 6th World Congress on Alternatives & Animal Use in the Life Sciences, Tokyo, Japan: 2007 Vol. 354.
121. Augustin C, Collombel C, Damour O. Use of dermal equivalent and skin equivalent models for identifying phototoxic compounds in vitro. Photodermatol Photoimmunol Photomed. 1997;13:27-36.
122. Lelievre D, Justine P, Christiaens F, et al. The EpiSkin phototoxicity assay (EPA): development of an in vitro tiered strategy using 17 reference chemicals to predict phototoxic potency. Toxicol In Vitro. 2007;21:977-95.
123. Bernard FX, Barrault C, Deguercy A, et al. Development of a highly sensitive in vitro phototoxicity assay using the SkinEthicTM reconstructed human epidermis. Cell Biol Toxicol. 2000;6:391-400.
124. Medina J, Elsaesser C, Picarles V, et al. Assessment of the Phototoxic Potential of Compounds and Finished Topical Products Using a Human Reconstructed Epidermis. In Vitr Mol Toxicol. 2001;14:157-68.
125. Bacqueville D, Mavon A. Comparative analysis of solar radiation-induced damage between *ex vivo* porcine skin organ culture and in vitro reconstructed human epidermis. Int J Cosmet Sci. 2009;31:293-302.
126. Kirkland D, Aardema M, Henderson L, et al. Evaluation of the ability of a battery of three in vitro genetoxicity tests to discriminate rodents carcinogens and non-carcinogens. Sensitivity, specificity and relative predictivity. Mut Res. 2005;584:1-256.
127. Flamand N, Marrot L, Belaidi JP, et al. Development of genotoxicity test procedures with Episkin, a reconstructed human skin model: towards new tools for in vitro risk assessment of dermally applied compounds? Mut Res. 2006;606:39-51.
128. Pfuhler S, Fellows M, van Benthem J, et al.In vitro genotoxicity test approaches with better predictivity: summary of an IWGT workshop. Mutat Res. 2011;723:101-7.
129. Reus AA, Reisinger K, Downs TR, et al. Comet assay in reconstructed 3D human epidermal skin models--investigation of intra- and inter-laboratory reproducibility with coded chemicals. Mutagenesis. 2013;28:709-20.
130. Schäfer-Korting M, Bock U, Diembeck W, et al. The use of reconstructed human epidermis for skin absorption testing: Results of the validation study. Altern Lab Anim. 2008;36:161-87.
131. Grégoire S, Patouillet C, Noé C, et al. Improvement of the experimental setup for skin absorption screening studies with reconstructed skin Episkin. Skin Pharmacol Physiol. 2008;21:89-97.
132. Gabbanini S, Lucchi E, Carli M, et al. In vitro evaluation of the permeation through reconstructed human epidermis of essentials oils from cosmetic formulations. J Pharm Biomed Ana. 2009;50:370-6.
133. Rozman B, Gasperlin M, Tinois-Tessoneaud E, et al. Simultaneous absorption of vitamins C and E from topical microemulsions using reconstructed human epidermis as a skin mode. Eur J Pharm Biophar. 2009;72:69-75.
134. Nohynek GJ, Duche D, Garrigues A, et al. Under the skin: biotransformation of para-aminophenol and para-phenylenediamine in reconstructed human epidermis and human hepatocytes. Toxicol Lett. 2006;158:196-212.
135. Pappinen S, Pryazhnikov E, Khirough L, et al. Organotypic cell cultures and two-photon imaging: Tools for in vitro and in vivo assessment of percutaneous drug delivery and skin toxicity. J Control Release. 2012;161:656-67.
136. Fleischli FD, Mathes S, Adlhart C. Label free non-invasive imaging of topically applied actives in reconstructed human epidermis by confocal Raman spectroscopy. Vibrational Spectroscopy. 2013;68:29-33.
137. Sok J, Pineau N, Dalko-Csiba M, et al. Improvement of the dermal epidermal junction in human reconstructed skin by c-xylopyranoside derivative. Eur J Dermatol. 2008;18: 297-302.
138. Vuillermoz B, Wegrowski Y, Contet-Audonneau JL, et al. Influence of aging on glycosaminoglycans and small leucine-rich proteoglycans production by skin fibroblasts. Mol Cell Biochem. 2005;277:63–72.
139. Shin JE, Oh JH, Kim YK, et al. Transcriptional regulation of proteoglycans and glycosaminoglycan chain-synthesizing glycosyltransferases by UV irradiation in cultured human dermal fibroblasts. J Korean Med Sci. 2011;26:417-24.
140. Vassal-Stermann E, Duranton A, Black AF, et al. A New C-Xyloside Induces Modifications of GAG Expression, Structure and Functional Properties. PLoS One. 2012;7:e47933.
141. Ruiz L, Benech F, Prunel A, et al. A new retinol against wrinkles. Poster: European Academy of Dermatology and Venereology Congress. 2009.
142. Michelet JF, Olive C, Rieux E, et al. The anti-ageing potential of a new jasmonic acid derivative (LR2412): *in vitro* evaluation using reconstructed epidermis Episkin™. Exp Dermatol. 2012;21:398-400.
143. Tran C, Michelet JF, Simonetti L, et al. *In vitro* and *in vivo* studies with tetra-hydro-jasmonic acid (LR2412) reveal its potential to correct signs of skin ageing. J Eur Acad Dermatol Venereol. 2014;28:415-23.
144. Pourzand C, Watkin RD, Brown JE, et al. Ultraviolet A radiation induces immediate release of iron in human primary skin fibroblasts: the role of ferritin. Proc Natl Acad Sci USA. 1999;96:6751-6.
145. Reelfs O, Eggleston I, Pourzand C. Skin protection against UVA-induced iron damage by multiantioxidants and iron chelating drugs/prodrugs. Curr Drug Metabol. 2010;11:242-9.
146. Séité S, Popovic E, Verdier MP, et al. Iron chelation can modulate UVA-induced lipid peroxidation and ferritin expression in human reconstructed epidermis. Photodermatol Photoimmunol Photochem. 2004;20:47-52.
147. Pygmalion MJ, Ruiz L, Popovic E, et al. Skin cell protection against UVA by Sideroxyl, a new antioxidant complementary to sunscreens. Free Radical Biol Med. 2010;49:1629-37.
148. Duval C, Schmdt R, Regnier M, et al. The use of reconstructed human skin to evaluate UV-induced modifications and sunscreen efficacy. Exp Dermatol. 2003;12:64-70.
149. Lejeune F, Christiaens F, Bernerd F. Valuation of sunscreen products using a reconstructed skin model exposed to simulated daily ultraviolet radiation: relevance of filtration profile and SPF value for daily photoprotection. Photodermatol Photoimmunol Photomed. 2008;24:249-55.
150. Bissett DL, Robinson LR, Raleigh PS, et al. Reduction in the appearance of facial hyperpigmentation by topical N-acetylglucosamine. J Cosmet Dermatol. 2007;6:20-6.
151. Imokawa G, Mishima Y. Loss of melanogenic properties in tyrosinases induced by glycosylation inhibitors within malignant melanoma cells. Cancer Res. 1982;42:1994-2002.
152. Bissett DL, Farmer T, McPhail S, et al. Genomic expression changes induced by topica N-acetyl Glucosamine in skin equivalent cultures. J Cosmet Dermatol. 2007;6:232-8.
153. Tomohiro Hakozaki, Tim Laughlin, Ashish Paradkar, et al. Undecylenoyl Phenylalanine Inhibits Stem Cell Factor Production in Human Keratinocytes. 22nd World Congress, Seoul Korea, Poster 1073.
154. Dumont, Khaiat et al. Sepicalm® VG, a new skin lightening enable to modulate melanogenesis-related genes and to prevent UV-induced pigmentation thanks to its soothing properties. Poster: Asian Societies of Cosmetic Scientists meeting. 2007.
155. Collin-Djangoné C, Sahuc F. et al. Potential use of RNAi on human skin. Poster: RANi Europe Meeting, 2008.

Chapter 4

Skin Color Types and Indian Skin Characteristics

Virginie Hourblin, *L'Oréal Research and Innovation, Aulnay-sous-Bois, France*
Suzy Cointereau-Chardon, *L'Oréal Research and Innovation, Chevilly-Larue, France*
Namita Misra, *L'Oréal Research and Innovation, Mumbai, India*
Frédéric Flament, *L'Oréal Research and Innovation, Chevilly-Larue, France*
Stéphanie Nouveau, *L'Oréal Research and Innovation, Aulnay-sous-Bois, France*
Maya Vedamurthy, *RSV Skin and Laser Centre and Apollo Hospitals, Chennai, India*
Shyam Verma, *Nirvana Skin Clinic, Vadodara, India*

INTRODUCTION

Defining Indian skin as "Asian skin" or "skin of color" may lack of accuracy[1] although India clearly pertains to Asia geographically. The Indian population shows a remarkable diversity with more than two thousand ethnic groups. In addition, great variations exist in terms of climate, diet and social parameters within the country. In this context, Indian skin shows a wide variability in color as well as some specificities. In particular pigmentary disorders are a major concern in India; of a great psychologic impact upon quality of life.[2]

Surprisingly, very few data are available on skin color diversities in India. Few studies specifically dedicated to Indian population have been performed to date. This chapter will mainly focus on a large typological study conducted in 2011, on 1,204 Indian women from different ages and different cities in India, Mumbai, Kolkata, Chennai and New Delhi.

INSIGHTS ON INDIAN SKIN COLOR BASED ON GENOME WIDE STUDIES

The evolutionary history of Indian ethnic groups and subsequent migration from central Asia, west Asia and southern China has resulted in a rich mosaic of socio-cultural, linguistic and biological diversities that also reflects in the variety of skin colors present on the Indian subcontinent. Broadly, Indians belong to Austro-Asiatic (AA), Tibeto-Burman (TB), Indo-European (IE) and Dravidian (DR) language families.[3] Distinct religious communities, hierarchical castes and sub-castes, and isolated tribal groups that comprise the people of India remain largely endogamous. The most comprehensive survey of genetic variations in India so far analyzed 405 single nucleotide polymorphisms (SNPs) in 55 groups and identified distinct clusters correlated to language and geography.[3]

Association between human skin color and genetic factors arose with the finding that zebrafish with a variation in the *SLC24A5* gene is a golden color and with fewer, smaller and lighter melanosomes than normal zebrafish.[4] Humans also harbor the *SLC24A5* gene and consulting HapMap, a free publicly accessible database of human genetic polymorphism, revealed that people of European ancestry as compared to Africans and East Asians have slightly different versions of the *SLC24A5* gene Africans and East Asians. Since, the genetic basis that underlies normal variation in the pigmentary traits of skin or hair and eye color has been the object of intense research aiming at understanding the diversity observed between and within human populations. Several approaches were undertaken, such as comparative genomics of candidate genes, identification of the human genome under positive selection and the genome-wide and specific allele association studies. Findings from these studies point towards independent selection for different pigmentation gene sets between Asian, European and African populations.[5]

At phenotypic level, human skin color is largely determined by two biological components, melanin and hemoglobin, and one major environmental component, that is exposure to sun ultraviolet (UV) rays. In East

Asians, additionally the skin adipose tissue or hypodermis may provide an additional yellowish tinge. A qualitative assessment of skin color variations on the Indian subcontinent represents the variation seen throughout the world. This is indeed reflected by genetic studies on Indian subpopulations. Four genes account for a major component of color variation amongst Indians: *SCL24A5* (ortholog of zebrafish golden), *TYR* (ortholog of mouse Albino gene), *SLC45A2* (ortholog of mouse Underwhite) and *MC1R*.[6,7] These genes have also been implicated in color variation between Europeans and Africans. Light skin in Europeans and dark skin in Africans is due to alternate alleles in the same genes. At least some of the same alleles responsible for this color difference between Europeans and Africans seem being involved in Indians. The *SLC45A2* SNP shows an allelic gradient from north to south in Europe.[5] Does this gradient also exists from North to South in India is a question of much sense. Indeed, a distinct genetic divergence is seen between Ancestral North Indians (ANI) and Ancestral South Indians (ASI) that may also manifest in skin colors of these two populations.[8] The region around the *SLC24A5* gene shows a considerable reduction in heterozygotes suggesting a major selective sweep of this light skinned allele through the population. Light skin in Indians and Central/ Western Eurasians have common origin independent of those in Asians, especially the contribution of *SLC24A5* allele. These results are more indicative of an ancestral origin rather than a selection sweep driven by sun UV-damage. On the other hand, the results also suggest that in South India and Sri Lanka natural selection may keep a low frequency of the 'light alleles', such as *SLC45A2*. Thus genomic variations associated with pigmentation in South Asian population reflect complex phenomenon of ancestral origin, migration and environmental factors.

Functional testing of variant alleles is paramount to connect phenotype correlations with biological differences. For instance, variant *MC1R* alleles show direct correlations between the biochemical signaling properties of the encoded receptor and the red-hair fair skin pigmentation phenotype. Direct testing of a range of clonal melanocyte cultures derived from donor skin tissue characterized for three causal SNPs within *SLC45A2*, *SLC24A5* and *OCA2* (blue-brown eye color) has assessed their impact upon melanin content and activity of tyrosinase. By culminating genetic and functional studies, it is apparent that genes that impact melanosome biogenesis or the melanin biosynthetic pathway are candidates to explain the diversity seen in human pigmentation that would also apply to Indian population.

SKIN COLOR EVALUATION METHODS

Colorimetry is a technology used to quantify color, and so describe objectively the color perception. It is similar to spectrophotometry, but is distinguished by its interest in reducing spectra to the physical correlates of color perception, most often the CIE 1931 XYZ color space tristimulus values and related quantities.

To assess and compare skin color *in vivo* some methods are available using calibration and standardization principles. We do not focus here on clinical tools but on the interest of objective, non-invasive and reproducible instrumental devices. Globally these instruments can be divided into two categories: one, such as Chromameter® or Spectrocolorimeter®, acquires color parameters and the other quantifies color by analyzing digital images in RGB model.[9,10]

Chromasphere® (Fig. 1) is a reference tool[11,12] for facial skin color assessment thanks to its stability, reliability and its capacity to use diffuse lighting systems that faithfully mimic sun natural daylight (CIE illuminant D65). The whole face is illuminated with a homogeneous light. Such

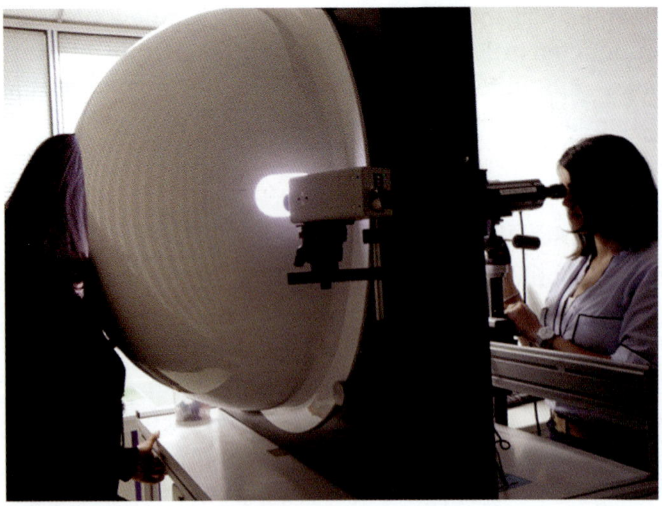

Figure 1: Chromasphere®
©L'Oréal Research and Innovation

a device is contact-free; avoiding any external pressure that could affect blood flow and induce change in skin color. Combining Chromasphere® with different equipments allows various color characteristics to be quantified.

Calibrated images can be obtained with charge-coupled device cameras, avoiding any drift in digital camera recording and thus allowing the operator to analyze data with different methods. The heterogeneity of skin color can be then assessed with coxellography index approach (co-occurrence matrix). Segmentation and image analysis allow carnation and pigmented spot areas to be detected and separated to obtain various parameters. Spots density, size or color could then be investigated. Meanwhile, colorimetric information is computed to describe complexion and contrasts between pigmented spots and surrounding areas.

Skin color can also be measured with a spectro-radiometer. This kind of device acquires reflectance of skin from 380 nm to 780 nm every 4 nm. The spectrum recorded on the visible field (400–700 nm) is expressed in the CIE 1976 standard colorimetric spaces L*a*b*C*h D65/10° (Fig. 2).

- The lightness L* uses a grey scale and accounts for more or less lightness and more or less darkness.
- The a* and b* are the color-opponent dimensions. These color axes are based on the fact that a color can not be both red and green, or both blue and yellow, because these colors oppose each other. On each axis the values run from positive to negative. On the a-a' axis, positive values indicate amounts of red while negative values indicate amounts of green. On the b-b' axis, yellow is positive and blue is negative. For both axes, zero is neutral grey.
- From the a* and b* values, the angle hue *h* and the chroma C* are calculated. The angle hue *h* correspond to the angle between the a* and b* axis and is the colored coordinate. It characterizes the color from red to yellow within the skin color space.
- The Chroma C* or saturation refers to the pureness or vividness. It refers to the intensity of the hue.

INDIAN SKIN OVERALL COMPLEXION

Color Skin Tone in India as Compared to Other Ethnicities

Previous works indicate that skin color of the Indian population is very diversified,[1,13,14] with phototypes III to VI, types IV and V being predominant.[15] Surprisingly, skin-related typology studies on Indian population are scarce. A few available papers being devoted to colorimetric characterization of Indian women skin and its specificities (age, homogeneities, etc). The differences of skin color across India, and its changes with geographical location were recently investigated.[16] In this article skin colors of 1,195 healthy Indian women from 18 to 85 years old originating from four cities were quantified using an objective colorimetric tool, Chromasphere®. Results showed a wide diversity of skin color within Indian women: the population covers a large range of skin colors, from very dark to light (Fig. 3).

The skin color of women from other ethnicities was previously evaluated[12,17,18] revealing a worldwide

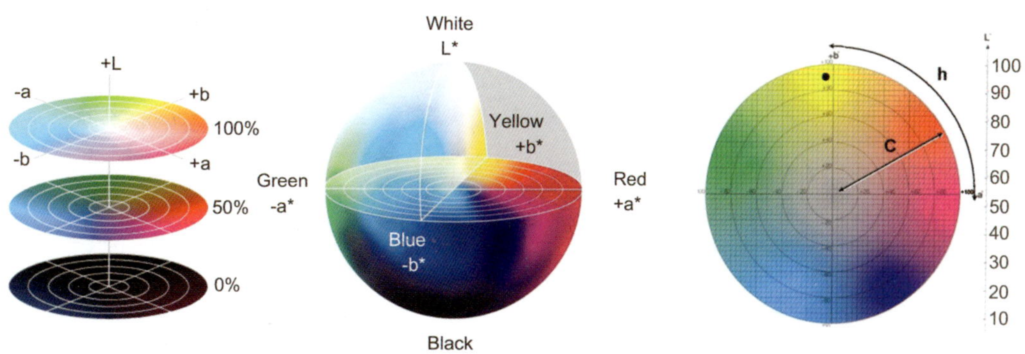

Figure 2: CIE L*a*b* and L*C*h color space
©L'Oréal Research and Innovation

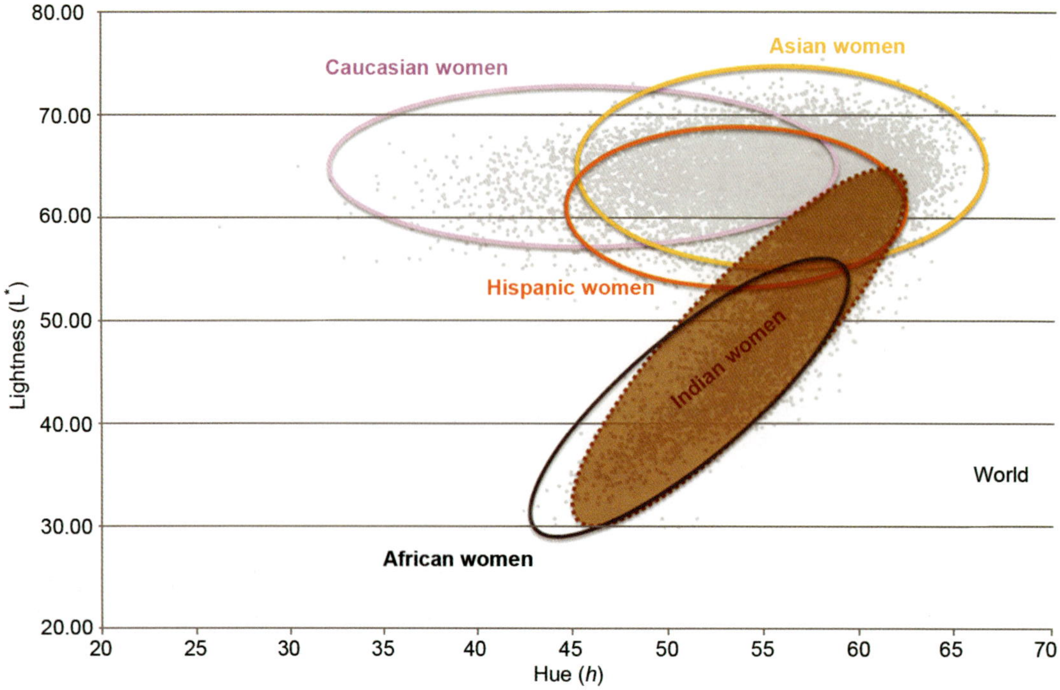

Figure 3: Skin color space in L* *h* plan measured by spectroradiometer in four different clusters of skin color: Caucasian, Asian, Hispanic and African (see Table 1). Projection of Indian women skin color in this worldwide skin color continuum
©L'Oréal Research and Innovation

continuum of skin color. The projection of Indian skin color space in this continuum is closed to the one of African women and women from African descent but with a larger range of lightness (Fig. 3). The Indian skin color space indeed overlaps those of Asian and Hispanic women. This data highlights the wide diversity of skin color in India as compared to other ethnicities.

Table 1: Skin color continuum studies; detailed studied population referring to Figure 3

Indian Women (n = 1195)	From Mumbai, Chennai, Kolkata and Delhi
Caucasian Women (n = 2054)	France: Paris Russia: Moscow USA: Chicago/New York
Asian Women (n = 4127)	China: Guangzhou, Shanghai, Beijing Japan: Tokyo Korea: Seoul Thailand: Bangkok France: Paris
Hispanic Women (n = 223)	USA: New York Brazil: Rio Mexico: Mexico
African and Women from African Descent (n = 853)	South Africa: Johannesburg France: Paris (with native of the French West Indies) USA: New York

Variation of Skin Color Tone within India: Differences Depending on Geographical Localization

Considering the diversity of climate/environment in India, the impact of geographical location on skin color has to be investigated. Results in Figure 3, arising from a recently published study, cover populations of four cities from north to south (Chennai and Delhi) and from west to the east (Mumbai and Kolkata).[16] Results of this study showed a huge variability in skin color among the four cities, suggesting an environmental impact upon skin color (Fig. 4).

The wider variations in skin color are found in Chennai. Instrumental measurements showed that the women living in this city present the largest hue range as well as the darkest, less saturated and reddest skin whatever the area of the face (Fig. 5). On a scale of

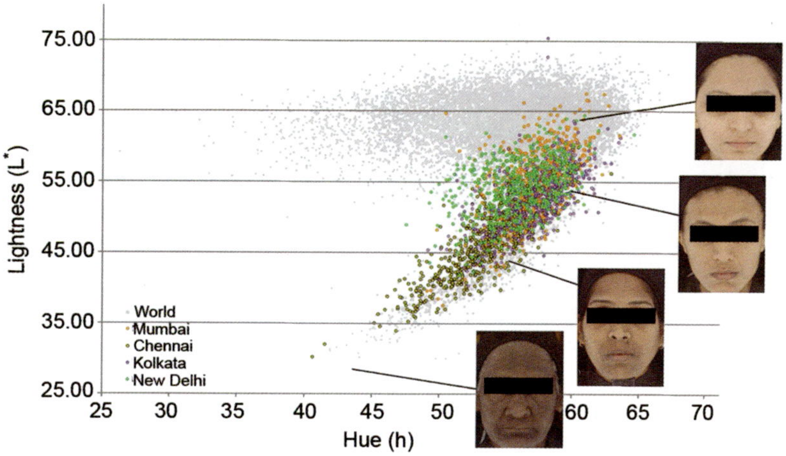

Figure 4: Indian skin tones in four cities: Mumbai, Chennai, Kolkata and New Delhi (lightness by hue)
©L'Oréal Research and Innovation

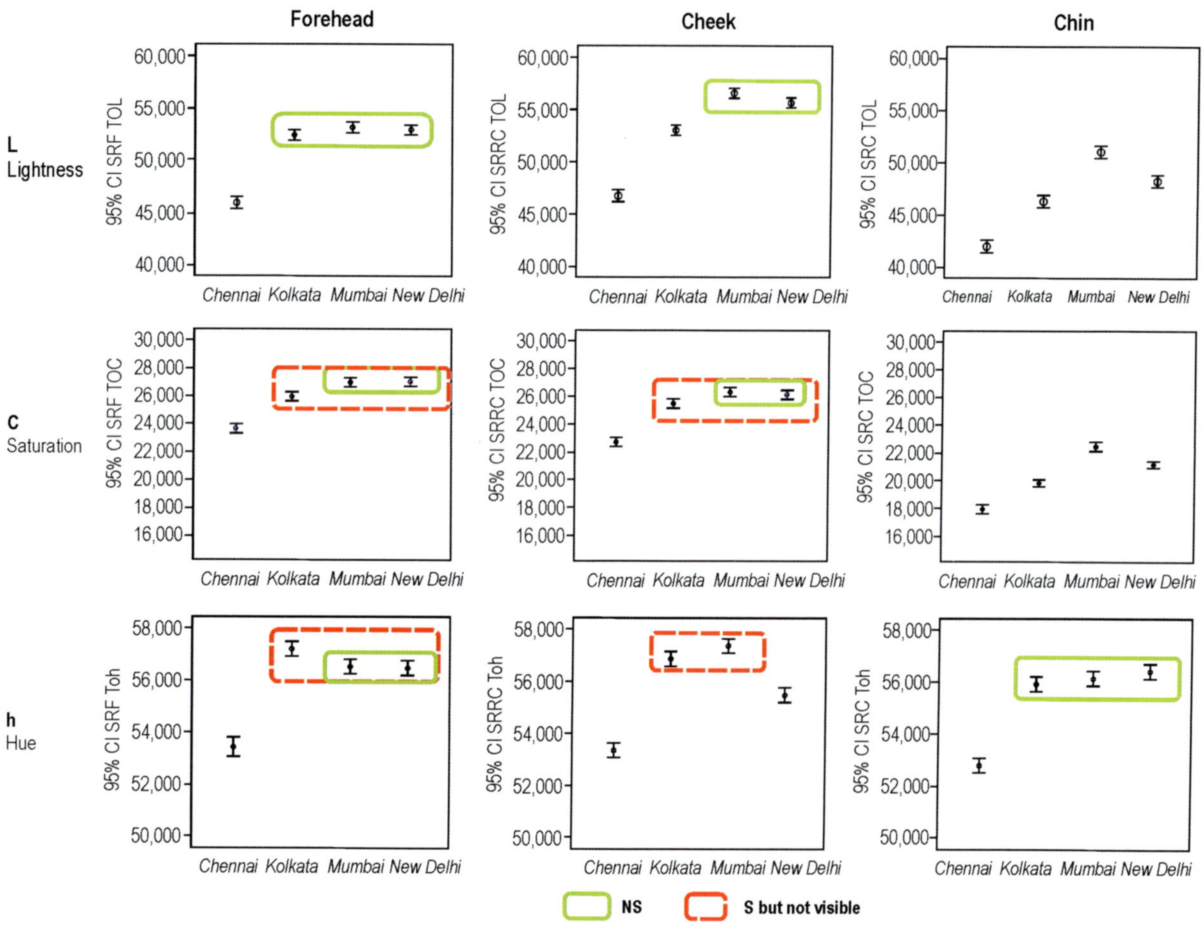

Figure 5: Comparison of skin color parameters per facial area in four Indian cities (Chennai, Kolkata, Mumbai, New Delhi) (n = 1,195 women)
©L'Oréal Research and Innovation

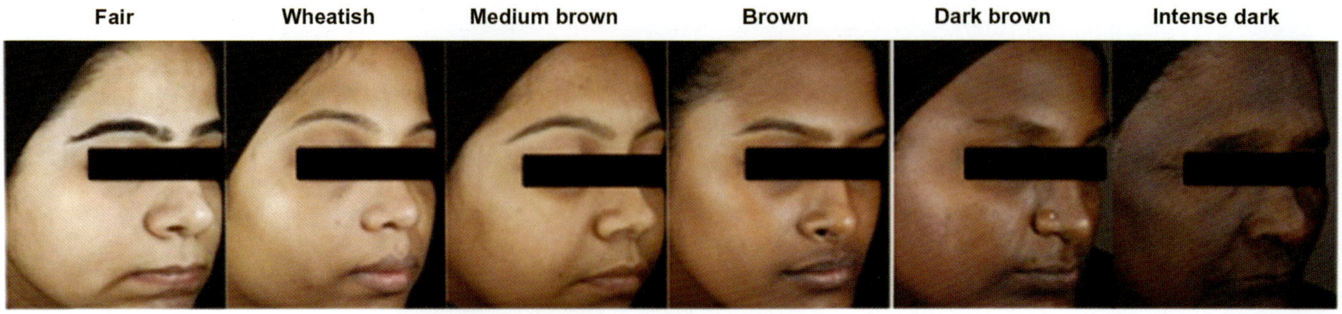

Figure 6: Indian skin complexion: Dermatologist assessment
©L'Oréal Research and Innovation

6 skin complexion types identified in India (Fig. 6), 74% of women skin colors are described as "brown" or "dark brown" by a dermatologist.[16]

The results for the three others cities are roughly similar with some noticeable particularities.

Kolkata shows the largest range of skin lightness and saturation. According to the graphic representation (Fig. 4), there is a strong link between lightness and hue: the darker the skin is, the redder and less vivid (less saturated) it is. Although skin color in Kolkata is quite darker as compared to Mumbai, hue or saturation is similar (Fig. 5). Skin colors of women from Mumbai and Delhi only differ by the hue component: cheeks are redder in Delhi than in Mumbai. Those differences of skin color complexion were confirmed clinically with a same rate (34%) of "medium brown" skin (Fig. 6) but different prevalence of "brown" and "wheatish" skin: 41% of "brown" and 21% of "wheatish" in Delhi versus 10% of "brown" and 45% "wheatish" in Mumbai.[16]

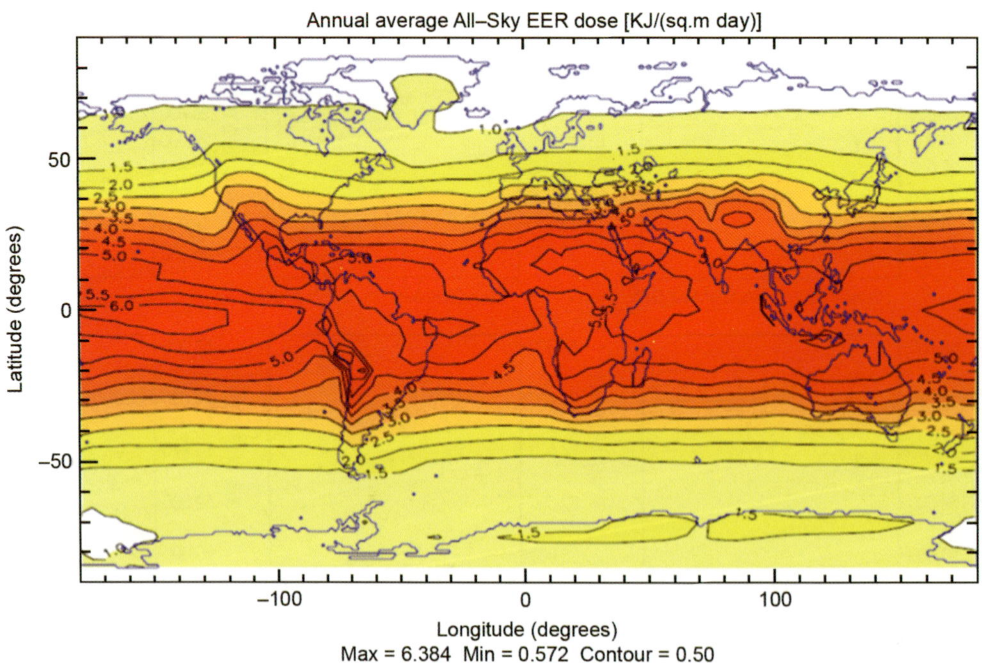

Figure 7: Annual average of sun exposure[19]
©L'Oréal Research and Innovation

The trends observed on cheek or forehead are more pronounced for the chin (perilabial area) (Fig. 5). This area is more discriminant since it allows the four cities to be differentiated in terms of lightness and saturation.

According to these results, it would appear that there is a latitude effect and an impact of the environment (sun UV exposure, life habits, pollution, etc) upon the skin color of Indian women. The skin colors of women from Chennai, located in the South of India, are very different from those of the Northern cities. India could then be split diagonally from South West to North East. The skin colors of the two cities of the East coast are darker whereas the skin colors of the two Western cities are lighter. This difference was also found in another study comparing Calicut and Delhi.[18] Several hypotheses could be proposed to explain this phenomenon. The importance of UV exposure during the year could be considered (Fig. 7). Chennai area indeed undergoes higher sun exposure than other cities.[19] Nevertheless, this hypothesis alone might not suffice to explain the huge variations observed in skin color. This might be also explained by the different flows of migration and the interbreeding of two distinct ancestral lineages: Dravidians and Indo-Europeans.[8]

Evolution of Indian Skin Color with Age

Skin darkening with age has been described in various populations, e.g. a Chinese group living in Chicago as reported by de Rigal et al.[20] However, such age-related changes were not observed in African-Americans, Caucasians, and Mexicans living in the same area.[20] A recent study on Chinese women living in China[21,22] showed a rather linear darkening with age along the life span. Another study conducted in eight Asian cities including two Indian cities (Calicut and Delhi) found that the melanin index increased with age while L* value decreased, indicating that skin darkens with age.[18]

The change in skin color with age in India was deeper investigated in the study previously mentioned.[16] Instrumental measurements showed that overall skin color darkens with age (Fig. 8). By comparing the changes in L* parameter with age between Indian women and women from other countries, it has been highlighted that Indian skin darkens at a different kinetics, i.e. twice slower than Asian skin and slightly faster than Caucasian skin.

But this age effect has different intensity depending on the Indian city (Fig. 9). Chennai is indeed the only city where the age effect is significant in the three color

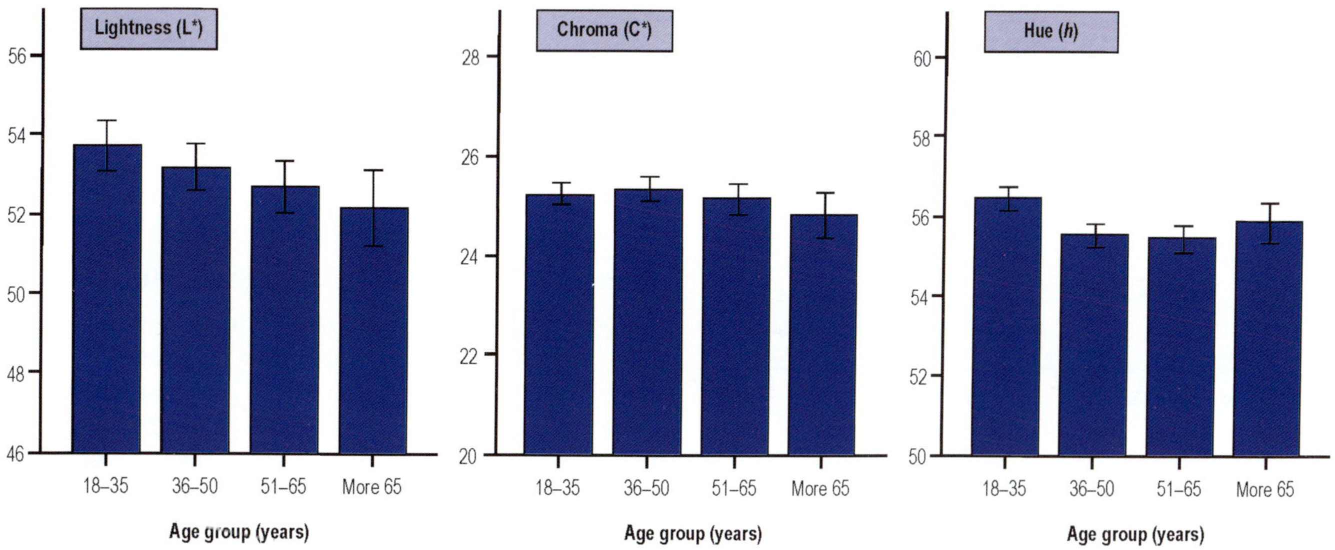

Figure 8: Average skin lightness, Chroma and Hue according to different age groups. Measured on cheek with spectroradiometer® (n = 1,195 Indian women)
©L'Oréal Research and Innovation

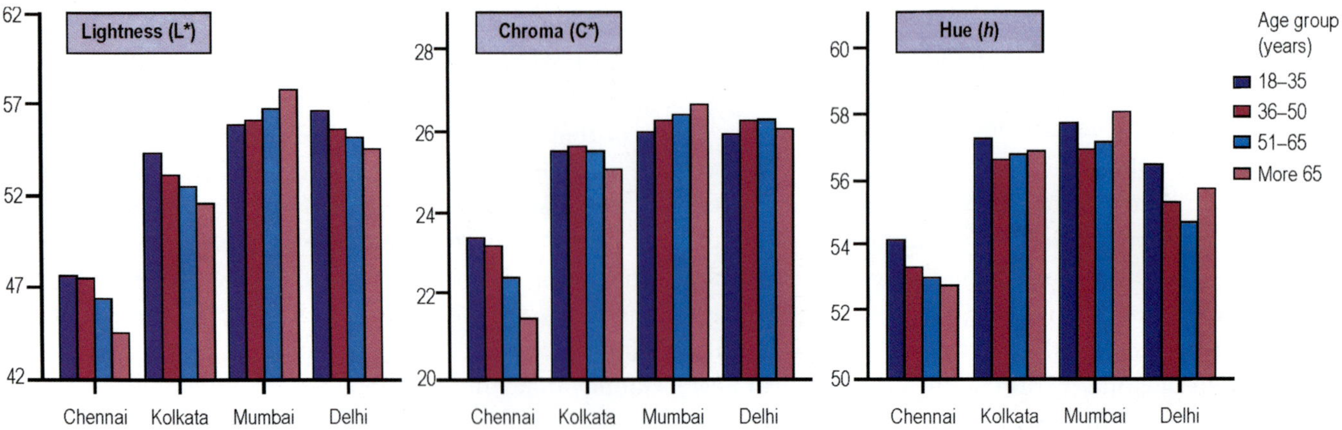

Figure 9: Average skin Lightness, Chroma and Hue according to different age groups in four Indian cities (Chennai, Kolkata, Mumbai, Delhi). Measured on cheek with Spectroradiometer® (n = 1,195 Indian women)

parameters with the highest darkening and a skin becoming redder and less saturated with age.

No significant change in skin color was found in Mumbai. Unlike Mumbai, skin color of women from Kolkata and Delhi darkens with age. This difference of age effect between those three cities could be related to the difference of skin color previously observed and by the specific environmental conditions of each city.

The difference of Indian skin color change with age between a rather photo-protected skin area (upper inner arm) and an exposed area (cheek) was also investigated (Fig. 10).[16] Chromameter® measurements showed that after 35 years, the skin becomes slightly fairer with age on the photo-protected area (Lightness increase by 6%), when it becomes barely darker on photo-exposed area (Lightness decrease by 2%). This may account for overall impression of facial darkening compared to the whole body for women, although facial darkening is of a low extent. This has been investigated in other populations in large cohorts of Caucasian's and Korean's (653 Caucasians and 497 Koreans).[23,24] In Caucasians, a significant darkening of exposed areas was observed after 20 years. Amongest Koreans, skin color alteration seems close to that found in the Indian study, the skin color remaining rather stable with age.

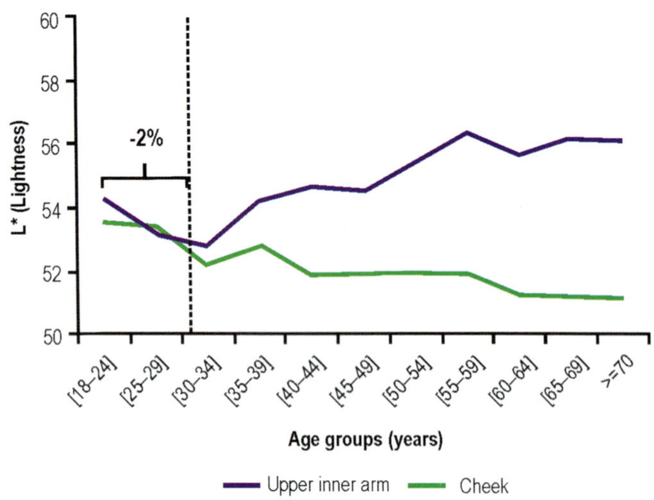

Figure 10: Average skin lightness in age groups (years) measured on cheek (photo-exposed area) and upper inner arm (photo-protected area) (n = 1,202)

SKIN COLOR UNEVENNESS IN INDIA

Overall Facial Skin Color Heterogeneity

Another issue concerning Indian skin color has emerged with regard to its heterogeneity. Coxellography index approach allows the overall color heterogeneity of the face to be evaluated taking into account the variations of color (hyperpigmented and hypopigmented spots, telangiectasies), and pores. Results showed that skin color heterogeneity of the cheek increased with age (Fig. 11), which could be explained by an increase in pigmentary disorders and hyperpigmented areas.

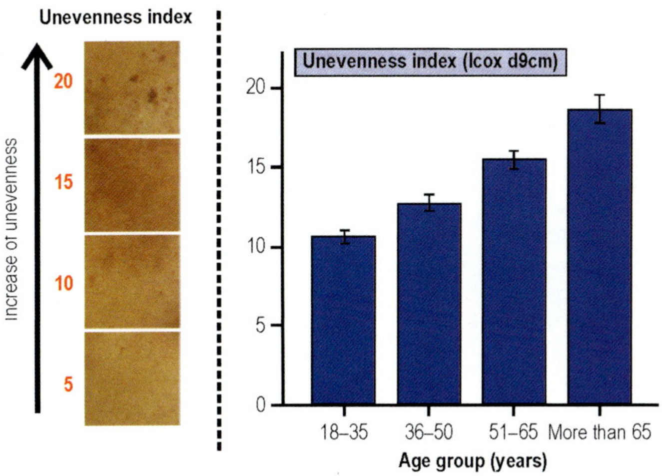

Figure 11: Overall skin color heterogeneity per age group in India (n = 1,195)
©L'Oréal Research and Innovation

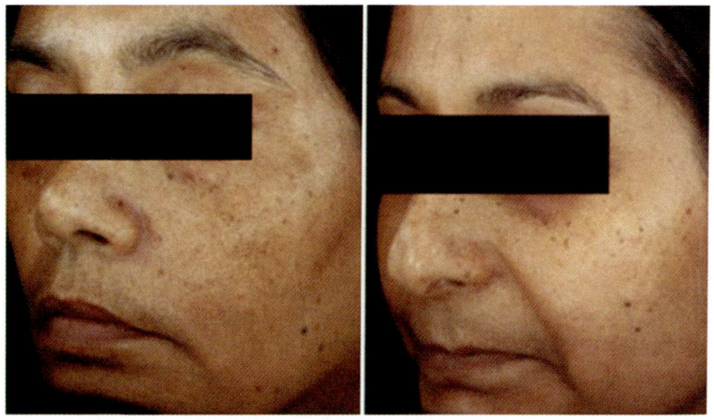

Figure 12: Hyperpigmented spots on two Indian women
©L'Oréal Research and Innovation

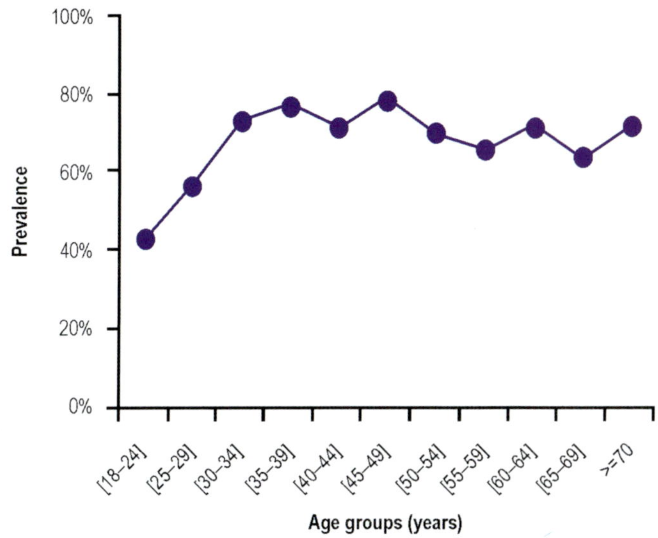

Figure 13: Prevalence of hyperpigmented spots (according to age group) assessed *in situ* by dermatologists (n = 1,204)
©L'Oréal Research and Innovation

Pigmentary Disorders

Few studies document the increased frequency of disorders characterized by hyperpigmentation in darker ethnic groups.[25-28] The importance of which is also reported as a frequent concern in Indian population. Some pigmentary disorders have been described in India,[29] hypopigmentary disorders, such as vitiligo, pityriasis alba or versicolor, and also hyperpigmentary disorders, such as melasma and some other facial melanoses.[30-33]

Hyperpigmented Spots

Hyperpigmented spots are a major concern with an early onset and an overall increase with age, well described in some other Asian countries. Several studies conducted in China showed that the early onset of marked pigmented spots is a characteristic of Asian skin aging.[34,35,22] Galzote et al.[18] also observed an increase in mottled pigmentation with age in different Asian populations, India included.

These results were confirmed in the Indian typology study:[16] more than 70% of women over 30 years show more than 10 small hyperpigmented spots on their face (Figs 12 and 13), increasing up to 80% in women over 50 years ($p < 0.0001$). Before 40 years, most of these small spots are post-inflammatory marks, in relation to the high prevalence of acne. From 30 years, dermatologists observed simplex lentigos and actinic lentigines in more than 80% of women, but differentiating them remain difficult. Many seborrheic keratoses were also observed (about 70% of women). Such a high prevalence and early onset of actinic lentigines and seborrheic keratoses (at around 30 years) in India are striking.

Instrumental methods confirmed these results. An individual analysis of pigmented spots with an automatic detection of colored objects revealed no change in the size of pigmented spots with age but an increase in their number and visibility (by contrast with the skin

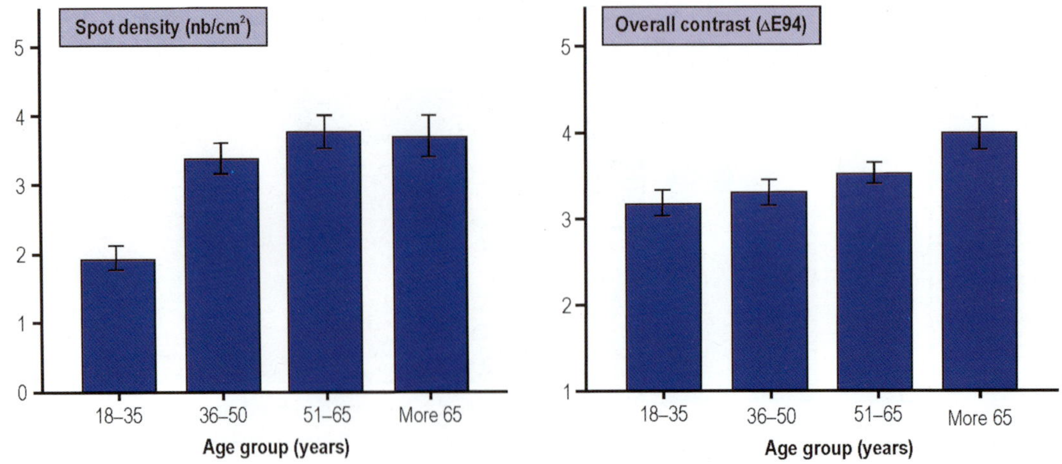

Figure 14: Density and overall contrast of facial spots according to age group in India
©L'Oréal Research and Innovation

complexion). Globally, the spots density increases significantly after 35 years, and shows no significant change after whereas the overall color contrast (ΔE94) between complexion and spots, i.e. the visibility of spots, increases significantly only from 50 years (Fig. 14).

Melasma and Patchily Hyperpigmented Macules

Melasma is a frequently described pigmentary disorder in the Indian population. The worldwide reported prevalence of melasma ranges from 8.8% among Latino females in the Southern United States[36] to 40% in Southeast Asian populations.[37] The Indian typology[16] confirmed the high prevalence of melasma in this country. The average age of women with melasma is 51 years with a prevalence of 19% in the studied population. A peak of melasma prevalence is observed *in situ* by dermatologists in about 30% of women aged from 40 years to 65 years (Figs 15 and 16).

However, melasma alone do not represent all the dyspigmented spread macules observed in this study. Dermatologists' assessments distinguish other ill-defined, patchily hyperpigmented macules on the face which differ from melasma. The prevalence of moderately to severely dyspigmented macules increases with age particularly on the malar area reaching 70% of women ($p < 0.0001$) (Fig. 17). Furthermore, the prevalence of spread macules steadily increases with age, unlike the bell curve distribution of melasma prevalence along life span.

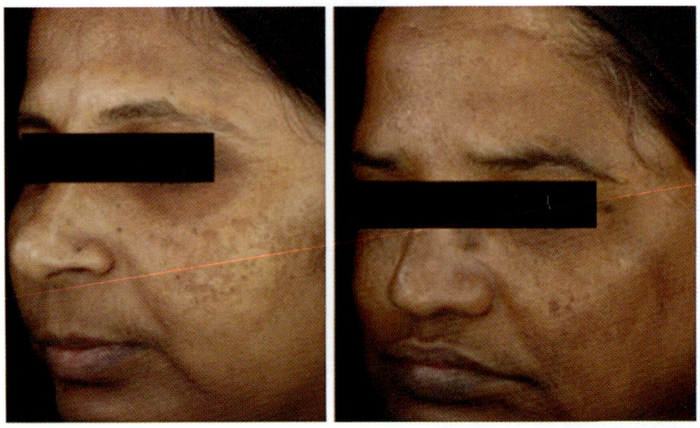

Figure 15: Melasma and dyspigmented macules observed in two Indian women
©L'Oréal Research and Innovation

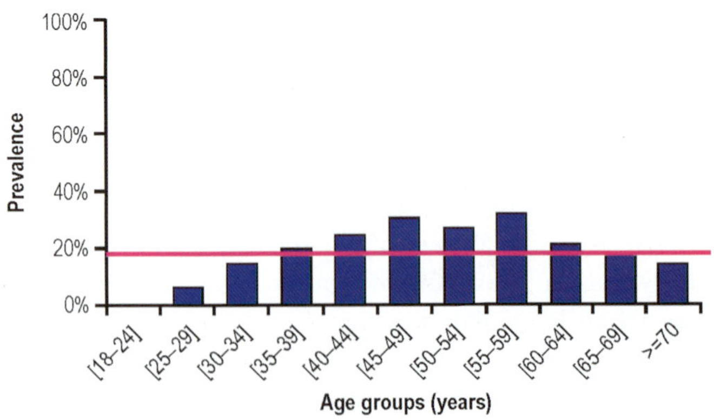

Figure 16: Prevalence of melasma (according to age group) assessed *in situ* by dermatologists (n = 1,204)

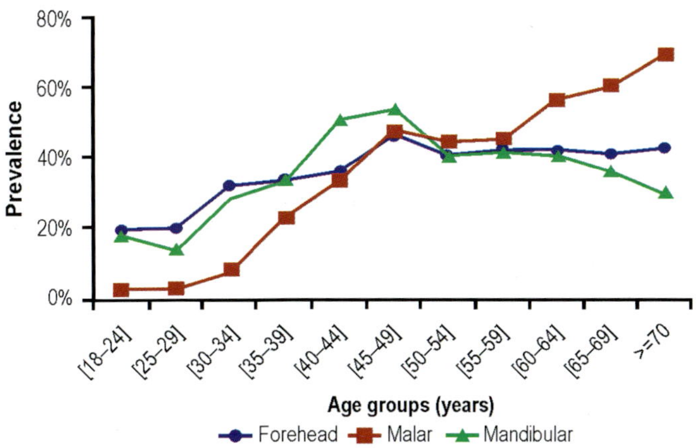

Figure 17: Prevalence of dyspigmented macules on forehead, malar or mandibular area (according to age group) assessed from photographs by dermatologists (n = 1,196)
©L'Oréal Research and Innovation

Hypopigmentary Disorders

The prevalence of vitiligo in India is often claimed higher, of a 0.46–8.8% range.[38] But according to a recent review focusing on the prevalence of vitiligo in the general population and excluding studies based on patients of dermatology clinics, the worldwide prevalence of vitiligo ranges 0.5–2%.[39] This appears consistent with the results from Hourblin et al.[16] who reported a low prevalence of vitiligo (0.9%), affecting less than 10% of women. The main diagnoses associated with hypopigmentary disorders were post-inflammatory hypopigmented marks and pityriasis alba. Some city-related effect (p <0.0001) was noticed, with hypopigmentary disorders prevalence varying from 5.2% in Chennai to 15.0% in Mumbai.

Hyperpigmented Areas

Dark Circles

Periorbital melanoses are very common dermatological disorders particularly in India. Despite its frequency, little is known about its etiology and management. Malakar et al.[33,40] describe them as a dark brown to black hyperpigmentation, usually bilaterally symmetrical, and define them as an extension of pigmentary demarcation lines (PDL) of the face. The recent Indian typology confirms the importance of this disorder in India,[16] with more than 50% of concerned women irrespective of age, and up to 80% beyond 35 years old. According to dermatologists' assessment, almost all women have dark circles on upper eyelid and on lower eyelid, of a different intensity with age (Fig. 18). The prevalence of women with moderate to severe dark circles on upper eyelid, increases with age from 50% up to 85%.

These clinical results are confirmed by instrumental measurements which quantify the dark circles color using Spectroradiometer® associated with Chromasphere®. The contrast with the cheek, i.e. their visibility, appears very important. The visibility of dark circles increases with the complexion lightness (Fig. 19); they are logically more visible on the lightest skin.

Facial Pigmentary Demarcation Lines

Pigmentary demarcation lines are physiological abrupt transition lines from areas of deeper pigmentation to lighter areas. They were first classified into five types on the whole body, A through E.[41] Then it was suggested that these lines can also occur on the face and lines F,

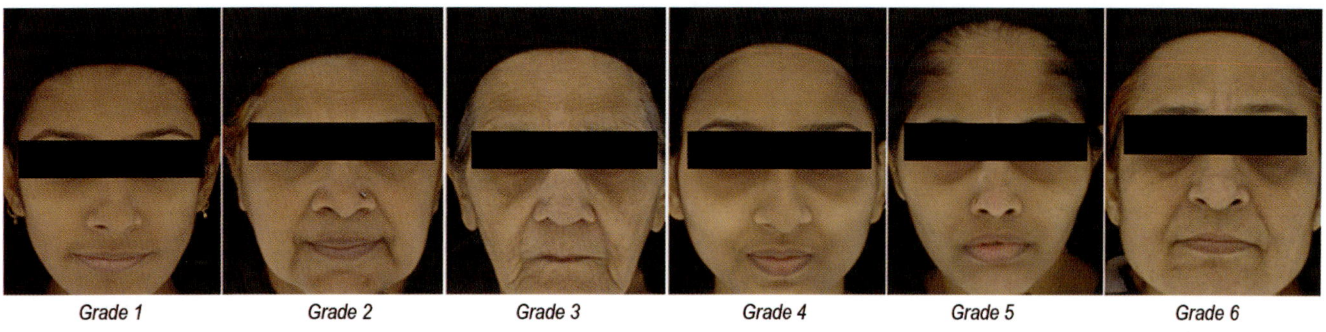

Figure 18: Atlas of dark circles color intensity
©L'Oréal Research and Innovation

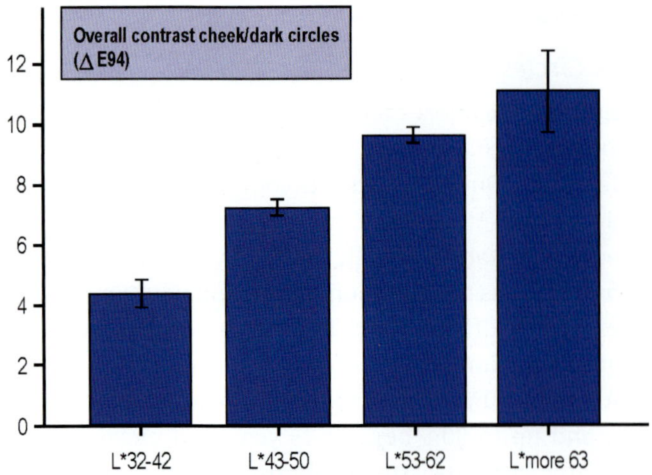

Figure 19: Overall contrast (ΔE94) between cheek and dark circles for each lightness complexion level
©L'Oréal Research and Innovation

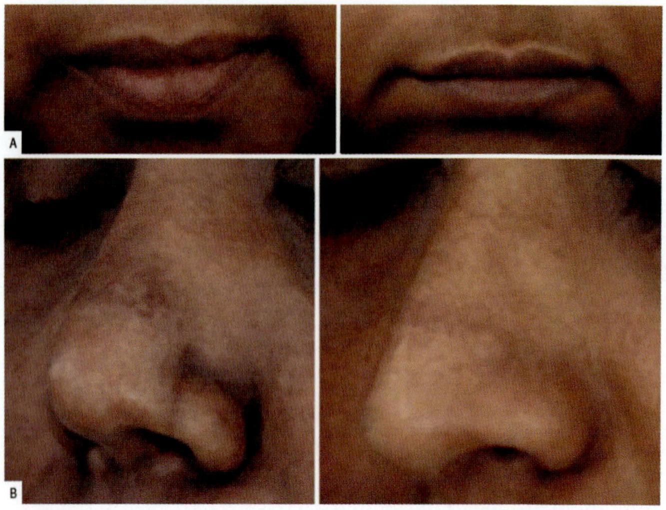

Figure 20: Specific hyperpigmented areas on Indian skin. **A**, Lip corners and **B**, Nose bridge
©L'Oréal Research and Innovation

G and H were added.[32] The facial lines differ from the rest of PDL since they present later, usually around puberty (lines A to E tend to present in early childhood), and they affect males less frequently.[42] The higher proportion of affected females may indicate hormonal influences. Pregnancy is associated with worsening of many pigmentary problems. These lines are almost always bilateral. In some people the lines merge with the periorbital pigmented circle.[40]

Other Specificities: Perilabial Pigmentation and Nose Bridge

As previously described,[32] Indian typology confirms that perilabial pigmentation is very frequent in Indian women. About 30% of women of all ages show moderately to severely pigmented upper lip. About 70% of women over 30 years have moderately to severely pigmented lip corners (Figs 20 and 21) whereas about 40% of women over 30 years present moderately to severely pigmented marionette lines.

A distinctive finding was pigmentation of the nose. About 50% of women of all ages showed pigmentation at the angles of the nose. In addition, 25% of women had a hyperpigmented line across the nose (42% of Mumbai women); in some of them, the line was broad and divided the nose into a darker area on top and a lighter area below (Figs 20 and 21). The prevalence of this disorder increased with age from 10 to 30%. Recent studies have described linear pigmentation across the nose associated with a grove or ridge, referred to as transverse nasal groove or nasal crease. The crease has been particularly emphasized in the case of the allergic salute.[43,44]

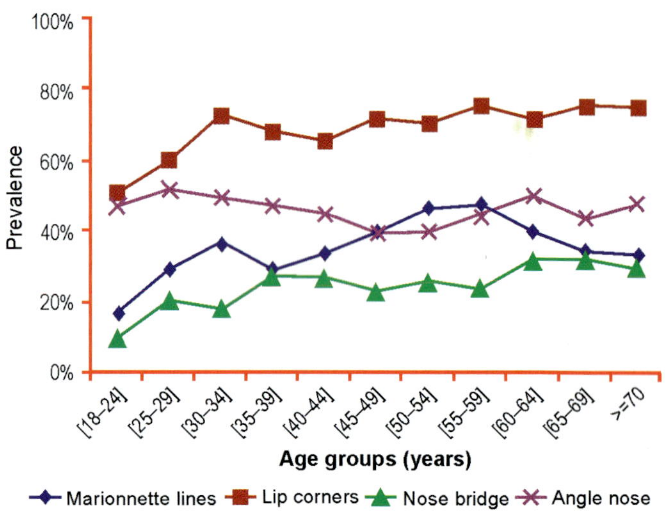

Figure 21: Prevalence of moderately to severely hyperpigmented areas (according to age group) assessed *in situ* by dermatologists (n = 1,204)
©L'Oréal Research and Innovation

Skin Color Contrasts of the Face

Thanks to the analysis of color contrasts between the different facial areas (forehead, cheek, chin and dark circles), five clusters (Fig. 22) were identified to illustrate the unevenness of the Indian women face. Dark circles play a big part in the segmentation due to their high frequence in India.

The cheek can be very light as compared to the rest of face leaving the forehead very dark comparatively (Group 4) or the chin can stand out by its darkness and lack of vividness (Group 2).

This again illustrates the importance of skin color heterogeneity in India with a wide diversity of skin color contrasts existing between the different parts of the face.

CONCLUSION

The color of the human skin results from complex mechanisms involving different genes, mainly related to melanin biosynthetic pathway. With its different flows of migration, India presents a wide range of biological diversity. This chapter highlights the uniqueness of Indian skin with its large diversity of color skin tone

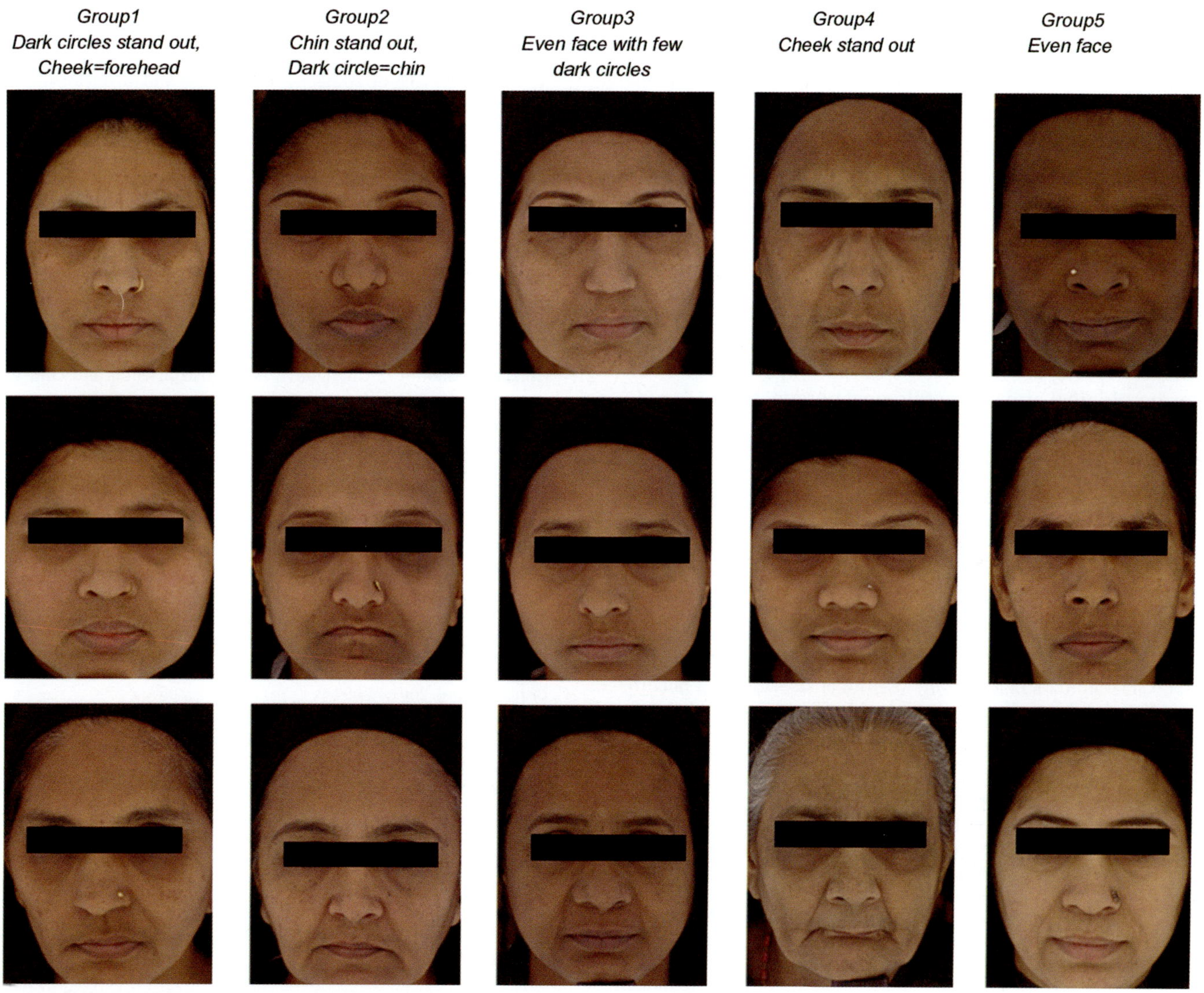

Figure 22: Facial skin color types based on the analysis of skin color contrasts ©L'Oréal Research and Innovation

covering a color scale from very dark to light. According to this parameter, the country could be split diagonally from South West to North East, with the darker skin in the South and East. Globally skin complexion appears not strongly affected by age compared to other Asian countries with a slight darkening of skin color with age particularly in the Southern region.

Skin color heterogeneity appears as a hallmark of Indian skin with an increase in facial skin color unevenness with age. This heterogeneity can be explained by an increase in pigmentary disorders, i.e. hyperpigmented spots and spread macules. These disorders occur at early stages and increase with age, contributing to overall facial unevenness. Indian facial skin also presents some original hyperpigmented areas, such as lip corners, marionette lines and nose bridges. In India, dark circles are the most prevalent hyperpigmented areas, darkening with age. This data raises the needs to further characterize and explore the mechanisms underlying the early onset and high prevalence of hyperpigmented spots, dyspigmented spread macules, and specific pigmented lines observed in the studied population.

These features are obviously of high concern for dermatological and cosmetological perspectives.

REFERENCES

1. Verma SB. Redefining colour of Indian skin. J Eur Acad Dermatol Venereol. 2008;22:1263-4.
2. Shenoi SD, Prabhu S. Role of cultural factors in the biopsychosocial model of psychosomatic skin diseases: an Indian perspective. Clin Dermatol. 2013;31:62-5.
3. Indian Genome Variation Consortium. Genetic landscape of the people of India: a canvas for disease gene exploration. J Genetics. 2008;87:3-20.
4. Lamason RL, Mohideen MA, Mset JR, et al. SLC24A5, a putative cation exchanger, affects pigmentation in zebrafish and humans. Science. 2005;310:1782-6.
5. Norton HL, Kittles RA, Parra E, et al. Genetic evidence for the convergent evolution of light skin in Europeans and East Asians. Mol Biol Evol. 2006;24:710-22.
6. Stokowski RP, Krishna Pant PV, Dadd T, et al. A genome wide association study of skin pigmentation in a South Asian Population. Am J Hum Genet. 2007;81:1119-32.
7. Mukherjee M, Mukerjee S, Sarkar-Roy N, et al. Polymorphism of four pigmentation genes (SLC45A2, SLC24A5, MC1R and TYRP1) among eleven endogamous population of India. J Genet. 2013;92:135-9.
8. Reich D, Thangaraj K, Patterson N, et al. Reconstructing Indian population history. Nature. 2009;461:489-94.
9. Malacara D. Color Vision and Colorimetry: Theory and Applications. Society of Photo-Optical Instrumentation Engineers, Bellingham, USA. 2002.
10. Schanda J, Editor. Colorimetry: Understanding the CIE System. John Wiley & Son, 2007.
11. de Rigal J, Abella ML, Giron F, et al. Development and validation of a new skin color chart. Skin Res Technol. 2007;13:101-9.
12. Caisey L, Grangeat F, Lemasson A, et al. Skin color and makeup strategies of women from different ethnic groups. Int J Cosmet Sci. 2006;28:427-37.
13. Jaswal IJ. Pigmentary variation in Indian populations. Acta Anthropogenet. 1983;7:75-83.
14. Jaswal IJ. Skin Colour in North Indian Populations. J Hum Evol. 1979;8:361-6.
15. Verma SB. Dermatology for the elderly: an Indian perspective. Clin Dermatol. 2011;29:91-6.
16. Hourblin V, Nouveau S, Roy N, et al. Skin complexion and pigmentary disorders in facial skin of 1204 women in 4 Indian cities. Indian J Dermatol Venereol Leprol. 2014;80:395-401.
17. Baras D, Caisey L. Skin, lips and lashes of different skins of color: typology and make-up strategies. In: AP Kelly and SC Taylor, (eds). Dermatology for Skin of Color. Mc Graw-Hill; Berkshire, UK: 2009. pp. 541-9.
18. Galzote C, Estanislao R, Suero MO, et al. Characterization of facial skin of various Asian populations through visual and non-invasive instrumental evaluations: influence of age and skincare habits. Skin Res Technol; 2014.
19. Christiaens F. Geographical distribution of harmful UV radiation. Poster 20th World Congress of Dermatology, Paris, France; 2002.
20. de Rigal J, Des Mazis I, Diridollou S, et al. The effect of age on skin color and color heterogeneity in four ethnic groups. Skin Res Technol. 2010;16:168-78.
21. Huixia Q, Xiaohui L, Chengda Y, et al. Instrumental and clinical studies of the facial skin tone and pigmentation of Shanghaiese women. Changes induced by age and a cosmetic whitening product. Int J Cosmet Sci. 2012;34:49-54.
22. Qiu H, Long X, Ye JC, et al. Influence of season on some skin properties: winter vs. summer, as experienced by 354 Shanghaiese women of various ages. Int J Cosmet Sci. 2011;33:377-83.
23. Lock-Anderson J, Knudstorp ND, Wulf HC. Facultative skin pigmentation in Caucasians: an objective biological indicator of lifetime exposure to ultraviolet radiation. Br J Dermatol. 1998;138:826-32.
24. Roh KY, Kim D, Ha SJ, et al. Pigmentation in Koreans: study of the differences from Caucasians in age, gender and seasonal variations. Br J Dermatol. 2001;144:94-9.
25. Halder RM, Grimes PE, McLaurin CI, et al. Incidence of common dermatoses in a predominantly black dermatologic practice. Cutis. 1983;32:388-90.
26. Sanchez MR. Cutaneous diseases in Latinos. Dermatol Clin. 2003;21:689-97.
27. Alexis A, Sergay AB, Taylor SC. Common dermatologic disorders of skin of colour; a comparative practice survey. Cutis. 2007;80:387-94.
28. Grimes PE. Management of hyperpigmentation in darker racial ethnic groups. Semin Cutan Med Surg. 2009;28:77-85.
29. Pasricha JS, Khaitan BK, Dash S. Pigmentary Disorders in India. Dermatol Clin. 2007;25:343-52.
30. Khanna N, Rasool S. Facial melanoses: Indian perspective. Indian J Dermatol Venereol Leprol. 2011;77:552-63.
31. Sarkar R, Puri P, Jain RK, et al. Melasma in men: a clinical,

aetiological and histological study. J Eur Acad Dermatol Venereol. 2010;24:768-72.

32. Somani VK, Razvi F, Sita VV. Pigmentary demarcation lines over the face. Indian J Dermatol Venereol Leprol. 2004;70:336-41.
33. Malakar S, Lahiri K, Banerjee U, et al. Periorbital melanosis is an extension of pigmentary demarcation line-F on face. Indian J Dermatol Venereol Leprol. 2007;73:323-5.
34. Nouveau-Richard S, Yang Z, Mac-Mary S, et al. Skin ageing: a comparison between Chinese and European populations. A pilot study. J Dermatol Sci. 2005;40(3):187-93.
35. Bazin R, Flament. Skin Aging Atlas volume 2. Asian type. Editions Puce et Plume, MED'COM publishing; France Paris: 2010.
36. Werlinger KD, Guevara IL, Gonzalez CM, et al. Prevalence of self-diagnosed melasma among pre-menopausal Latino women in Dallas and Fort Worth, Tex. Arch Dermatol. 2007;143:424-5.
37. Sivayathorn A. Melasma in Orientals. Clin Drug Investig. 1995;10: 24-40.
38. Shah H, Mehta A, Astik B. Clinical and sociodemographic study of vitiligo. Indian J Dermatol Venereol Leprol. 2008;74(6):701.
39. Krüger C, Schallreuter KU. A review of the worldwide prevalence of vitiligo in children/adolescents and adults. Int J Dermatol. 2012;51:1206-12.
40. Malakar S, Dhar S. Pigmentary demarcation lines over the face. Dermatology. 2000;200(1):85-6.
41. Selmanowitz VJ, Krivo JM. Pigmentary demarcation lines. Comparison of Negroes with Japanese. Br J Dermatol. 1975;93:371-7.
42. Al-Samary A, Al Mohizea S, Bin-Saif G, et al. Pigmentary demarcation lines on the face in Saudi women. Indian J Dermatol Venereol Leprol. 2010;76(4):378-81.
43. Sathyanarayana BD, Basavaraj HB, Nischal KC, et al. Appraisal of transverse nasal groove: A study. Indian J Dermatol Venereol Leprol. 2012;78:439-42.
44. Myers WA. The "nasal crease". A physical sign of allergic rhinitis. JAMA. 1960;174:1204-6.

Chapter 5

Physiology of Pigmentation: New Biological Concepts Associated with Skin and Hair Pigmentation

Manoj K Tembhre, *All India Institute of Medical Sciences, New Delhi, India*
Somesh Gupta, *All India Institute of Medical Sciences, New Delhi, India*
Stéphane Commo, *L'Oréal Research and Innovation, Aulnay-sous-Bois, France*

INTRODUCTION

All organisms, from simple invertebrates to complex human beings, exist in different colors, which arise from the unique distribution of pigments throughout the integument. Skin and hair pigmentation is an important part of human phenotypes, affording visual characteristics of a large range of natural variations, depending on people origins and their geographic-related distributions. Skin and hair color primarily rely on the presence of melanins, of which both the amount and type are responsible for the color diversity. Pigmentation is indeed a complex process which involves an intricate biological network regulated by genetic, environmental, and endocrine factors. Although the natural diversity of pigmentation mainly relies upon genetic background, skin and hair color changes occur throughout life due to physiological (e.g. aging), pathological and environmental conditions.

The knowledge of the physiology of skin and hair pigmentation is of strong importance to identify the regulatory factors responsible for skin and hair color, and to identify safe and efficient approaches to correct dyspigmentation problems for possibly meeting people expectation. This chapter proposes an update of the current knowledge and concepts on the physiology of skin and hair pigmentation.

HISTOLOGY OF THE MELANIN UNITS

Melanocytes are dendritic melanin-producing cells derived from the neural crest through migration and differentiation processes. Hence, during the embryonic development the melanocyte precursors called melanoblasts migrate along a dorsal lateral pathway to reach the skin at early fetal development stage. Finally, they take position within the basal layer of epidermis and, later on, enter within the hair follicle when the latter develops.

Melanocytes rest on the basement membrane and present long cellular extensions called dendrites that allow them to transfer produced melanins to the surrounding keratinocytes. The functional organization that links melanocytes with the recipient keratinocytes is called the "epidermal melanin unit" (EMU) in the skin[1] and, by analogy, the "hair follicle melanin unit" (HFMU) in the case of hair follicle (Fig. 1).

Melanocytes are distributed throughout the skin of the human body. There is an average 800–1,000 melanocytes/mm^2 with no difference between ethnics. Melanocyte density, however, varies according to body area: the highest density is found in genital area and the lowest in palms and soles, whereas with age, a 10% decrease in the number of skin melanocytes occurs every decade. In the human hair follicle, melanin-producing melanocytes are located in the hair bulb, lying upon the basal membrane surrounding the dermal papilla, where they transfer melanins to cortical keratinocytes of the hair shaft. In addition to the bulb area, the permanent part of the outer root sheath (ORS) of human hair follicle also contains melanocytes, albeit in an inactive state with regard to melanogenesis[2-4] (Fig. 1). It is assumed that these amelanotic melanocytes represent a reservoir of melanocyte precursors or melanocyte stem cells that can be stimulated resulting in skin re-pigmentation of vitiligo lesions following ultraviolet (UV) exposure.[5]

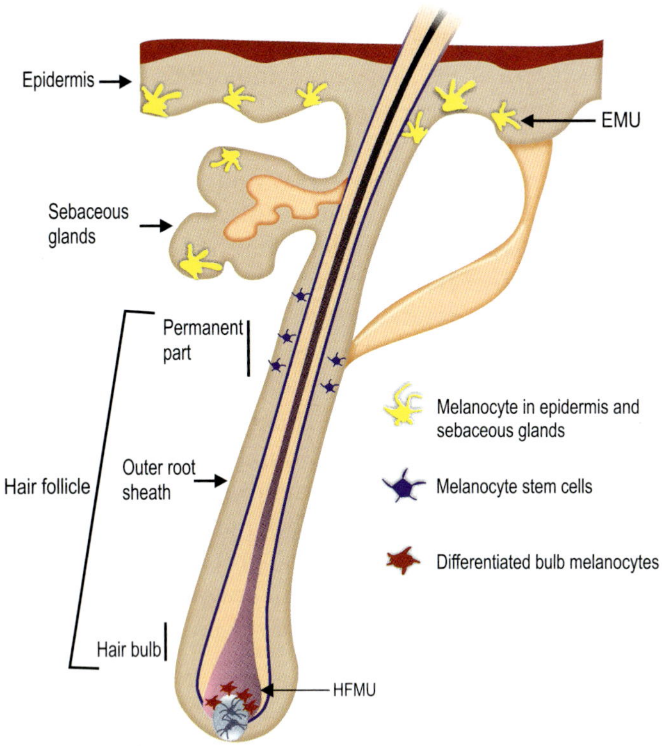

Figure 1: Histology of the melanin units
©L'Oréal Research and Innovation
Abbreviations: EMU, epidermal melanin unit; HFMU, hair follicle melanin unit.

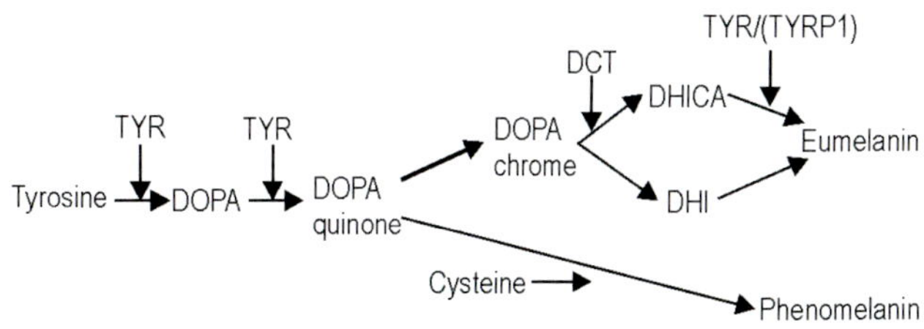

Figure 2: Melanogenesis pathway
©L'Oréal Research and Innovation
Abbreviations: TYR, Tyrosinase: DCT, Dopachrome tauto-merase; DOPA, 3, 4- dihydroxyphenylalanine; DHICA, 5,6-dihydroxy-indole-2-carboxylic acid; DHI, 5, 6-dihydroxyindole; TYRP1, Tyrosinase related protein-1.

MELANOGENESIS

Melanins are complex biopolymer pigments that give color to skin, hairs and eyes. Melanins comprise eumelanins (brown to black pigments) and pheomelanins (yellow to red pigments) in various amount, produced through a metabolic pathway involving at least three distinct enzymes, namely, tyrosinase (Tyr, EC 1.14.18.1), tyrosinase-related protein 1 (TYRP1; EC 1.14.18.-) and tyrosinase-related protein 2 (DCT, EC 5.3.3.12), encoded at the TYR, TYRP1 and DCT loci, respectively.

Melanogenesis implies the conversion of tyrosine into DOPA quinone in a two-step reaction controlled by tyrosinase, the rate-limiting enzyme for melanin synthesis (Fig. 2).[6] In the absence of thiol compounds (e.g. cysteine), dopaquinone undergoes intramolecular cyclization into cyclodopa that becomes rapidly oxidized into dopachrome, a relatively stable intermediate.[7,8] DCT induces l-dopachrome conversion into 5,6-dihydroxy-indole-5-carboxylic acid (DHICA).[9] In the absence of DCT, dopachrome would spontaneously decarboxylate and give rise to 5,6-dihydroxyindole (DHI). The dihydroxyindoles DHI and DHICA are further oxidized to produce eumelanin polymers. Oxidative polymerization of DHI and DHICA is directly catalyzed by tyrosinase or indirectly by dopaquinone.[10,11] In the presence of cysteine, pheomelanin synthesis proceeds through cysteine thiol addition to dopaquinone producing cysteinyldopas, which further undergo oxidation, giving rise to benzothiazine intermediates and eventually pheomelanin polymers.[12] Although TYRP1 is required for full melanin production, e.g. genetic TYRP1 polymorphisms being responsible for oculocutaneous albinism 3 (OCA3), the precise activity and function of TYRP1 are still controversial.

Melanin biosynthesis occurs in specialized, melano-cyte specific organelles called melanosomes (Fig. 3).

Melanosomes originate from the trans-Golgi network and progressively evolve into mature, melanin containing melanosomes.[13,14] Melanosomes are typically divided into four maturation stages (I–IV) determined by their structure and the amount, quality, and arrangement of melanin produced. Stage I melanosomes are spherical vacuoles lacking tyrosinase activity with no internal structural components. The presence of Pmel17/gp100, an important melanosomal structural protein, determines the transformation of stage I melanosomes into elongated, fibrillar organelles known as stage II melanosomes,[15,16] which contain tyrosinase and exhibit minimal deposition of melanin. In stage III, melanin synthesis increases and the pigment is uniformly deposited on the internal

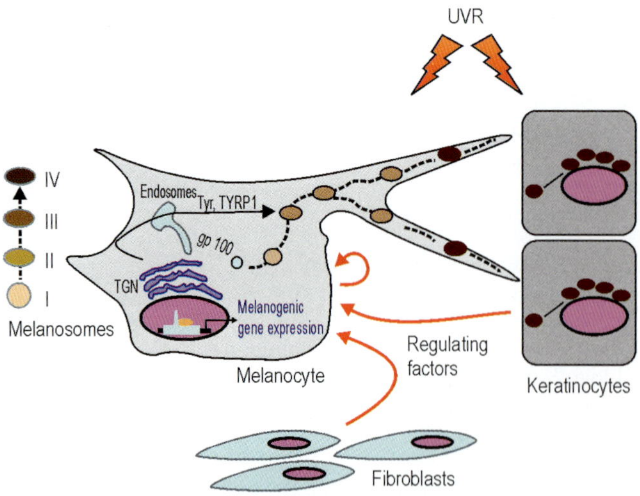

Figure 3: Diagram showing melanosome maturation
©L'Oréal Research and Innovation
Abbreviations: UVR, Ultraviolet rays; TGN, trans-Golgi network; Tyr, tyrosinase; TYRP1, tyrosinase-related protein 1; gp100, glycoprotein 100.

protein fibrils. In the last developmental stage (IV), melanosomes are electron-opaque due to complete melanization, with a minimal tyrosinase activity. The developmental stages detailed above refer mainly to eumelanosomes. The melanosome permits the melanin biosynthesis to take place in the absence of direct interaction with the cytoplasm, many of the melanin synthesis intermediates being highly reactive and potentially toxic to the melanocyte.[17,18] The demonstration that melanosomes contain more than 600 different proteins[19] suggests that the fine tuning of melanin production likely involves a complex network of proteins, whose particular contributions are still to be identified. As an illustration, melanin synthesis is affected by melanosomal pH, with tyrosinase being more active at neutral pH. It was shown that melanosomes have a lower pH in lightly pigmented melanocytes of Caucasian origin than that of melanosomes from darkly pigmented melanocytes of African origin.[20] Although the precise molecular mechanism is not identified yet, it is likely that melanosomal pH is governed by V-ATPases in combination with the melanosomal pink protein.[21]

In parallel to maturation, melanosomes progressively move towards the melanocyte membrane to be transferred to neighboring keratinocytes. Mechanisms governing melanosome routing and transfer to keratinocytes are partly described.[22,23] Yet some important aspects still remain unclear, melanosomes movement towards dendrite ends would involve a microtubule-dependent transport and a myosin 5A- and actin-dependent capture at the tip of dendrites. This process likely also involves myosin X, the small GTPase Rab27a along with melanophilin. Finally, melanosomes are transferred to surrounding keratinocytes. This later process was suggested to be regulated by the keratinocyte membrane receptors PAR 2 (Protease-activated receptor).[24]

Altogether, melanosome biogenesis, routing and transfer, along with melanosomal protein trafficking require numerous protein complexes, and while those proteins are not directly involved in melanin biosynthesis, changes in the efficiency of these protein complexes are responsible for pigmentary phenotypes, e.g. genetic variations responsible for Hermanski-Pudlak syndromes, Griscelli syndromes.

Once within the keratinocytes, melanosomes are found either individually distributed or in clusters composed of membrane-bound melanosome aggregates depending on skin phenotype. Melanin is thus distributed throughout the lower epidermis and mostly in basal keratinocytes (Fig. 4). Generally, within the basal keratinocytes, melanosomes are located at the apical surface, forming photo-protective cap to the nucleus. It is generally assumed that the protein structure of melanosomes is degraded by lysosomal enzymes as the keratinocytes differentiate and move upward to the stratum corneum, leading to the observation of "melanin dust" in the upper layers of the epidermis. In dark skin, however, some melanosomes are not degraded in the

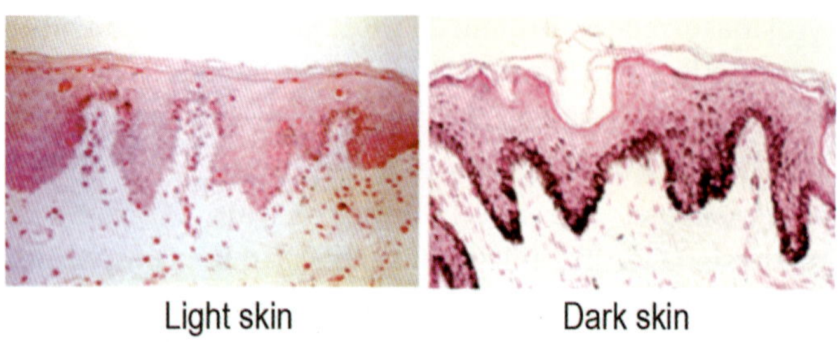

Figure 4: Light and dark human skins: Melanin stained by Fontana Masson
©L'Oréal Research and Innovation

stratum corneum. Ultimately, melanin is released from the epidermis by corneocyte desquamation.

Specificities of Hair Pigmentation

Hair follicles display a cyclical activity, transiting under a stochastic way from an active steady state (the anagen phase) to a dormant steady state (the telogen phase), each of these steady states showing clear distinct mean duration[25] (see Chapter 12: New Insights in Hair Research). The transition from the active to the dormant steady state is characterized by a follicle degradation process (the catagen phase), a short phase involving an abrupt and early cessation of matrix cell proliferation and arrest of inner root sheath (IRS) specific proteins synthesis.[26] The transition from the dormant to the active steady state is characterized by a neomorphogenesis process (the neogen phase).[27]

In the anagen hair follicle, melanocytes are divided into two distinct subpopulations (Fig. 1):

(1) The first population is located in the permanent part of the hair follicle. It is a pool of melanocyte stem cells that re-populate the new hair bulb with melanocytes at the onset of the neogen phase.
(2) The second population is located in the hair matrix above the dermal papilla and actively produces melanin during the anagen phase.

Due to successive cycles of growth, the HFMU must also be renewed cyclically during life (Fig. 1). The hair follicle pigmentary machinery present in the bulb region regenerates cyclically and is synchronized with the hair follicle during hair cycle.[4] It has been demonstrated that melanogenic activity of the follicular melanocytes is strictly coupled with the anagen stage due to anagen phase-coupled tyrosinase and TYRP1 expression in bulb melanocytes.[4] Noteworthy, hair follicle melanocytes are distinct from epidermal melanocytes due to the lack of DCT expression in bulbar melanocytes,[28] responsible for a reduced DHICA melanin content in human hair.[29]

REGULATION OF PIGMENTATION

Pigmentation is a complex process regulated by numerous physiological (intrinsic) and exogenous factors. This paragraph gives an overview of pigmentation regulating factors. The reader should, however, keep in mind that numerous other factors are involved the activity of which being sometimes still a matter of debate.

Microphthalmia-associated Transcription Factor

Microphthalmia-associated transcription factor (MITF) is assumed to be the "master regulator" of melanocytes, and it plays a pivotal role in the regulation of mammalian pigmentation providing positive regulation of transcription of TYR, TYRP1 and DCT genes through interaction with M and E boxes which is a prerequisite for production of melanin pigment. Dominant mutations at human MITF locus lead to Waardenburg syndrome type 2A (characterized by patchy depigmentation of hairs and skin, hearing loss and heterochromia iridisin) and Tietze's syndrome (characterized by generalized albinism, profound deafness, and hypoplasia of eyebrows). Thus clinical, genetic and experimental observations clearly demonstrate that MITF is essential for the development and function of melanocytes both in skin and hair.

α-MSH, ACTH and MC1R

The observation that polymorphisms in the melanocortin 1 receptor gene (MC1R) are associated with fair skin and red hair phenotypes demonstrated the major role of MC1r signaling in pigmentation.[30] MC1r is a seven transmembrane domain Gs-protein-coupled receptor for α-MSH that is highly expressed in melanocytes. α-MSH is derived from the proopiomelanocortin (POMC) prohormone, and in the skin, is produced mainly by keratinocytes. The binding of α-MSH to MC1R triggers a "melanogenic cascade" that starts with the activation of adenylate cyclase that results in the stimulation of cyclic adenosine monophosphate (cAMP) synthesis,[31,32] activation of the cAMP-dependent protein kinase A (PKA), phosphorylation of nuclear CREB transcription factor, increased MITF expression and finally increased tyrosinase and related proteins expression. The increased expression of tyrosinase and related proteins will favor the synthesis of eumelanin. Other agonists for MC1r have been demonstrated, such as the POMC-derived peptide ACTH, with propigmentation property.

It has been demonstrated that the systemic administration of α-MSH, β-MSH or ACTH in humans stimulates skin pigmentation, predominantly in sun-exposed areas.[33,34] Clinical observations have also shown that the pathologically increased levels of plasma ACTH in Addison disease, or the excessive ACTH production by tumors (Nelson syndrome) are accompanied with hyperpigmentation and skin atrophy.[35,36] The demonstration that MC1r polymorphisms are associated with the red hair phenotype[30] clearly points out for a role of α-MSH and MC1r signaling in the control of hair pigmentation. Surprisingly, although α-MSH/MC1r controls the pheomelanin/eumelanin ratio and hair color in humans, MC1r loss of function mutation is not associated with loss of tyrosinase and TYRP1 expression in human hair bulb,[37] in contrast with what is observed in mice.[38] This observation demonstrates that although α-MSH/MC1r controls the switch between eumelanins and pheomelanins in human hair, melanocyte differentiation and melanogenic enzyme expression in human hair bulb do not primarily require α-MSH/MC1r signaling.[37]

Beta (β)-Endorphin

β-endorphin belongs to the opioid peptide family comprising enkephalins and dynorphins. β-endorphin originates from the cleavage of POMC prohormone and is a strong agonist for μ and δ opiate receptors. Endorphins are implicated in the pathogenesis of several dermatoses. As an example, elevated β-endorphin plasma levels have been reported in vitiligo, psoriasis and atopic dermatitis. The β-endorphin/μ-opiate receptor system is expressed in human epidermal melanocytes and *in vitro* studies have demonstrated that β-endorphin upregulates both melanocyte dendricity and proliferation and stimulates melanin synthesis.[39]

Endothelins

Endothelins (ETs) are endothelium-derived peptides with potent vasoconstrictor activity, detected in a broad range of tissues including skin. ETs comprise three isopeptides ET-1, ET-2 and ET-3. ET-3 stimulates melanoblast proliferation and the differentiation of neural crest progenitors into fully mature pigmented melanocytes and acts synergistically with stem cell factor (SCF; steel factor). ET-1 stimulates tyrosinase activity via binding to endothelin receptors and the subsequent activation of protein kinase C (PKC), elevation of cAMP and activation of protein kinase K (PKA).[40] In addition, ETs have also been implicated in the development of melanocyte dendricity. In the skin, ET-1 is secreted by keratinocytes and its expression is stimulated by UVB rays, leading to melanocyte proliferation and stimulation of melanogenesis.[41]

Stem Cell Factor

Stem cell factor, also known as mast cell growth factor (MGCF), c-kit ligand (KL), or steel factor (SLF), is a growth factor/cytokine. Normal skin keratinocytes constitutively produce SCF which signals via the c-kit receptors that are expressed on various cell types including melanocytes.[42] The SCF/c-kit interaction is critical for melanocyte survival. Mutations in the c-kit receptor have been identified within a continuous range of human piebaldism phenotypes. The role of SCF/c-kit has been implicated in many disease conditions, such as alopecia areata and vitiligo with melanocytes in the perilesional skin of vitiligo patients exhibiting reduced c-kit expression.[43,44] Participation of SCF/c-kit signaling has also been reported in melanoma progression.[45]

Eicosanoids

Eicosanoids are arachidonic acid-derived second messengers that include prostaglandins, leukotrienes and thromboxane. Prostaglandins and leukotrienes are inflammatory mediators which signal through various G protein-coupled seven-transmembrane receptors that differ in their G protein specificity. It has been clinically observed that most dermatitis (inflammatory dermatoses) are associated with striking changes in melanocyte function. Eicosanoids were the first inflammatory mediators investigated for their effects on melanocyte function, since their levels are increased in skin after sunburn, atopic dermatitis associated acute inflammation, contact dermatitis, psoriasis, and urticaria pigmentosa. It has been reported that eicosanoids modulate the normal melanocyte function by increasing pigmentation (LTB4, LTC4, PGD2, PGE2), growth (LTC4), differentiation (LTC4), and motility (LTC4) of melanocytes.[46]

In particular, prostaglandin F2α was shown to darken eyelashes, as revealed by a secondary effect of latanoprost treatment for glaucoma.[47] Later on, several *in vitro* studies carried out on normal human melanocytes demonstrated the ability of prostaglandins E2 and F2α to stimulate tyrosinase expression and melanin synthesis, along with dendrite development.[48-50] Indeed human hair follicles express the enzymes necessary for PGE2 and PGF2α production.[51] Moreover, a full repertoire of prostaglandin receptors was identified in the bulb of human hair follicle.[52] Altogether, these results strongly suggest that PGE2 and PGF2α, along with their cognate receptor signaling, play a role in melanin production in human hair.

Histamine

Histamine (β-imidazolylethylamine) exhibits a broad range of activities since acting on various tissues, including immune cells, stomach and nervous systems, and plays a role in the regulation of cell proliferation/differentiation, neurotransmission and immunomodulation. Histamine is generated by enzymatic decarboxylation of histidine by L-histidine decarboxylase and is stored within cell granules. Histamine has been demonstrated in several skin compartments including mast cells, blood vessels, eccrine gland, hair follicles and epidermis.[53] Several clinical observations point out the contribution of histamine in pigmentation conditions. The increased skin pigmentation associated with urticaria pigmentosa and systemic mastocytosis appears to result from increased local concentrations of histamine. Close association has been found between melanin-containing cells and mast cells in the lesions of nodular mastocytosis.[54] With other respects, Kim[55] demonstrated that the expression levels of the H_2 receptor was significantly decreased in depigmented compared to normally pigmented epidermis in patients with vitiligo. On a molecular point of view, the ability of histamine to stimulate melanin synthesis and expression of tyrosinase and related proteins has been demonstrated *in vitro*.[56] This *in vitro* H_2-mediated histamine effect likely occurs through signaling cascades involving ERK, CREB and Akt activation, eventually stimulating both melanocyte migration and proliferation along with melanin synthesis. In addition, studies on experimental models suggested that histamine and H_2 receptor contributed to UV-induced pigmentation.[57] On another hand, histamine and H_2 receptor agonists also increased survival of vitiliginous, but not normal keratinocytes, with NF-κB activation. Therefore, histamine may have also a role on keratinocyte survival.

Steroid Hormones

Estrogens are steroid hormones that have significant effects upon many aspects of skin physiology and pathophysiology,[58] including skin aging, pigmentation, hair growth, sebum production, and skin cancer. The contribution of steroid hormones in pigmentation was evidenced a long time ago,[59] and increased skin pigmentation during pregnancy on some specific sites, e.g. areolae and genitalia and appearance of the linea nigra on the belly[60,61] were attributed to increased secretion of estrogen and progesterone. In addition, *in vitro* studies have evidenced that both 17-estradiol and androgen stimulate tyrosinase activity *in vitro*.[62,63] The multiple estrogen actions are mediated mainly by two estrogen receptors (ER): ERα and Erβ,[64] and melanocytes were shown to express androgen and estrogen receptors.[63,65] ERβ is preferentially expressed in human epidermis, blood vessels, and dermal fibroblasts. In the hair follicle, ERβ expression is localized to nuclei of ORS, epithelial matrix, and dermal papilla cells. ERα is not clearly detected in the epidermis or hair follicles.

Ultraviolet Rays

Ultraviolet rays (UVR) are among the major environmental determinants in regulating pigmentation (Fig. 5, see also "Facultative Pigmentation" section).

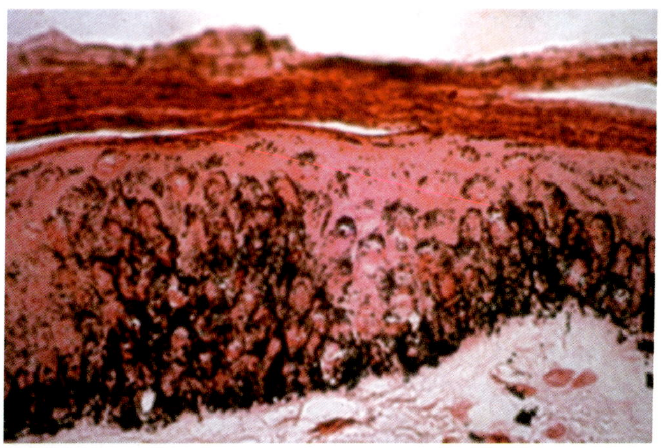

Figure 5: Skin histology showing melanogenesis process after UVR exposure
©L'Oréal Research and Innovation

UVR trigger pigmentation in distinct manners, depending on the duration and intensity of exposure. With long and intense exposure, UVR increases pigmentation through the regulation of gene expressions, including POMC, MITF, TYR, TYRP1 and DCT, and numerous other factors among ET-1 and SCF, all of which contributing to the increase in melanin synthesis, melanocyte dendricity and melanocyte density.[66-69] This UVR-induced pigmentation involves keratinocyte and fibroblast response since UVR induce the expression of melanogenic factors both in keratinocytes and fibroblasts. UVR also enhances levels of proteinase-activated receptor 2 (PAR2) which stimulates melanosome transfer and distribution within epidermal keratinocytes.[70]

NATURAL VARIATIONS OF PIGMENTATION IN HUMANS

Diversity of Human Skin and Hair Pigmentation

Human hair and skin display a large range of natural colors depending on people origin and somehow illustrates their geographic-related distribution.

Using an objective colorimetric tool, the Chromasphere®, the skin color of 8,452 women from different worldwide origins was evaluated revealing a wide diversity of skin colors around the world, even within groups of same ethnic origin. In particular, this data highlighted the diversity of skin color in India. (See chapter 4 for more details).

In the same idea, a recent worldwide study carried out on more than 4,000 persons over the five continents, provided quantitative demonstration of hair color diversity.[71] While 50% of the overall population worldwide was shown to have very dark and dark brown hair: Asians, Melanesians and Africans exhibiting the darkest hair color and the smallest diversity of shades, the blond hair phenotype was essentially limited to the northern and eastern Europeans.

In other respects, the identification of the "chemical phenotype" of pigmented tissues has greatly progressed, thanks to the development of chemical methods dealing with melanin analysis. These methods are based upon the assessment of specific degradation products of melanin: pyrrole-2,3,5-tricarboxylic acid (PTCA) as a specific degradation product of DHICA-derived units in eumelanins, pyrrole-2,3-dicarboxylic acid (PDCA) as a specific degradation product of DHI-derived units in eumelanins, and 4-amino-3-hydroxyphenylalanine (4-AHP) as a specific marker of pheomelanins.[72] The PDCA/PTCA ratio appears being most important to describe the eumelanin biosynthetic pathway involved between DHI vs DHICA eumelanins.

The variation in skin color among various ethnic origins is mainly determined by the number, melanin content, and distribution of melanosomes produced and transferred by each melanocyte to a cluster of keratinocytes surrounding it.[73,74] Keratinocytes in fair skin tend to cluster their poorly pigmented melanosomes above the nuclei, whereas in dark skin the heavily pigmented melanosomes are distributed individually in keratinocytes, thus maximizing their absorption of light.

Melanin analysis in a large sample of hair of various colors demonstrated that hair color, from black to blond, mainly relies on eumelanin content, black hair containing the higher eumelanin amount.[72] No variation in the pheomelanin level could be shown in this range of hair colors. By contrast, red hair was characterized by an elevated content of pheomelanin in comparison with all other hair colors. Regarding eumelanin, it was shown that East Asian hair contained higher PDCA/PTCA ratio as compared to Caucasian and African-American hairs.[29] In addition, in African-American and in Caucasian hairs, PDCA/PTCA ratios similarly increased with age and, in the elderly, individuals tend to reach the constant ratio measured in Asian hair. These observations suggest a chronological change in melanocyte phenotype in human hair, e.g. a decrease in the dopachrome tautomerase expression.

Natural variations of hair color and melanin content in hair are genetically controlled. Polymorphisms associated with normal pigmentary phenotypes have been identified through examining genetic variations. Hence, beyond the longstanding identified MC1r polymorphisms overrepresented in Northern Europeans and associated with red hair, fair skin and freckles, genomic studies enriched the list of gene polymorphisms which are associated with normal variation of pigmentation, e.g. IRF4, Slc24a4 , Slc24a5, TPCN2 and new genetic variations associated with normal pigmentation diversity were identified in the four genes already associated with oculocutaneous albinism, TYR (OCA1), OCA2, TYRP1 (OCA3) and Slc45a2 (OCA4).[75-79] Noteworthy, some of the SNPs were overly represented in subpopulations and exhibited geographic-specific distribution. For instance, A111G variation in Slc24a5 (rs1426654) was shown to have allele frequency differences, with Thr111 being over 90% in Europeans while Ala111 reached at least 90% in African and East Asian populations.[80] Similarly, the 374G allele (rs16891982) of MATP (Slc45a2) showed almost 90% frequency in Europeans while being below 10% in African and East Asian populations.[80]

The function and the role of most of the genes newly identified to contribute to normal variation of pigmentation are not known. Cook et al. analyzed cultured human melanocytes bearing allele variants of Slc45a2 and Slc24a5.[81] The authors could demonstrate an increase in melanin content along with higher tyrosinase activity in melanocytes with either Slc45a2-L374 or Slc24a5-A111 variant, each associated with dark hair and skin. Although the study does not afford clues to refine the precise function of both proteins in pigmentation, results demonstrate that both Slc45a2 and Slc24a5 act within melanocytes. Interestingly, most genes identified so far as contributing to natural variation of pigmentation in humans appear being genes expressed in melanocytes, suggesting that although melanocyte activity is controlled by paracrine factors and melanocyte environment, it is mainly melanocyte acting genes that clearly control normal pigmentation traits.

Surprisingly, in humans, only one SNP has been identified for DCT, the third tyrosine related enzyme, specifically in East Asian population with no particular pigmentary phenotype.[82] Similarly, no SNP has been reported for pMel17/gp100 in humans, while both DCT and silver mutations have been reported in mice and are responsible for pigmentation trait.

Is There a Correlation between Skin, Hair and Eye Color?

Although skin, hair and eye colors are generally correlated, numerous observations strongly suggest that constitutive pigmentation in the three tissues is somehow distinctly regulated in humans. In this respect, Caucasians with fair skin and blue eyes along with black/dark hair can be easily seen. This weak correlation between skin, hair and eye color in Caucasians, with the exception of those with red hair, was exemplified in a Danish cohort.[83] Likewise, Chinese and African (sub-Saharian) individuals exhibit hair of similar color,[71] while each population have distinct skin colors, with Chinese skin being lighter in color, with lower melanin content.[84] Another striking example is the age-dependent graying of hair which is not concomitant to whitening of the skin, in any body location. These observations suggest that constitutive pigmentation in human skin and hair harbor some specific characteristics in each and a few illustrations can already be emphasized.

First of all, the hair pigmentary system primarily relies on a melanocyte stem cell pool that is cyclically activated, as previously discussed earlier in this chapter. Such melanocyte reservoir has not been described in epidermis. Premature exhaustion of this melanocyte reservoir with age occurs in hair follicle and is responsible for hair graying, while melanocytes in the adjacent epidermis area are not affected.[85] Hence, factors involved in melanocyte stem cells maintenance in hair follicle are critical factors for hair pigmentation while they would be of little importance for skin pigmentation in adult.

Another striking difference is that pigmentation is both constitutive and inducible in skin while hair pigmentation is constitutive only and linked to hair cycle, being active only during the anagen phase. In this respect, melanogenic enzyme expression, e.g. tyrosinase, TYRP1, is observed in hair bulb melanocytes only during the anagen phase of hair.[4] Thus, in a given genetic background, hair follicle melanocytes require anagen hair bulb structures to be endowed with melanogenic capabilities. It is thus likely that the regulating factors, e.g. paracrine factors or cell-cell interactions that commit hair melanocytes into melanin producing cells arise from the hair bulb itself. Whether or not these regulating factors differ in hair bulb and in skin is unclear, however one might expect some differences if we consider differences between skin and hair color that may occur in a given individual. This different behavior is also strongly supported by the observation that hair follicle melanocytes do not express the melanogenic enzyme DCT, whereas DCT is expressed in all melanocytes in the epidermis.[28] The lack of DCT was observed in eumelanic hair from individuals of various origins and in red hair. Though the cause of the lack of DCT expression is unclear, it is, however, obviously linked to melanocyte environment within the hair follicle since once hair follicle melanocytes are isolated from hair follicle and grown *in vitro*, they do express DCT.[28]

Noteworthy, the lack of DCT expression appears specific to human hair follicle since DCT is expressed in melanocytes in human eyelash,[86] and in mice hair. The demonstration that DCT is not expressed in human hair bulb melanocytes was further supported by melanin assays carried out on several distinct human hair samples showing that human hair melanin contains a low level of the DHICA-derived compound PTCA as compared to melanins of other origins.[72]

Finally, one should simply note that hair bulb melanocytes have a high melanin production activity compared to skin melanocytes, as evidenced by the strong melanin deposition in hair bulb as compared to epidermis, and thus hair bulb melanocytes do possess an entire machinery particularly efficient for melanin production.

Facultative Pigmentation

Sunlight, and mostly its UV waveband, is the major natural stimulus that increases the basal level of skin pigmentation, being called "facultative pigmentation".

Three types of facultative pigmentations are observed: (i) a rapid and short-lived darkening called immediate pigment darkening (IPD); (ii) a rapid and lasting darkening called persistent pigment darkening (PPD) and (iii) a delayed tanning (DT).

Immediate Pigment Darkening and Persistent Pigment Darkening

Immediate pigment darkening is a blue-gray pigmentation that develops immediately during skin exposure to UVA rays, with the most efficient wavelength being between 320 nm and 340 nm. This transient pigmentation fades rapidly within 1 hour post exposure and loses its blue component within the second hour. When skin is exposed to higher UVA doses, a stable persistent darkening pigmentation (PPD) develops and remains for up to several days. IPD is more easily seen in subjects with phototypes III and IV.

Immediate pigment darkening could result from photo-oxidation and polymerization of pre-existing melanin intermediates. In addition, spatial rearrangement of melanosomes in melanocytes, and/or keratinocytes may also contribute to this transient skin darkening.[87]

Delayed Tanning

Prolonged exposure to UV or sunlight triggers DT after 2–3 days. DT is characterized by a brownish increase of skin color that persists for 1 month after UV exposure and that decreases with corneocyte desquamation. DT relies on complex alterations affecting not only melanocytes, but also other cells of the skin. In melanocytes, activation of gene expression occurs and involves upregulation of regulatory transcription factors, such as MITF-M and USF-1, and subsequently an increase in their melanogenic target gene expression, e.g. tyrosinase and related proteins.[88,89] Altogether, this orchestrated regulation of gene expression lead to an increase in melanin synthesis with an enrichment of black eumelanin (DHI melanin) in photoexposed skin.[74,84] In addition, the density of melanocytes increases, melanocytes become hypertrophic and dendrite number and length increase as well as the transfer of melanosomes into keratinocytes. In skin keratinocytes, POMC gene is activated, in a p53 dependent manner, leading to an increase in α-MSH release and subsequent melanocyte activation. DT is maximally stimulated by wavelengths of the erythemal spectrum, i.e. essentially UVB range (290–320 nm) and to a lesser extent UVA and visible radiation (320–700 nm). However, UVA tan lasts longer than UVB-induced tan.[90]

Hair Graying

Hair graying is a natural feature in human beings. The graying of hair is characterized by the lack of melanin pigment in hair shaft. Global graying of the scalp has been described as a gradual and progressive process occurring over more than 15 years in men.[91] The study by Panhard et al.[71] recently revisited the "50" rule of thumb from Keogh and Walsh[92] according to which at age 50, 50% of people have 50% of gray hair and in contrast, the authors showed that by 50 years, 63% of individuals worldwide had gray hair, with an average rate of 19% of gray hair. Indeed, an age-dependent increase in both the frequency and the rate of gray hair was observed in 91% of individuals showing 40% of gray hair in the age range of 61–65 years. Noteworthy, the authors evidenced that men have slightly more often gray hair with higher rate than women, with topological specific features since temples steadily showed significantly more gray hair in men. In addition, ethnical or geographical differences were found in African individuals showing both lower frequency and lower rate of gray hair, as compared to Caucasians.[71,93,94]

From a biological point of view, hair graying is due to a gradual and progressive depletion of the melanocyte stem cell pool located in the ORS of hair follicles.[85] The absence of melanocyte stem cells leads to the development of a bulb devoid of melanocytes at the telogen to neogen transition and to the production of a white hair shaft with no melanin. Thus, maintenance of a melanocyte stem cell pool in the ORS of hair follicle is a prerequisite for the hair pigmentation unit renewal and the growth of pigmented hair. The molecular process that causes premature exhaustion of these melanocyte stem cells is not precisely revealed. However, some clues seem emerging.

In mice, several experimental models and genetic mutations have highlighted the particularly high sensitivity of melanocyte stem cells to oxidative stress-associated DNA damage, responsible for the exhaustion of these cells and eventually hair graying.[95-98] Although of strong interest for a mechanistic knowledge, neither the identified genes nor the triggering events responsible for hair graying in these models were shown to be relevant for natural human hair graying and it is still unknown whether they hold for the cause of the natural graying in humans.

In humans, compiling observations also point out towards an oxidative-stress related process responsible for melanocyte stem cell depletion during hair graying. In that respect, gray hair contains higher level of the mitochondrial "common" deletion than pigmented and white hair.[99] The same authors also demonstrated that hair follicle melanocytes showed a higher sensitivity to exogenous stress than other hair follicle cells. A decrease in catalase expression and activity have also been observed in epidermal and hair follicle melanocytes isolated from old donors which might account for higher sensitivity to oxidative stress.[100] On the other hand, unlike melanocytes in epidermis, human hair follicle melanocytes do not express the melanocyte enzyme DCT,[28] which beside its role in melanin synthesis, was shown to provide a beneficial effect towards oxidative stress in various models, including melanocytes.[101-103] Altogether, these results strongly suggest that the lack of DCT expression in hair follicle melanocytes may contribute to some extent to their particular sensitivity to oxidative stress. Study on hair of various origins and from people at different ages also evidenced that DCT expression could decrease with age in human hair.[29] This chronological change in DCT expression would contribute to specific melanocyte exhaustion within hair follicle and eventually to hair graying.

It is thus likely that unlike epidermal melanocytes, human hair follicle melanocytes undergo chronological changes leading to a decrease in expression of proteins that have the ability to protect melanocytes stem cells from oxidative stress, e.g. DCT. Indeed, genetic determination, as well as systemic factors, would also undoubtedly affect the incidence and the rate of hair graying.

CONCLUSION

Pigmentation is a complex process that results from an intricate network of cellular and molecular connections between numerous cell populations in the skin, the key players being fibroblasts, keratinocytes and melanocytes. In the recent years, comprehensive advances have been made in the understanding of human pigmentation thanks to comparative genomic approaches, experimental researches and clinical observations. Human skin and hair color is clearly a multifactorial trait with a number of major determinant genes, several modifier genes and environmental influences, such as exposure to sun UV rays, and gender effects. Although the contribution of some major pigmentation genes, e.g. POMC, MC1R, tyrosinase, DCT, MITF, have been thoroughly described, more comprehensive molecular, cellular and genetic studies are still required. They hopefully should confirm and shed light on the precise role of many other pigmentation genes recently pointed out towards a better understanding of pigmentation related disorders. This upgraded knowledge is a prerequisite to improve the treatment of dyspigmented or unesthetically pigmented conditions.

REFERENCES

1. Seiji M, Shimao K, Birbeck MS, et al. Subcellular localization of melanin biosynthesis. Ann N Y Acad Sci. 1963;100:497-533.
2. Starico RG. Amelanotic melanocytes in the outer sheath of the human hair follicle. J Invest Dermatol. 1959;33:295-7.

3. Horikawa T, Norris DA, Johnson TW, et al. DOPA-negative melanocytes in the outer root sheath of human hair follicles express premelanosomal antigens but not a melanosomal antigen or the melanosome-associated glycoproteins tyrosinase, TRP-1, and TRP-2. J Invest Dermatol. 1996;106:28-35.
4. Commo S, Bernard BA. Melanocyte subpopulation turnover during the human hair cycle: an immunohistochemical study. Pigment Cell Res. 2000;13:253-9.
5. Ortonne JP, Schmitt D , Thivolet J. PUVA-induced repigmentation of vitiligo: scanning electron microscopy of hair follicles. J Invest Dermatol. 1980;74:40-2.
6. Simon JD, Peles D, Wakamatsu K, et al. Current challenges in understanding melanogenesis: bridging chemistry, biological control, morphology, and function. Pigment Cell Melanoma Res. 2009;22:563-79.
7. Ito S, Wakamatsu K. Chemistry of mixed melanogenesis--pivotal roles of dopaquinone. Photochem Photobiol. 2008;84:582-92.
8. Land EJ, Ito S, Wakamatsu K et al. Rate constants for the first two chemical steps of eumelanogenesis. Pigment Cell Res. 2003;16: 487-93.
9. Aroca P, Garcia-Borron JC, Solano F, et al. Regulation of mammalian melanogenesis. I: Partial purification and characterization of a dopachrome converting factor: dopachrome tautomerase. Biochim Biophys Acta. 1990;1035:266-75.
10. Edge R, D'ischia M, Land EJ, et al. Dopaquinone redox exchange with dihydroxyindole and dihydroxyindole carboxylic acid. Pigment Cell Res. 2006;19:443-50.
11. Olivares C, Jimenez-Cervantes C, Lozano JA, et al. The 5,6-dihydroxyindole-2-carboxylic acid (DHICA) oxidase activity of human tyrosinase. Biochem J. 2001;354:131-9.
12. Wakamatsu K, Ohtara K, Ito S. Chemical analysis of late stages of pheomelanogenesis: conversion of dihydrobenzothiazine to a benzothiazole structure. Pigment Cell Melanoma Res. 2009;22: 474-86.
13. Hearing VJ. Biochemical control of melanogenesis and melanosomal organization. J Invest. Dermatol Symp Proc. 1999;4:24-8.
14. Raposo G, Marks MS. Melanosomes—dark organelles enlighten endosomal membrane transport. Nat Rev Mol Cell Biol. 2007;8: 786-97.
15. Kushimoto T, Basrur V, Valencia J, et al. A model for melanosome biogenesis based on the purification and analysis of early melanosomes. Proc Natl Acad Sci USA. 2001;98:10698-703.
16. Berson JF, Harper DC, Tenza D, et al. Pmel17 initiates premelanosome morphogenesis within multivesicular bodies. Mol Biol Cell. 2001;12:3451-64.
17. Pawelek J, Korner A, Bergstrom A, et al. New regulators of melanin biosynthesis and the autodestruction of melanoma cells. Nature. 1980;286:617-9.
18. Urabe K, Aroca P, Tsukamoto K, et al. The inherent cytotoxicity of melanin precursors: a revision. Biochim Biophys Acta. 1994;1221:272-8.
19. Chi A, Valencia JC, Hu ZZ, et al. Proteomic and bioinformatic characterization of the biogenesis and function of melanosomes. J Proteome Res. 2006;5:3135-44.
20. Fuller BB, Spaulding DT, Smith DR. Regulation of the catalytic activity of preexisting tyrosinase in black and Caucasian human melanocyte cell cultures. Exp Cell Res. 2001;262:197-208.
21. Ancans J, Tobin DJ, Hoogduijn MJ, et al. Melanosomal pH controls rate of melanogenesis, eumelanin/phaeomelanin ratio and melanosome maturation in melanocytes and melanoma cells. Exp Cell Res. 2001;268:26-35.
22. Singh SK, Kurfurst R, Nizard C, et al. Melanin transfer in human skin cells is mediated by filopodia--a model for homotypic and heterotypic lysosome-related organelle transfer. FASEB J. 2010;24:3756-69.
23. Wasmeier C, Hume AN, Bolasco G, et al. Melanosomes at a glance. J Cell Sci. 2008;121:3995-9.
24. Wolff K. Melanocyte-keratinocyte interactions *in vivo*: the fate of melanosomes. Yale J Biol Med. 1973;46:384-96
25. Halloy J, Bernard BA, Loussouarn G, et al. Modeling the dynamics of human hair cycles by a follicular automaton. Proc Natl Acad Sci USA. 2000;97:8328-33.
26. Commo S, Bernard BA. Immunohistochemical analysis of tissue remodelling during the anagen-catagen transition of the human hair follicle. Br J Dermatol. 1997;137:31-8.
27. Bernard BA. The human hair follicle, a bistable organ? Exp. Dermatol. 2012;21:401-3.
28. Commo S, Gaillard O, Thibaut S, et al. Absence of TRP-2 in melanogenic melanocytes of human hair. Pigment Cell Res. 2004b;17:488-97.
29. Commo S, Wakamatsu K, Lozano I, et al. Age-dependent changes in eumelanin composition in hairs of various ethnic origins. Int J Cosmet Sci. 2012;34:102-7.
30. Rees JL. The melanocortin 1 receptor (MC1R): more than just red hair. Pigment Cell Res. 2000;13:135-140.
31. Chhajlani V, Wikberg JE. Molecular cloning and expression of the human melanocyte stimulating hormone receptor cDNA. FEBS Lett. 1992;14:309:417-20
32. Mountjoy KG, Robbins LS, Mortrud MT, et al. The cloning of a family of genes that encode the melanocortin receptors. Science. 1992;28:257:1248-51.
33. Lerner AB, McGuire J. Effect of alpha- and beta-melanocyte stimulating hormones on the skin color of mean. Nature. 1961;189:176-9.
34. Levine N, Sheftel SN, Eytan T, et al. Induction of skin tanning by subcutaneous administration of a potent synthetic melanotropin. JAMA. 1991;266:2730–6.
35. Fitzpatrick TB, Eisen AZ, Wolff K, et al. Dermatology in General Medicine. New York: McGraw-Hill, 1997.
36. Slominski A, Wortsman J. Neuroendocrinology of the skin. Endocr Rev. 2000;21:457-87.
37. Commo SF, Gaillard O, Rees JL, et al. Impact of homozygosity of R151C variant of MC1r in human hair follicle melanocytes. J Invest Dermatol. 2008;128:1319-22.
38. Kobayashi T, Vieira WD, Potterf B, et al. Modulation of melanogenic protein expression during the switch from eu- to pheomelanogenesis. J Cell Sci. 1995;108:2301-9.
39. Kauser S, Schallreuter KU, Thody AJ, et al. Regulation of human epidermal melanocyte biology by betaendorphin. J Invest Dermatol. 2003;120:1073-80
40. Imokawa G, Kobayashi T, Miyagishi M, et al. The role of endothelin-1 in epidermal hyperpigmentation and signaling mechanisms of mitogenesis and melanogenesis. Pigment Cell Res. 1997;10:218-28.
41. Imokawa G, Miyagishi M, Yada Y. Endothelin-1 as a new melanogen: coordinated expression of its gene and the tyrosinase gene in UVB-exposed human epidermis. J Invest Dermatol. 1995;105:32-7.
42. Broudy VC. Stem cell factor and hematopoiesis. Blood. 19997;90:1345-64.
43. Norris A, Todd C, Graham A, et al. The expression of the c-kit receptor by epidermal melanocytes may be reduced in vitiligo. Br J Dermatol. 1996;134:299--06
44. Kitamura R, Tsukamoto K, Harada K, et al. Mechanisms underlying the dysfunction of melanocytes in vitiligo epidermis: role of SCF/

KIT protein interactions and the downstream effector, MITF-M. J Pathol. 2004;202:463-75.
45. Huang S, Luca M, Gutman M, et al. Enforced c-KIT expression renders highly metastatic human melanoma cells susceptible to stem cell factor-induced apoptosis and inhibits their tumorigenic and metastatic potential. Oncogene. 1996;13:2339-47.
46. Norris DA, Morelli JG, Fujita M. Melanocytes interactions in skin. In: The Pigmentary System, edited by Nordlund JJ, Biossy RE, Hearing VJ, King RA, and Ortonne J-P. New York: Oxford Univ. Press; 1998, pp. 123–133
47. Johnstone MA. Hypertrichosis and increased pigmentation of eyelashes and adjacent hair in the region of the ipsilateral eyelids of patients treated with unilateral topical latanoprost. Am J Ophthalmol. 1997;124 544-7.
48. Scott G, Leopardi S, Printup S, et al. Proteinase-Activated Receptor-2 Stimulates Prostaglandin Production in Keratinocytes: Analysis of Prostaglandin Receptors on Human Melanocytes and Effects of PGE and PGF on Melanocyte Dendricity. J Invest Dermatol. 2004;122:1214-24.
49. Scott G, Jacobs S, Leopardi S, et al. Effects of PGF2alpha on human melanocytes and regulation of the FP receptor by ultraviolet radiation. Exp Cell Res. 2005;304:407-16.
50. Starner RJ, McClelland L, Abdel-Malek Z, et al. PGE(2) is a UVR-inducible autocrine factor for human melanocytes that stimulates tyrosinase activation. Exp Dermatol. 2010;19:682-4.
51. Colombe L, Vindrios A, Michelet JF, et al. Prostaglandin metabolism in human hair follicle. Exp Dermatol. 2007;16:762-9.
52. Colombe L, Michelet JF, Bernard BA. Prostanoid receptors in anagen human hair follicles. Exp Dermatol. 2008;17:63-72.
53. Malaviya R, Morrison AR, Pentland AP. Histamine in human epidermal cells is induced by ultraviolet light injury. J Invest Dermatol. 1996;106:785-9.
54. Okun MR, Bhawan J. Combined melanocytoma-mastocytoma in a case of nodular mastocytosis. J Am Acad Dermatol. 1979;1:338-47.
55. Kim NH, Lee AY. Histamine effect on melanocyte proliferation and vitiliginous keratinocyte survival. Exp Dermatol. 2010;19:1073-9.
56. Lee HJ, Park MK, Lee EJ, et al. Histamine receptor 2-mediated growth-differentiation factor-15 expression is involved in histamine-induced melanogenesis. Int J Biochem Cell Biol. 2012;44:2124-8.
57. Anbar TS, Westerhof W, Badawy NA, et al. The effect of H_1 and H_2 receptor antagonists on melanogenesis. Indian J Dermatol Venereol Leprol. 2012;78:64-7.
58. Thornton MJ. The biological actions of estrogens on skin. Exp Dermatol. 2002;11:487-502.
59. Hamilton JB, Hubert G. Photographic nature of tanning of the human skin as shown by studies of male hormone therapy. Science. 1938;88:481.
60. Esteve E, Saudeau L, Pierre F, et al. [Physiological cutaneous signs in normal pregnancy: a study of 60 pregnant women]. Ann Dermatol Venereol. 1994;121:227-31.
61. Wong RC, Ellis CN. Physiologic skin changes in pregnancy. J Am Acad Dermatol. 1984;10:929-40
62. McLeod SD, Ranson M, Mason RS. Effects of estrogens on human melanocytes in vitro. J Steroid Biochem Mol Biol. 1994;49:9-14.
63. Tadokoro T, Itami S, Hosokawa K, et al. Human genital melanocytes as androgen target cells. J Invest Dermatol. 1997;109:513-7.
64. Greene GL, Gilna P, Waterfield M, et al. Sequence and expression of human estrogen receptor complementary DNA. Science. 1986;231:1150-4.
65. Jee SH, Lee SY, Chiu HC, et al. Effects of estrogen and estrogen receptor in normal human melanocytes. Biochem Biophys Res Commun. 1994;199:1407-12.
66. Corre S, Mekideche K, Adamski H, et al. In vivo and ex vivo UV-induced analysis of pigmentation gene expressions. J Invest Dermatol. 2006;126:916-8.
67. Miyamura Y, Coelho S. G, Wolber R, et al. Regulation of human skin pigmentation and responses to ultraviolet radiation. Pigment Cell Res. 2007;20:2-13.
68. Kadekaro AL, Kavanagh RJ, Wakamatsu K, et al. Cutaneous photobiology. The melanocyte vs. the sun: who will win the final round? Pigment Cell Res. 2003;16:434-47.
69. Scott G, Deng A, Rodriguez-Burford C, et al. Protease-activated receptor 2, a receptor involved in melanosome transfer, is upregulated in human skin by ultraviolet irradiation. J Invest Dermatol. 2001;117:1412-20.
70. Imokawa G. Autocrine and paracrine regulation of melanocytes in human skin and in pigmentary disorders. Pigment Cell Res. 2004;17:96-110
71. Panhard S, Lozano I, Loussouarn G. Greying of the human hair. A worldwide survey, re-visiting the "50" rule of thumb. Br J Dermatol. 2012;167:865-73.
72. Ito S, Nakanishi Y, Valenzuela RK, et al. Usefulness of alkaline hydrogen peroxide oxidation to analyze eumelanin and pheomelanin in various tissue samples: application to chemical analysis of human hair melanins. Pigment Cell Melanoma Res. 2011;24:605-13.
73. Tadokoro T, Yamaguchi Y, Batzer J, et al. Mechanisms of skin tanning in different racial/ethnic groups in response to ultraviolet radiation. J Invest Dermatol. 2005;124:1326-32.
74. Alaluf S, Heath A, Carter N, et al. Variation in melanin content and composition in type V and VI photoexposed and photoprotected human skin: the dominant role of DHI. Pigment Cell Res. 2001;14:347.
75. Han J, Kraft P, Nan H, et al. A genome-wide association study identifies novel alleles associated with hair color and skin pigmentation. PLoS Genet. 2008;4e1000074.
76. Lamason RL, Mohideen MA, Mest JR, et al. SLC24A5, a putative cation exchanger, affects pigmentation in zebrafish and humans. Science. 2005;310:1782-6.
77. Sturm RA. Molecular genetics of human pigmentation diversity. Hum Mol Genet. 2009;18:9-17.
78. Sulem P, Gudbjartsson DF, Stacey SN, et al. Two newly identified genetic determinants of pigmentation in Europeans. Nat Genet. 2008;40:835-7.
79. Sulem P, Gudbjartsson DF, Stacey SN, et al. Genetic determinants of hair, eye and skin pigmentation in Europeans. Nat Genet. 2007;39:1443-52.
80. Norton HL, Kittles RA, Parra E, et al. Genetic evidence for the convergent evolution of light skin in Europeans and East Asians. Mol Biol Evol. 2007;24:710-22.
81. Cook AL, Chen W, Thurber AE, et al. Analysis of cultured human melanocytes based on polymorphisms within the SLC45A2/MATP, SLC24A5/NCKX5, and OCA2/P loci. J. Invest Dermatol. 2009;129:392-405.
82. Lao O, de Gruijter JM, van DK, et al. Signatures of positive selection in genes associated with human skin pigmentation as revealed from analyses of single nucleotide polymorphisms. Ann Hum Genet. 2007;71:354-69.
83. Lock-Andersen J, Wulf HC, Knudstorp ND. Interdependence of eye and hair colour, skin type and skin pigmentation in a Caucasian population. Acta Derm Venereol. 1998;78:214-9.

84. Alaluf S, Atkins D, Barrett K, et al. Ethnic variation in melanin content and composition in photoexposed and photoprotected human skin. Pigment Cell Res. 2002;15:112-8.
85. Commo S, Gaillard O, Bernard BA. Human hair greying is linked to a specific depletion of hair follicle melanocytes affecting both the bulb and the outer root sheath. Br J Dermatol. 2004a;150:435-43.
86. Thibaut S, De Becker, Caisey L, et al. Human eyelash characterization. Br J Dermatol. 2010;162:304-10
87. Routaboul C, Denis A, Vinche A. Immediate pigment darkening: description, kinetic and biological function. Eur J Dermatol. 1999;9:95-9
88. Corre S, Mekideche K, Adamski H, et al. *In vivo* and *ex vivo* UV-induced analysis of pigmentation gene expressions. J Invest Dermatol. 2006;126:916-8.
89. Miyamura Y, Coelho S. G, Wolber R, et al. Regulation of human skin pigmentation and responses to ultraviolet radiation. Pigment Cell Res. 2007;20:2-13.
90. Chardon A, Cretois I, Hourseau C. Color changes induced on various skin categories by repeated exposures to UV rays. In Urbach F, eds. Biological responses to UVA radiation. Overland Park: ValdenMar Publishing Co;1992. pp.159-78.
91. Burch PR, Murray JJ, Jackson D. The age-prevalence of arcus senilis, greying of hair, and baldness. Etiological considerations. J Gerontol. 1971;26:364-72.
92. Keogh EV, Walsh RJ. Rate of greying of human hair. Nature. 1965;207:877-8.
93. Boas F, Michelson N. The greying of hair. Am J Phys Anthropol. 1932;17:213-28.
94. Straile WEA. A study of the hair follicle and its melanocytes. Dev Biol. 1964;10:45-70.
95. Cao L, Li W, Kim S, et al. Senescence, aging, and malignant transformation mediated by p53 in mice lacking the Brca1 full-length isoform. Genes Dev. 2003;17:201-13.
96. Inomata K, Aoto T, Binh NT, et al. Genotoxic stress abrogates renewal of melanocyte stem cells by triggering their differentiation. Cell. 2009;137:1088-99.
97. Rudolph KL, Chang S, Lee HW, et al. Longevity, stress response, and cancer in aging telomerase-deficient mice. Cell. 1999;96:701-12.
98. Yamamura K, Kamada S, Ito S, et al. Accelerated disappearance of melanocytes in bcl-2-deficient mice. Cancer Res. 1996;56:3546-50.
99. Arck PC, Overall R, Spatz K, et al. Towards a "free radical theory of graying": melanocyte apoptosis in the aging human hair follicle is an indicator of oxidative stress induced tissue damage. FASEB J. 2006;20:1567-9.
100. Kauser S, Westgate GE, Green MR, et al. Human hair follicle and epidermal melanocytes exhibit striking differences in their aging profile which involves catalase. J Invest Dermatol. 2011;131:979-82.
101. Michard Q, Commo S, Belaidi JP, et al. TRP-2 specifically decreases WM35 cell sensitivity to oxidative stress. Free Radic Biol Med. 2008a;44:1023-31.
102. Michard Q, Commo S, Rocchetti J, et al. TRP-2 expression protects HEK cells from dopamine- and hydroquinone-induced toxicity. Free Radic Biol Med. 2008b;45:1002-10.
103. Sendoel A, Kohler I, Fellmann C, et al. HIF-1 antagonizes p53-mediated apoptosis through a secreted neuronal tyrosinase. Nature. 2010;465:577-83.

Chapter 6

Pigmentary Disorders, Prevention, Treatment and Cosmetics Contributions

Jean-Paul Ortonne, *University Hospital of Nice, Nice, France*
Thierry Passeron, *University Hospital of Nice, Nice, France*
Chakaravarthi Srinivas, *PSG Institute of Medical Sciences and Research, Coimbatore, India*

INTRODUCTION

Human skin color is the most striking polymorphic feature of humans. The color of the skin is a subtle mix of pigments that included melanins, but also hemoglobin or carotenoids. Any variation in these pigments or abnormal accumulation of other endogenous or exogenous pigments will cause pigmentary changes in the skin. However, the wide skin color gradient is mainly due to melanin pigments produced by highly specialized epidermal cell, the melanocytes, and normally confined in the epidermis. Melanin production is genetically determined. However, over- or underproduction of melanin is the cause of hyper or hypopigmented lesions. The precise etiology of these conditions is still unknown. Pigmentary disorders are troublesome in a cosmetic point of view and have a considerable impact on the quality of life of affected people. Pigmentary disorders can cause psychological and emotional distress and can pose a negative impact on a person's health-related quality of life.

Multiple studies now document the increased frequency of disorders characterized by hyperpigmentation in people with darker skin.

This chapter constitutes an update of current knowledge on skin pigmentation and will focus on the three main hyperpigmentary disorders:

1. Actinic lentigo
2. Melasma
3. Postinflammatory hypopigmentation and hyperpigmentation.

ACTINIC LENTIGO

Definition and Epidemiology

Solar lentigines (SLs, also called as age spots, liver spots, actinic lentigos or senile lentigines) are macular hyperpigmented lesions, induced by chronic sun exposure, which evolve slowly over years (Fig. 1). SLs are viewed as an early sign of aging. The incidence of SLs formation increases with age and is more abundant upon high exposure to sunlight or to tanning devices.

The relationship between SL, age and ultraviolet (UV) exposure was confirmed in an epidemiological study.[1]

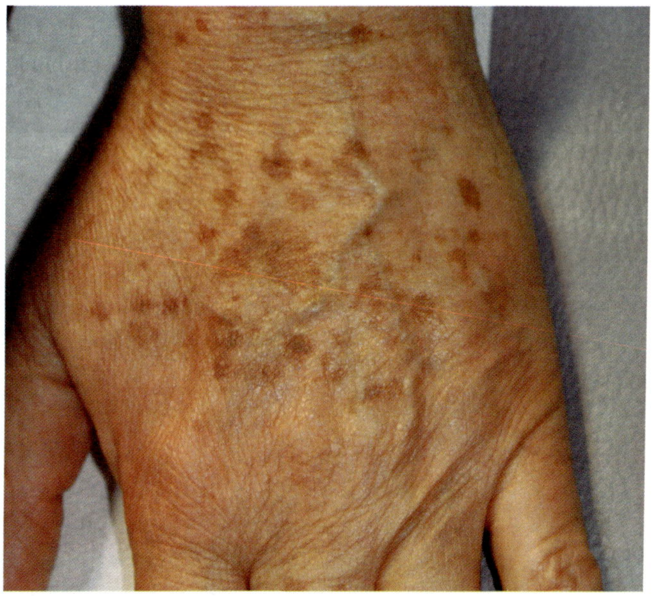

Figure 1: Patient with solar lentigines on the hand
Courtesy: Prof. Thierry Passeron, Nice, France

In this study, the presence of SLs in the face and on the back was assessed on 577 patients with skin cancer and 385 individuals without a history of skin cancer (Leiden Skin cancer Study). Epidemiological and environmental data were collected. The results showed a strong positive association of SL with age. SL on the back were positively associated with cumulative ($p = 0.01$) and intermittent ($p = 0.0002$) sun exposure, with a history of sunburns before the age of 20 years ($p = 0.0003$) and the number of sunburns in childhood ($p = 0.002$). SLs in the face were significantly associated with cutaneous signs of photodamage, i.e. elastosis and actinic keratosis. Interestingly, this study had not found an association between SL and skin type and/or hair color, however the study only includes skin types from I to IV.

A case control study focused on identifying some epidemiological factors related to multiple senile lentigos of the face.[2] The study was conducted in France in individuals aged between 60 years and 80 years, comparing cases (n = 118) with a very high number of SLs on the face for their age, and controls (n = 118) with no or very few SLs for their age. The results showed that multiple senile lentigo of the face preferentially affected old dark-skinned Caucasians who have repeatedly received intermittent and intense solar irradiations during all their life, and have developed multiple lentigos of the upper back often earlier in life.

More recently, multiple SLs of the upper back and shoulders (MSLBS) have been demonstrated as being associated with intense sunburns in the past and with cutaneous melanoma of the back.[3] This study conducted in France on 125 adult patients followed up for cutaneous melanoma, showed that 37.6% of them have MSLBS.

All those studies confirmed that chronic sun exposure, which is inevitably related to increasing age, plays an important role in the pathogenesis of SLs.

Differential Diagnosis

The differential diagnosis of SLs includes ephelides, macular seborrheic keratoses, simple lentigines, pigmented actinic keratoses, lentigo maligna, junctional melanocytic nevi and large cell acant homas. There is a continuum expanding from solar lentigo to macular varieties of seborrheic keratosis. Demonstration of a keratotic surface with horn cysts is consistent with seborrheic keratosis. Pigmented actinic keratosis is more likely to have a scaly, rough surface. Lentigo maligna often exhibits greater variation in pigmentation and irregularity of borders compared with SL. Simple lentigines are often smaller and more heavily pigmented than SLs, and arise in childhood with less relationship to UV exposure. Ephelides (freckles) are also located on sun-exposed areas, but they usually begin in childhood. They do not affect palms, soles and mucous membrane, and they tend to fade or disappear during the winter season. Small palmar cafe-au-lait spots is often seen in Von Recklinghausen Disease (Premlata Yesudian).

Histopathological Characteristics and New Insights in Solar Lentigo Pathogenesis

Histological hallmarks of SL lesions are hyperpigmentation of basal keratinocytes and elongation of the epidermal rete ridges. In general, SLs have both keratinocytic and melanocytic hyperplasia, but no melanocyfic atypia and no nests of melanocytes.

Andersen et al. showed in 1997[4] that compared with normal photoexposed facial skin, lentigines from the face often had a flattened epidermis. They also had a mean 2.1-fold increase in melanocytes, a 2.1-fold increase in epidermal area and a 2.2-fold increase in epidermal melanin content. In their study, SL of the face frequently lacked the rete ridge hyperplasia classically associated with lentigines from other anatomic sites.

In vivo reflectance confocal microscopy (RCM) examination of SLs show features that correlate well with histologic findings, such as supranuclear melanin caps. A recent report gave new insights on the dynamic pathomechanisms of SLs by studying dendritic melanocytes inside and at the outer rim of SL lesional areas.[5] Using RCM, the study showed that dendritic melanocytes were rarely seen in the center of a SL, but were seen at a very high frequency in the outer rim of a SL. This suggests that the melanocytes are more active at the edge of a SL, produce more melanin and often spread their dendrites widely in a horizontal direction.

Despite the association of SL to ultraviolet (UV) exposure, the mechanisms underlying the development of these spots are not completely defined.

A gene expression profiling analysis of SL in relation to immunohistochemical characteristics demonstrated an upregulation of genes related to inflammation, fatty-acid metabolism and melanocytes and a downregulation of cornified envelope-related genes.[6] This suggest that SL is induced by the mutagenic effect of repeated UV light exposures in the past, leading to the characteristic enhancement of melanin production, together with decreased proliferation and differentiation of lesional keratinocytes on the background of chronic inflammation.

Cutaneous pigmentation is regulated by a complex melanogenic network in which both keratinocytes and fibroblasts synthesize growth factors and cytokines. Various factors, such as α-melanocyte-stimulating hormone, endothelin-1 or stem cell factor (SCF) are involved in the onset and maintenance of the increased pigmentation.

Because of the potential role of endothelin as a paracrine cytokine in the activation of epidermal melanocytes, the role of the epidermal endothelin cascade in hyperpigmentation mechanism of SL was investigated.[7] Kadono et al. found in SL lesional skin: a twofold increase of tyrosine-positive melanocytes of the dermal/epidermal interface, a relatively stronger staining of endothelin-1 antibodies and an accentuated expression of transcripts for endothelin-1 and endothelin-B receptor, compared to the perilesional epidermis. Their findings suggested an accentuation of the epidermal endothelin cascade, especially with respect to expression of endothelin and the endothelin B receptor, in the mechanism involved in the hyperpigmentation of SLs.

Lin et al. studied the potential role of keratinocyte growth factor (KGF) in the development of SL.[8] They found on human skin biopsies an increase in tyrosinase TYR-positive cells and expression throughout SL progression, as compared to normal skin. The levels of KGF, KGFR, SCF, proliferation marker Ki67 and protease-activated receptor-2 (PAR-2) varied during SL progression. Ki67, K15 and KGF/KGFR were significantly upregulated at early-mid SL stages. The latest-stage SLs expressed the lowest levels of KGF, KGFR, SCF, Ki67 and PAR-2. The upregulation of KGF/KGFR might induce the formation of rete ridges and hyperpigmentation. The reduced levels of all examined proteins (except TYR and K15) suggest a possible inactive status (dormancy or quiescence) of advanced lesions.

In parallel to the cross-talk between keratinocytes and melanocytes, increasing evidence underlines the crucial role exerted by the dermal cells and interactions between mesenchymal and epithelial cells in the control of skin pigmentation through the release of fibroblast-derived growth factors. An increased number of melanophages, identified as factor XIIIa+ dermal dendrocytes, was found in SL affected skin compared with unaffected skin from the same subject.[9] This suggests that these cells may contribute to the alteration of the melanin/melanocyte balance in the epidermis and promote SL development.

In another study, the involvement of the fibroblast-derived growth factors, hepatocyte growth factor (HGF), KGF and SCF in SL hyperpigmentation were investigated.[10] The results showed a positive staining for HGF, KGF and SCF in the upper dermis of SL lesions indicating that the dermis is an important source of these cytokines. A strong staining for HGF and KGF on papillary dermis was also found, revealing that these growth factors may also play a key role in the paracrine stimulation of melanocytes in SL. These data underline the contribution of fibroblasts to the hyperpigmentation of SL in addition to the well-documented involvement of keratinocyte-derived cytokines. Fibroblasts may be persistently activated by UV exposure to release melanogenic growth factors; this inducible cytokine network may act both directly and indirectly through keratinocytes and contribute to the hyperpigmentation of SL.

Treatment

Laser Therapy

Solar lentigines are effectively treated with Q-switched (QS) lasers and intense pulsed light. The treatment with QS laser has been proven to be the most effective approach, especially if the lesions are numerous but it remains more expensive as compared to other approaches.[11] One or two laser sessions are sufficient.[11] While 694 and 755 nm are usually preferred is most cases, light lentigos are better treated with 532 nm QS lasers.[12] More recently, the thulium laser in fractionated mode was reported to improve SLs.[13] The 1927 nm wavelength of this laser has a strong affinity for water. At the contrary of QS lasers that will selectively target the melanin, the thulium laser approach has best to be considered for a more global photoaging care.

Cryotherapy

Melanocytes are particularly susceptible to freezing, and hence they should be avoided in dark-skinned people because of the risk of permanent depigmentation. The freezing agent must be applied gently to avoid blistering and skin necrosis. Cryotherapy with liquid nitrogen is commonly used successfully to treat SL. Although satisfactory results are common, cryotherapy can lead to hypopigmentation, hyperpigmentation atrophy, scarring and/or frequent recurrence.

Chemical Stripping

Chemical stripping agents, such as trichloroacetic acid with a concentration of 30%, trichloroacetic acid with a concentration of 50–70%, used alone or in combination, can achieve some effects.

Preventive Measures: Use of Sunscreens

As we know the strong association between UV and SL, sun protection all through the year is very crucial for preventing from SL. Patients should avoid sun exposure between 10:00 in the morning and 3:00 in the afternoon. If they have to go out, then they should use an umbrella or wear a hat to protect from sun. Meanwhile, they should also apply sunscreen agents that can block not only UVB but also UVA radiation to protect the skin from UV-induced damage since reported studies have given clear evidence of the very significant contribution of UVA in skin pigmentation. The broad spectrum sunscreen should be chosen in accordance with the season and the environment.

As SL tend to recur,[14] a maintenance treatment associated with the sun protection measures can be very useful.

MELASMA

Introduction and Epidemiology

Melasma is a common, acquired disorder, characterized by symmetric, hyperpigmented patches with an irregular outline that occur most commonly on the face. It is most prevalent among young to middle-aged women who are Indian, Hispanic, Asian or of African or Middle Eastern descent, i.e. darker skin phototypes. Melasma also tends to persist longer in those with more darkly pigmented skin.[15]

Melasma in men is much less common than in women. The percentage of men among melasma patients is reported to be approximately 26% in Indian, 14.5% in Latino, 10% in Caucasian and 4% in Korean.[16-18]

Classically, exacerbating factors include pregnancy, oral contraceptives and sun exposure.

Clinical Features

Light to dark brown or brown-gray patches with irregular borders appear primarily on the face. The areas of hypermelanosis are distributed symmetrically in three classic patterns: (1) centrofacial, (2) malar and (3) mandibular. The centrofacial pattern is most commonly observed, with involvement of the lateral forehead, cheeks, nose, upper lip (sparing the philtrum) and chin.

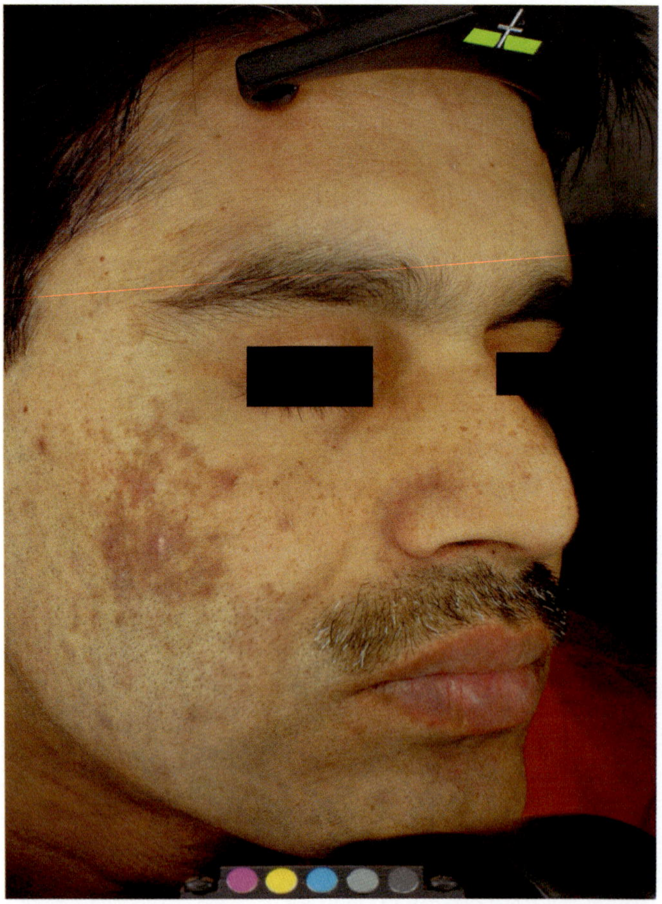

Figure 2: Classical presentation of facial melasma in an Indian man
Courtesy: Prof. Jean-Paul Ortonne, Nice, France

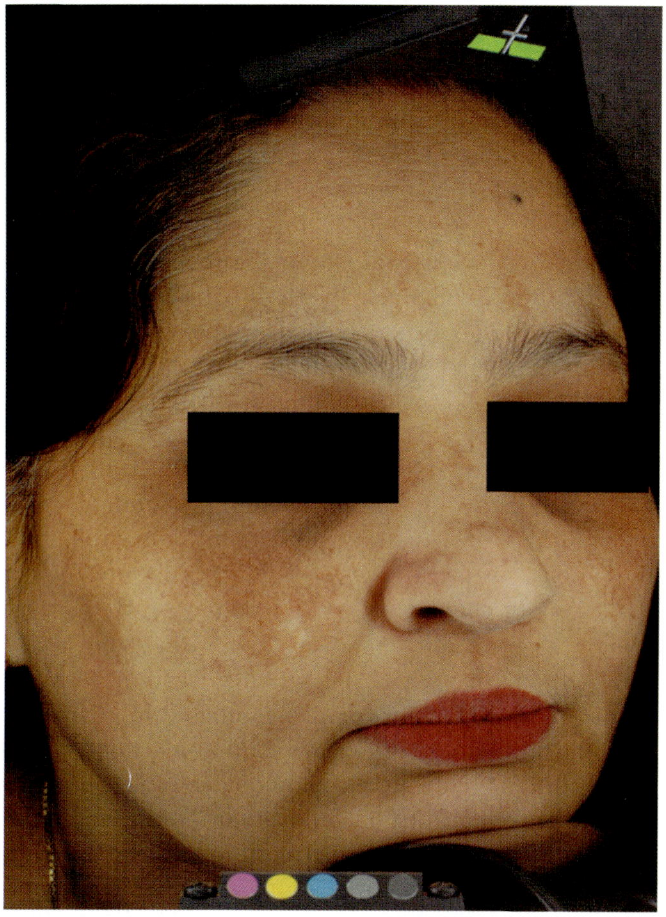

Figure 3: Classical presentation of facial melasma in an Indian woman
Courtesy: Prof. Jean-Paul Ortonne, Nice, France

In the malar and mandibular forms, the distribution is more limited, i.e. cheeks plus nose and mandibular ramus, respectively (Figs. 2 and 3).

Additional sites of involvement include the extensor forearms and the mid upper chest. Few studies have attempted to address those extrafacial melasma. Recently, Ritter et al. conducted a case-control study to evaluate the clinical characteristics of patients with this pigmentary disorder.[19] They observed that the most common location of lesions was the arms (95%) followed by the forearms (80%), chest (46.6%) and back (11.1%). Extrafacial melasma appears to be related to menopause, family history and personal history of facial melasma. However, the term of extra-facial melasma and the link with those hyperpigmented lesions with melasma is still under debate.

Melasma lesions fade during the winter months and they frequently either first appear or are accentuated following exposure to UV irradiation or during pregnancy. In lightly pigmented individuals, the "mask of pregnancy" often diminishes or disappears after parturition, whereas it may persist in women with more darkly pigmented skin.

Differential Diagnosis of Melasma

Disorders that can be confused for melasma[20] include postinflammatory pigmentation, solar lentigines, ephelides, drug-induced pigmentation, actinic lichen planus, facial acanthosis nigricans, frictional melanosis, acquired bilateral nevus of Ota-like macules (Hori's nevus), nevus of Ota and other facial hyperpigmentation with a melasma-like presentation, e.g. pigment demarcation lines.[21]

Histopathological Characteristics, Etiology and Pathogenesis of Melasma

Histological Characteristics

The histopathological pattern of melasma is primarily an increase of melanin deposition in the epidermis. Interestingly, the number of melanocytes is not increased in melasma suggesting that the hyperpigmentation is most likely the result of abnormal melanin production or distribution. The melanocytes within lesional skin are larger with prominent dendrites than melanocytes in unaffected skin, suggesting that melanocytes are very active in melasma. The protein levels of melanogenesis-associated factors (TYR, TYRP1, DCT and SILV) were increased in melasma lesions, indicating higher melanogenic activity in lesional skin.[22] The presence of pendulous melanocytes is also a characteristic of melasma.[23] Some melanocytes have shown the feature of protruding into the dermis. This feature has been described not only melasma, but also in other hyperpigmentary disorders, such as café-au-lait spots and senile lentigo and in the intense UV-A irradiated skin even in normal black skin, suggesting that pendulous melanocytes occur in epidermal hypermelanosis related to hyperactivity of the melanocytes. It is speculated that chronic sun exposure may increase MMP2 expression, which loose basement membrane in melasma.[24,25] These would be responsible for the pendulous change of melanocytes in melasma. The additional histological distinguishing characteristics of melasma are those of photodamage skin, such as solar elastosis, collagen degeneration and increased vascularity. A control study performed on 27 skin samples of patients with melasma also showed that lesional skin had abundant elastotic material compared with nonaffected skin.[26] Mast cells were also more prominent in the elastotic areas of melasma skin. Melasma could be a result of a cumulative sun exposure, in a microenvironment of cutaneous photoaging in which inflammatory cells, particularly mast cells, play a key role.

Sarvjot et al. confirmed the histopathological features of melasma on 43 patients in New Delhi.[27] The study showed that solar elastosis (55.8%) was the single most common histological finding apart from increased melanin concentration, epidermal flattening and dermal lymphomononuclear inflammation. Ritter et al. found similar histopathological pattern for extra-facial melasma, with signs of solar degeneration and a similar number of melanocytes compared to nonlesional skin.[19]

Reflectance confocal microscopy application to skin imaging allows great advance in melasma comprehension.[28-30] *In vivo* RCM is a noninvasive, repetitive imaging tool that provides real-time images at nearly cellular histological resolution. RCM images of melasma showed characteristic significantly increased hyper refractile cobblestone pattern at the level of basal cell layer in lesional skin compared with perilesional normal skin, corresponding to epidermal hyperpigmentation. Dendritic cells and plump bright dermal cells corresponding to activated melanocytes and melanophages, respectively, were also observed in some patients. RCM images showed variable degree of solar elastosis characterized by hypo refractile, lacy, ragged structures in the superficial dermis suggesting the existence of chronic solar damage in the melasma.

This leads to the common hypothesis that the areas with melasma had been affected because they were subject to the greatest degree of exposure to sunlight and actinic damage.

Etiology

Multiple etiological factors have been implicated in the pathogenesis of melasma, which include UV radiation exposure, pregnancy, contraceptive pills, hormonal replacement therapy and cosmetics, phototoxic and anti-seizure medications.

A large-scale survey of 324 melasma-affected women suggested that a combination of known triggers, such as pregnancy, hormonal birth control, a family history, and sun exposure affect the onset of melasma.[31] However, this study reports a weak impact of contraceptive pills on the spontaneous evolution of melasma, especially if patients have a familial history of melasma. It also shows that only 20% of melasma begin in the pregnancy period and that almost 10% of cases have an onset during the menopausal period. A recent survey conducted among 302 Brazilian women with melasma[32] reported that pregnancy induced melasma was associated to early disease onset and number of pregnancies. Childbearing was correlated to melasma extension. Interestingly, both studies showed that older disease onset age was associated to darker skin phototypes.

Melasma in men is definitely less common than in women, but shares the same clinicohistopathological characteristics as in women. The main causative factors among the male patients appeared to be sun-exposure and family history.[33] A recent histopathological study confirmed that the main factor involved in the development of male melasma may be sun exposure.[34] This study showed that increased vascularity, the SCF in the epidermis and dermis, and its receptor, c-kit, might play an important role in the mechanism associated with the hyperpigmentation in male melasma. Those findings suggest that the dermal changes associated with chronic UV exposure might be the most important factor associated with the development of male melasma.

Pathogenesis

The pathogenesis of melasma is far to be fully understood, and different mechanisms involving different biological signaling pathways are still under investigations.

A large-scale gene expression profiling was performed to investigate the pathogenesis of melasma.[22] The results showed that in melasma lesions, melanogenesis in melanocytes is activated at least partially at the transcriptional level. This study showed the alteration of the expressions of some genes associated with UV exposure, confirming the role of sun exposure in melasma. Furthermore, several signaling pathways, including the Wnt signaling and lipid metabolism pathways, were identified to be potentially involved in the development of melasma lesions. Most lipid metabolism-associated genes were found down-regulated in lesional skin. This finding was supported by an impaired barrier function in melasma.

The impairment of the barrier function was confirmed recently by an analysis of skin biophysical characteristics of 16 Korean women with melasma.[35] The results showed a normal hydration state and sebaceous gland activity in melasma skin. However, stratum corneum thickness was reduced in the lesional skin and it positively correlated with the barrier recovery rate. Interestingly, a negative correlation was found between melanin index and barrier recovery rate, meaning that patients with severe melasma may be having poor stratum corneum function. The mechanisms underlying abnormal barrier function in melasma are unclear, but down-regulated lipid metabolism-associated genes may be a causal factor of the impairment of epidermal barrier function in melasma. Improving stratum corneum function should be considered in treating melasma.

The Wnt signaling pathway in the hyperpigmentation occurring in melasma was further investigated by Kim et al.[36] They showed that the expression of Wnt inhibitory factor-1 (WIF-1) gene was significantly reduced in the hyperpigmented skin from melasma patients, but not in healthy controls. WIF-1 downregulation, which may occur in epidermal keratinocytes and in dermal fibroblasts, is involved in melasma development because of the stimulation of melanogenesis and melanosome transfer through upregulation of the canonical and the noncanonical Wnt signaling pathway.

Recent studies also suggest the involvements of dermal factors in the pathogenesis of melasma. The increased solar elastosis in melasma may suggest that accumulated sun exposure is necessary for the development of melasma. And the process of solar damage to the dermis may influence the development of hyperpigmentation in the overlying epidermis. Kang et al. conducted a study on 60 skin samples obtained from lesional and nonlesional facial skin of Korean women with melasma to investigate the expression of SCF and c-kit since those factors are highly implicated in hyperpigmentation mechanism.[37] They found that the dermal SCF and its receptor c-kit are overexpressed in melasma, suggesting that they play an important role in the mechanism of hyperpigmentation in melasma. The overexpression of SCF and c-kit in melasma lesional skin was confirmed by Torres-Alvarez et al.[24]

Other Signaling Pathways Investions

Activation of the inducible nitric oxide synthase (iNOS)/nitric oxide (NO) pathway in keratinocytes has been reported to be associated with the pathogenesis of melanogenesis. Thus iNOS expression in human melasma lesion was studied,[38] and showed an elevated expression, indicating that NO production may play an important role in the mechanism of hyperpigmentation in human facial melasma.

A neural involvement in the pathogenic mechanisms of pigmentation was also considered since characteristic clinical features of melasma are symmetry of hyperpigmentation and distribution related to trigeminal nerves.[39] The study showed that lesional skin of melasma expresses neuropeptides, such as nerve growth factor receptor (NGFR) and neural endopeptidase (NEP) more than the surrounding nonlesional skin. The results suggest that neuroactive molecules, including NGF, may be critical factors for the pathogenesis of melasma that may directly affect the microenvironment around melanocytes via a NGFR-IR nerve fiber pathway, and that greater NEP expression in melasma has an important role in regulation of melanogenesis.

Management of Melasma

One purpose of the treatment of melasma is to avoid the above-mentioned causative and aggravating factors. The other purpose is to reduce the size of the diseased skin and correct the facial defects by inhibiting the pigment producing activity of melanocyte, destroying and removing melanosomes, and preventing or diminishing relapse.

Exposure to the sun is a major cause and aggravating factor of melasma, so patients should be warned against such exposure (see the content below: Sun-blocking products). At the same time, they should not take light-sensitive drugs and use improperly-made cosmetics. Discontinuation of oral contraceptive pills should be discussed if they were introduced during the year of the onset or worsening of the melasma. Currently, a large variety of skin care products are available on the market. First of all patients should choose appropriate whitening cosmetics according to their skin type and restore skin barrier function in diseased areas under the guidance of a dermatologist. As melasma is a long lasting disorder, the induction treatment, usually given for 3–4 months, has to be associated with a maintenance therapy and a strict photoprotection in order to maintain the results and to reduce the relapses.

Local Treatment

The gold standard treatment for melasma is topical bleaching agents.

Hydroquinone

It prevents the dopa from converting into melanin through inhibiting tyrosinase activity and destroys melanocyte through inhibiting DNA and RNA synthesis. Commonly used concentration of the drug is 2–5%. As it gets easily oxidized in the air and in sunlight, it is better to apply the drug in the night and store it in an airtight container away from light. Also, patients should pay attention to the potential side effects of the drug like skin irritation, contact dermatitis, etc.

Tretinoin

It is believed that tretinoin is effective in preventing the enzymatic transformation through inhibiting tyrosinase mediated oxidation of dopa and thus it can hold up the synthesis of melanin. Tretinoin has also a positive effect by increasing the epidermal turn over, thus enhancing the elimination of the melanin contained in keratinocytes. The commonly used concentration is from 0.05% to 0.1%. The side effects of the drug include erythema, desquamation, and post-inflammatory pigmentation. The 0.1% tretinoin cream is commonly used.

Azelaic acid

It prevents melanocyte proliferation and has toxic effects on these cells. It inhibits the activity of the mitochondrial oxidation reduction enzyme and the synthesis of DNA and slightly inhibits tyrosinase *in vitro*. The commonly used concentration is 20%. Side effect is slight skin irritation.

Combination approaches

In order to improve curative effects and decrease adverse drug reaction, the above mentioned drugs can be used in combination. Kligman has recommended a triple combination (TC) for treatment of hyperpigmentation: hydroquinone/hydrocortisone/retinoic acid triad.[40] The use of tretinoin in combination with arbutin and ammonium glycyrrhizinate has been reported to be effective in treating melasma with fewer and less severe side effects than hydroquinone used alone or any other external application drug.

Evidence-based literature still focuses entirely on TC creams and its rational use is one of the most cost-effective interventions.[41] TC creams was now also associated with superficial peelings, in particular in darker skin individuals.[42] A TC of 4% hydroquinone, 0.05% Tretinoin and 0.1% mometasone furoate cream associated with glycolic acid peels was recently studied on 10 Indian patients with melasma.[43] The patients were instructed to apply medication all over the face at night, and physical sunscreen of SPF 19 was used in the morning. Serial glycolic acid peels were used at three weekly intervals. The results were noted after four peels. More than 50% improvement in pigmentation was noted in 5 out of 10 patients. Two patients showed more than 75% improvement. The remaining three patients showed between 20% and 49% of improvement. The triple cream appeared suitable for Indian skin, and the addition of glycolic acid peels enhances the overall improvement in melasma.

Whitening products

Patients can choose appropriate cosmetic products that have whitening effects as an adjunctive therapy for the treatment of melasma to improve the condition and the color of the skin. Cosmetic skin whitening agents with an efficacy comparable to hydroquinone but with a better safety profile have been developed. For example, a topical formulation with kojic acid, emblica extract and glycolic acid has been evaluated in a double blind study versus 4% hydroquinone.[44] Eighty participants from various ethnic origins based on Fitzpatrick skin classification (White, Hispanic, Asian, Middle Eastern and light to medium skin tone black individuals) were enrolled in this study. The results showed that the formulation

PIH. As for melasma, a combination of topical creams and gels, chemical peels, and photoprotection products, including the use of sunscreens, may be necessary for significant improvement. The use of broad-spectrum sunscreens may hasten the fading process and help prevent further hyperpigmentation secondary to sun exposure. Avoidance of exposure to UV light is an essential component of all treatment regimens for PIH, although in some cases, postinflammatory response could appear on sun protected area (i.e. *Tinea cruris*).

In particular, treatment of PIH in patients with Fitzpatrick skin types IV–VI is often difficult, and treatment-related irritation may actually exacerbate PIH. In this high-risk group of patients, prevention is an essential management strategy. Dermatologists should identify patients at higher risk for PIH, treat potential precipitating diseases swiftly and avoid unnecessary surgery and cosmetic procedures. These patients should also be advised to avoid and protect against sun exposure.

Therapeutic and cosmetics options are similar to melasma (see section III), the standard treatment for PIH being hydroquinone. Hydroquinone is the most commonly used therapy for PIH. It is used for the treatment of epidermal hyperpigmentation at concentrations of 2–4%. Prolonged treatment periods extending for 6–12 months may be required.

Combination products containing hydroquinone, retinoids and sunscreens appear to be the most beneficial treatment options, although there are few evidence-based studies for PIH.[74,75] For example, an encapsulated formulation of hydroquinone 4% plus retinol 0.15% entrapped in microsponge reservoirs was developed for the treatment of melasma and PIH.[76] Grimes saw improvements in subjects with moderate photodamage as early as 4 weeks. Treatments were generally well tolerated, with only minimal or mild burning, itching, or irritation, usually during the first 4 weeks. However, clearing of PIH was seen only in one patient in this series.

Postinflammatory Hypopigmentation

Postinflammatory hypopigmentation represents an acquired partial or total loss of cutaneous melanin. Its distribution (localized vs widespread) is related to the cause and extent of the inflammation. The same inflammatory cutaneous disorders that lead to hyperpigmentation in one individual can result in hypopigmentation in another. When there is severe inflammation of the skin, a loss rather than a dysfunction of melanocytes can be seen which results in achromia. The primary cutaneous disorders that can cause postinflammatory hypopigmentation are listed in Table 1.

Postinflammatory hypopigmentation usually appears as hypochromic more than achromic macules or patches, often asymptomatic and in the configuration and distribution of the inflammatory dermatosis. In the patients with a decrease, but not complete loss of pigment, it may be difficult to predict whether the hypopigmentation will persist or gradually disappear. For example, slightly hypochromic macules, such as those secondary to atopic dermatitis usually disappear in a few weeks whereas achromic macules left by scleroderma, lupus erythematosus or pinta may be permanent.

Because of the color contrast, postinflammatory hypopigmentation is more obvious in darkly of feathered margins, helps to distinguish postinflammatory hypomelanosis from other achromic dermatoses, such as vitiligo. In addition, Wood's lamp examination accentuates the hypopigmented lesions in fair-skinned individuals and helps the clinician determine whether there is achromia or hypochromia.

The next step in the evaluation of the patient is to attempt to establish the primary cutaneous disorder that is responsible. A good clinical history is followed by an observation of clinical features, such as distribution and size of lesions as well as associated secondary changes, e.g. scale.

The differential diagnosis includes hypopigmentation from previous therapies, in particular, the use of potent topical steroids.

The treatment of hypopigmentation remains a challenge. Undoubtedly, in the majority of cases, time is the most effective means of improvement. Slightly hypopigmented areas usually recover within a few weeks, whereas severely hypopigmented areas may take years to repigment. Sun exposure or exposure to UVA or UVB light in moderate amounts may help to restore pigmentation when the melanocytes within the affected area are still functional.

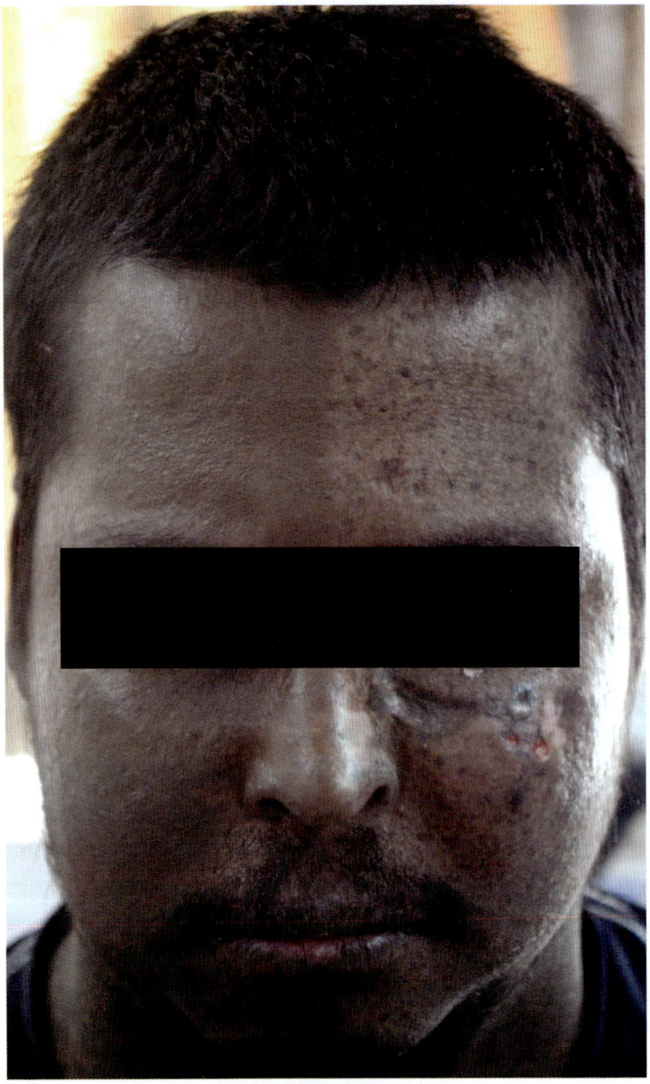

Figure 4: Cosmetic camouflage in a xeroderma pigmentosum patient with freckles, depigmentation, hyperpigmentation
Courtesy: Prof. Srinivas Chakravarthi

In order to avoid enhancing color contrast, care should be taken not to tan the normal surrounding skin. In this respect, the use of targeted phototherapy, such as excimer laser or lamp can be useful. In achromic lesions with a total loss of melanocytes, epidermal or melanocytic grafting is a therapeutic option.

Both postinflammatory hyper- and hypopigmention can be managed by use of camouflage (Fig. 4) which possibly has sunscreen properties as well. Carefully applied orange color is effective in masking hyperpigmented lesions.

REFERENCES

1. Bastiaens M, Hoefnagel J, Westendorp R, et al. Solar lentigines are strongly related to sun exposure in contrast to ephelides. Pigment Cell Res. 2004;17:225-9.
2. Monestier S, Gaudy C, Gouvernet J, et al. Multiple senile lentigos of the face, a skin ageing pattern resulting from a life excess of intermittent sun exposure in dark-skinned caucasians: a case-control study. Br J Dermatol. 2006;154:438-44.
3. Reguiaï Z, Jovenin N, Bernard P, et al. Melanoma, past severe sunburns and multiple solar lentigines of the upper back and shoulders. Dermatology. 2008;216:330.
4. Andersen WK, Labadie RR, Bhawan J. Histopathology of solar lentigines of the face: a quantitative study. J Am Acad Dermatol. 1997;36:444-7.
5. Nakajima A, Funasaka Y, Kawana S. Investigation by *in vivo* reflectance confocal microscopy: melanocytes at the edges of solar lentigines. Exp Dermatol. 2012;21:18-21.
6. Aoki H, Moro O, Tagami H, et al. Gene expression profiling analysis of solar lentigo in relation to immunohistochemical characteristics. Br J Dermatol. 2007;156:1214-23.
7. Kadono S, Manaka I, Kawashima M, et al. The role of the epidermal endothelin cascade in the hyperpigmentation mechanism of lentigo senilis. J Invest Dermatol. 2001;116:571-7.
8. Lin CB, Hu Y, Rossetti D, et al. Immuno-histochemical evaluation of solar lentigines: The association of KGF/KGFR and other factors with lesion development. J Dermatol Sci. 2010;59:91-7.
9. Unver N, Freyschmidt-Paul P, Hörster S, et al. Alterations in the epidermal-dermal melanin axis and factor XIIIa melanophages in senile lentigo and ageing skin. Br J Dermatol. 2006;155:119-28.
10. Kovacs D, Cardinali G, Aspite N, et al. Role of fibroblast-derived growth factors in regulating hyperpigmentation of solar lentigo. Br J Dermatol. 2010;163:1020-7.
11. Todd MM, Rallis TM, Gerwels JW, et al. A comparison of 3 lasers and liquid nitrogen in the treatment of solar lentigines: a randomized, controlled, comparative trial. Arch Dermatol. 2000;136:841-6.
12. Tanzi EL, Lupton JR, Alster TS. Lasers in dermatology: four decades of progress. J Am Acad Dermatol. 2003;49:1-31.
13. Polder KD, Harrison A, Eubanks LE, et al. 1,927-nm fractional thulium fiber laser for the treatment of nonfacial photodamage: a pilot study. Dermatol Surg. 2011;37:342-8.
14. Passeron T. Lasers. Ann Dermatol Venereol. 2012;139:S159-65.
15. Grimes PE. Melasma. Etiologic and therapeutic considerations. Arch Dermatol 1995;131:1453-7.
16. Vazquez M, Maldonado H, Benmaman C, et al. Melasma in men: a clinical and histologic study. Int J Dermatol. 1988;27:25-7.
17. Sarkar R, Jain RK, Puri P. Melasma in Indian males. Dermatol Surg. 2003;29:204.
18. Pichardo R, Vallejos Q, Feldman SR, et al. The prevalence of melasma and its association with quality of life in adult male Latino migrant workers. Int J Dermatol. 2009;48:22-6.
19. Ritter CG, Fiss DV, Borges da Costa JA, et al. Extra-facial melasma: clinical, histopathological, and immunohistochemical case-control study. J Eur Acad Dermatol Venereol. 2013;27(9):1088-94.
20. Sheth VM, Pandya AG. Melasma: a comprehensive update: part I. J Am Acad Dermatol. 2011;65:689-97
21. Malakar S, Dhar S. Pigmentary demarcation lines over the face. Dermatology. 2000;200:85-6.
22. Kang HY, Suzuki I, Lee DJ, et al. Transcriptional profiling shows altered expression of wnt pathway- and lipid metabolism-related genes as well as melanogenesis-related genes in melasma. J Invest Dermatol. 2011;131:1692-700.

23. Lee DJ, Park KC, Ortonne JP, et al. Pendulous melanocytes: a characteristic feature of melasma and how it occurred. Br J Dermatol. 2012;166:684-96.
24. Torres-Álvarez B, Mesa-Garza IG, Castanedo-Cázares JP, et al. Histochemical and immunohistochemical study in melasma: evidence of damage in the basal membrane. Am J Dermatopathol. 2011;33:291-5.
25. Choi JR, Won CH, Oh ES, et al. Does altered basement membrane of melasma lesion affect treatment outcome in Asian skin? Am J Dermatopathol. 2013;35:137-8.
26. Hernández-Barrera R, Torres-Alvarez B, Castanedo-Cazares JP, et al. Solar elastosis and presence of mast cells as key features in the pathogenesis of melasma. Clin Exp Dermatol. 2008;33:305-8.
27. Sarvjot V, Sharma S, Mishra S, et al. Melasma: a clinicopathological study of 43 cases. Ind J Pathol Microbiol. 2009;52:357-9.
28. Kang HY, Bahadoran P, Ortonne JP. Reflectance confocal microscopy for pigmentary disorders. Exp Dermatol. 2009;19:233-9.
29. Kang HY, Bahadoran P, Suzuki I, et al. *In vivo* reflectance confocal microscopy defects pigmentary changes in melasma at a cellular level resolution. Exp Dermatol. 2010;19:228-33.
30. Liu H, Nie W, Chen X, et al. Histological classification of melasma with reflectance confocal microscopy: a pilot study in Chinese patients. Skin Res Technol. 2011;17:398-403.
31. Ortonne JP, Arellano I, Berneburg M, et al. A global survey of the role of ultraviolet radiation and hormonal influences in the development of melasma. J Eur Acad Dermatol Venereol. 2009;23:1254-62.
32. Tamega A, Miot LD, Bonfietti C, et al. Clinical patterns and epidemiological characteristics of facial melasma in Brazilian women. J Eur Acad Dermatol. 2013;27:151-6.
33. Sarkar R, Puri P, Jain RK, et al. Melasma in men: a clinical, etiological and histological study. J Eur Acad Dermatol Venereol. 2010;24:768-72.
34. Jang YH, Sim JH, Kang HY, et al. The histopathological characteristics of male melasma: comparison with female melasma and lentigo. J Am Acad Dermatol. 2012;66:642-9.
35. Lee DJ, Lee J, Ha J, et al. Defective barrier function in melasma skin J Eur Acad Dermatol Venereol. 2012;26:1533-7.
36. Kang HY, Hwang JS, Lee JY, et al. The dermal stem cell factor and c-kit are overexpressed in melasma. Br J Dermatol. 2006;154:1094-9.
37. Kim JY, Lee TR, Lee AY. Reduced WIF-1 expression stimulates skin hyperpigmentation in patients with melasma. J Invest Dermatol. 2013;133:191-200.
38. Jo HY, Kim CK, Suh IB, et al .Co-localization of inducible nitric oxide synthase and phosphorylated Akt in the lesional skins of patients with melasma. J Dermatol. 2009;36:10-6.
39. Bak H, Lee HJ, Chang SE, et al. Increased expression of nerve growth factor receptor and neural endopeptidase in the lesional skin of melasma. Dermatol Surg. 2009;35:1244-50.
40. Kligman AM, Willis I. A new formula for depigmenting human skin. Arch Dermatol. 1975;111:40-8.
41. Hurley ME, Guevara IL, Gonzales RM, et al. Efficacy of glycolic acid peels in the treatment of melasma. Arch Dermatol. 2002;138:1578-82.
42. Sarkar R, Kaur C, Bhalla M, et al. The combination of glycolic acid peels with a topical regimen in the treatment of melasma in dark-skinned patients: a comparative study. Dermatol Surg. 2002;28: 828-32.
43. Godse KV, Sakhia J. Triple combination and glycolic acid peels in melasma in Indian patients. J Cosmet Dermatol. 2011;10:68-9.
44. Draelos ZD, Yatskayer M, Bhushan P, et al. Evaluation of a kojic acid, emblica extract, and glycolic acid formulation compared with hydroquinone 4% for skin lightening. Cutis. 2010;86:153-8.
45. Saraswat A, Lahiri K, Chatterjee M, et al. Topical corticosteroid abuse on the face: a prospective, multicenter study of dermatology outpatients. Indian J Dermatol Venereol Leprol. 2011;77:160-6.
46. Lakhdar H, Zouhair K, Khadir K, et al. Evaluation of the effectiveness of a broad-spectrum sunscreen in the prevention of chloasma in pregnant women. J Eur Acad Dermatol Venereol. 2007;21:738-42.
47. Cho HH, Choi M, Cho S, et al. Role of oral tranexamic acid in melasma patients treated with IPL and low fluence QS Nd:YAG laser. J Dermatolog Treat. 2013;24:292-6.
48. Wu S, Shi H, Wu H, et al. Treatment of melasma with oral administration of tranexamic acid. Aesthetic Plast Surg. 2012;36:964-70.
49. Tse TW, Hui E. Tranexamic acid: an important adjuvant in the treatment of melasma. Cosmet Dermatol. 2013;12:57-66.
50. Rokhsar CK, Fitzpatrick RE. The treatment of melasma with fractional photothermolysis: a pilot study. Dermatol Surg. 2005;31:1645-50.
51. Tannous ZS, Astner S. Utilizing fractional resurfacing in the treatment of therapy-resistant melasma. J Cosmet Laser Ther. 2005;7:39-43.
52. Lee HS, Won CH, Lee DH, et al. Treatment of melasma in Asian skin using a fractional 1,550-nm laser: an open clinical study. Dermatol Surg. 2009;35:1499-504.
53. Karsai S, Fischer T, Pohl L, et al. Is non-ablative 1550-nm fractional photothermolysis an effective modality to treat melasma? Results from a prospective controlled single-blinded trial in 51 patients. J Eur Acad Dermatol Venereol. 2012;26:470-6.
54. Sardana K, Chugh S, Garg VK. Which therapy works for melasma in pigmented skin: Lasers, peels, or triple combination creams? Indian J Dermatol Venereol Leprol. 2013;79:420-2.
55. Sardana K, Chugh S, Garg V. Are Q-switched lasers for Nevus of Ota really effective in pigmented skin? Indian J Dermatol Venereol Leprol. 2012;78:187-9.
56. Kar HK, Gupta L, Chauhan A. A comparative study on efficacy of high and low fluence Q-switched Nd: YAG laser and glycolic acid peel in melasma. Indian J Dermatol Venereol Leprol. 2012;78:165-71.
57. Ortonne JP, Passeron T. Melanin pigmentary disorders: treatment update. Dermatol Clin. 2005;23:209-26.
58. Wattanakrai, P, Mornchan R, Eimpunth S. Low-fluence Q-switched neodymium-doped yttrium aluminum garnet (1,064 nm) laser for the treatment of facial melasma in Asians. Dermatol Surg. 2010;36:76-87.
59. Li YH, Chen JZ, Wei HC, et al. Efficacy and safety of intense pulsed light in treatment of melasma in Chinese patients. Dermatol Surg. 2008;34:693-700.
60. Konishi N, Kawada A, Kawara S, et al. Clinical effectiveness of a novel intense pulsed light source on facial pigmentary lesions. Arch Dermatol Res. 2008;300:S65-7.
61. Chan HH, Kono T. The use of lasers and intense pulsed light sources for the treatment of pigmentary lesions. Skin Therapy Lett. 2004;9:5-7.
62. Chan H. The use of lasers and intense pulsed light sources for the treatment of acquired pigmentary lesions in Asians. J Cosmet Laser Ther. 2003;5:198-200.
63. Wang CC, Hui CY, Sue YM, et al. Intense pulsed light for the treatment of refractory melasma in Asian persons. Dermatol Surg. 2004;30:1196-200.
64. Moreno Arias GA, Ferrando J. Intense pulsed light for melanocytic lesions. Dermatol Surg. 2001;27:397-400.
65. Niwa Massaki AB, Eimpunth S, Fabi SG, et al. Treatment of melasma with the 1,927-nm fractional thulium fiber laser: a retrospective analysis of 20 cases with long-term follow-up. Lasers Surg Med. 2013;45:95-101.

66. Kang WH, Yoon KH, Lee ES, et al. Melasma: histopathological characteristics in 56 Korean patients. Br J Dermatol. 2002;146:228-37.
67. Passeron T, Fontas E, Kang HY, et al. Melasma treatment with pulsed-dye laser and triple combination cream: a prospective, randomized, single-blind, split-face study. Arch Dermatol. 2011;147:1106-8.
68. Lee HI, Lim YY, Kim BJ, et al. Clinicopathologic efficacy of copper bromide plus/yellow laser (578 nm with 511 nm) for treatment of melasma in Asian patients. Dermatol Surg. 2010;36:885-93.
69. Ruiz-Maldonado R, de la Luz Orozzo-Covarrubias M. Postinflammatory hypopigmentation an hyperpigmentation. Semi Cutaneous Med Surg. 1997;16:36-43.
70. Chua-Ty G, Goh CL, Koh SL. Pattern of skin diseases at the national skin centre (Singapore) from 1989–1990. Int J Dermatol. 1992;31:555-9.
71. Taylor SC, Cook-Bolden F, Rahman Z, et al. Acne vulgaris in skin of color. J Am Acad Dermato. 2002;46:S98-106.
72. Tomita Y, Maeda K, Tagami H. Melanocyte-stimulating properties of arachidonic acid metabolites: Possible role in postinflammatory pigmentation. Pig Cell Res. 1992;5:357-61.
73. Ortonne JP. Retinoic acid and pigment cells: A review of in *in-vitro* and in-vivo studies. Br J Dermatol. 1992;127:43-7.
74. Taylor S, Grimes P, Lim J, et al. Postinflammatory hyperpigmentation. J Cutan Med Surg. 2009;13:183-91.
75. Grimes PE. Management of hyperpigmentation in darker racial ethnic groups. Semin Cutan Med Surg. 2009;28:77-85.
76. Grimes PE. A microsponge formulation of hydroquinone 4% and retinol 0.15% in the treatment of melasma and postinflammatory hyperpigmentation. Cutis. 2004;74:362-8.

Chapter 7

Ultraviolet-induced Skin Damage and Its Prevention with Sunscreen

Françoise Bernerd, *L'Oréal Research and Innovation, Aulnay-sous-Bois, France*
Dominique Moyal, *L'Oréal Research and Innovation, Asnières, France*
Sathish B Pai, *Kasturba Medical College, Manipal University, Manipal, India*
Chakaravarthi Srinivas, *PSG Institute of Medical Sciences and Research, Coimbatore, India*

INTRODUCTION

Solar Ultraviolet Rays

The electromagnetic spectrum of sun radiation ranges from very short cosmic rays to very long radio waves and beyond (Fig. 1). Within this spectrum, ultraviolet (UV) rays account for 9%, of which three different ranges are commonly distinguished, i.e. UVC, B and A. UVC rays, the shortest in wavelength and the highest in photon associated energy, extend from 100 nm to 290 nm. However, no ray of wavelength below 290 nm reaches the earth's surface since blocked by the ozone layer. In contrast, UVB (290–320 nm) and UVA (320–400 nm) rays reach the earth's surface and are responsible for cutaneous photobiological events. UVA can be further subdivided into longer wavelengths, UVA1 (340–400 nm) and shorter wavelengths, UVA2 (320–340 nm). Most cutaneous changes induced by sunlight result from the impact of UV rays.

Solar UV irradiance also depends on geo-orbital and environmental parameters. With regard to the elliptical orbit of the earth around the sun, the distance between the sun and the earth varies by about 3.4% along the year. This results in a variation of approximately 7% in intensity and in slightly higher levels of UV rays in summer in the southern as compared to the northern hemisphere. Both quality (spectrum) and quantity (intensity) of terrestrial UV rays vary with sun elevation above the horizon, or solar altitude. The latter depends on the time of the day, day of year, and geographical location (latitude and

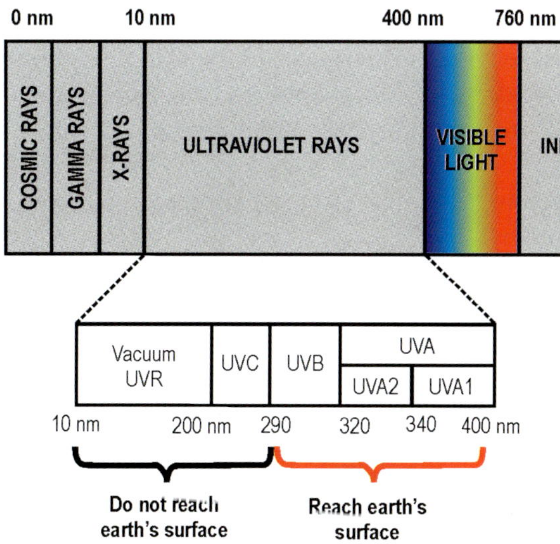

Figure 1: Electromagnetic spectrum of sun radiation

longitude). By a summer day, the UV energy received (daily dose) includes approximately 3.5% UVB and 96.5% UVA.[1] As shown by Jablonski et al.[2] the highest UVB intensities are found near the equator with important variations mostly due to latitude and the corresponding atmospheric scattering and absorption. Comparative levels of UVA are higher than those of UVB and are less influenced by latitude. The resulting exposure to both UVB and UVA over the year in India should, therefore, be considered among the highest in the world.

Balasaraswathy et al. showed that both UVA and UVB reached a peak between 11.30 am and 1.30 pm in Coimbatore, India.[3] In addition, UVB rays were much less intense than UVA's at the morning and evening. This study also showed that, in Coimbatore, compared to the average irradiance found between March and October, UVB intensity decreased in November, December, January and February by 24%, 40%, 19% and 12%, respectively, whereas UVA's diminished by 13%, 22%, 18% and 13%, respectively. This data clearly indicates that UVA irradiance is less affected by seasons, and decreases to a lesser extent than UVB in winter.

Environmental parameters can also influence UV exposure. They include the ozone total column and the ozone vertical atmospheric profile, clouds, pollutants, dusts, aerosols and albedo [reflection of ultraviolet radiation (UVR) from the ground].[4] Absorption by ozone, in addition to cutting off UVC rays, has a dramatic influ-ence on the amount of UVB rays reaching the ground.[5-10] Since aerosols and dusts are less concentrated at high altitudes, UV irradiance values are higher in mountains than at sea level. Finally, a highly reflecting environment, such as white sand, fresh snow or, to a lesser extent, white broken clouds acting as reflectors, can significantly increase UV irradiance.[11]

Division between UVB and UVA originally came from glass manufacturers defining B as the UV part blocked by glass and A that able to cross it. Hence, by definition the major part of UVA radiation is not absorbed by standard glass: car windows, verandas, conservatories, and windows in general fail to protect against UVA as they do from UVB rays. Thus, high UVA doses may be received while erythemal UVB is filtered out.

The contribution of diffuse UV rays is also important and should not be underestimated. Indeed, a recent study suggests that diffuse rays may explain a large part of the cumulative annual exposure dose.[12]

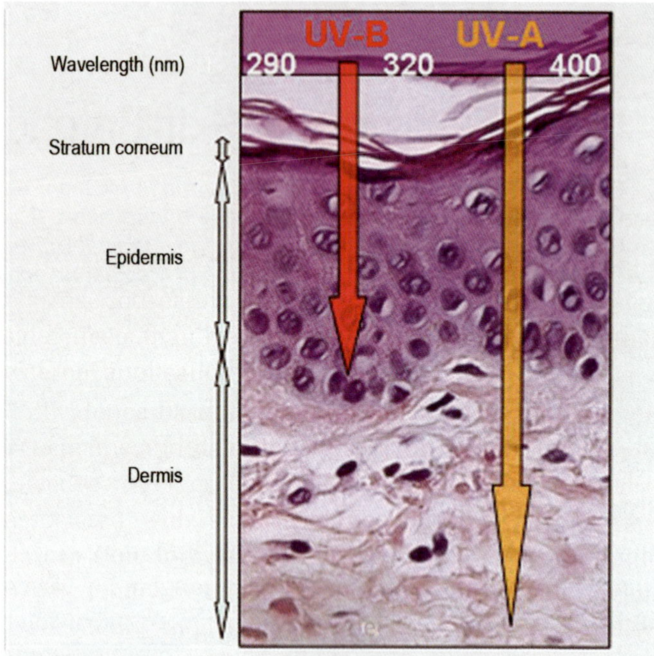

Figure 2: Depth of ultraviolet rays penetration into skin ©L'Oréal Research and Innovation

Ultraviolet Rays and Skin

Seventy percent of UVB rays reaching the skin are absorbed by the stratum corneum, 20% reach viable epidermis, and only 10% penetrate the upper part of the dermis. On the other hand, UVA rays are far more penetrating than UVB's. UVA rays are partly absorbed by epidermis and 20–30% of these can actually reach deep dermis (Fig. 2). In the skin, UV photons are absorbed by cell chromophores, most being nucleic acids, aromatic amino acids and melanin.

CLINICAL ASPECTS OF UV-INDUCED SKIN DAMAGE

Visible changes of sun exposed skin result its response to UV's according to normal or abnormal molecular absorption (Fig. 3).

Photodermatoses

Photodermatoses encompass a group of cutaneous disorders reflecting abnormal or overexpressed skin reaction in response to UV radiation. Despite a better resistance to sunburn reaction thanks to a higher

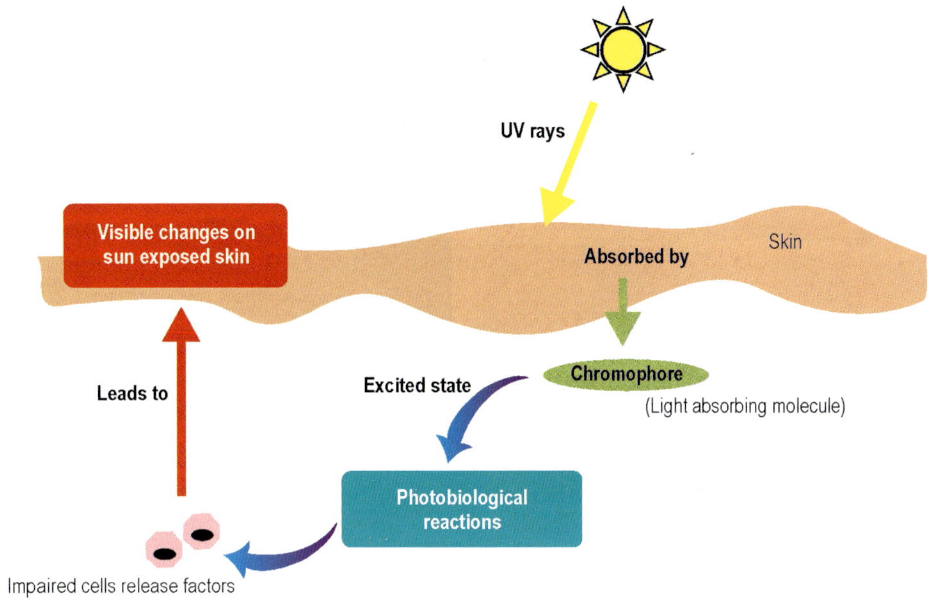

Figure 3: Diagrammatic representation of photobiological response of skin ©L'Oréal Research and Innovation

melanin content, photodermatoses remain common in dark-skinned people with some variations in their clinical spectrum.[13] The occurrence of photodermatoses is common in India owing to tropical weather, lack of knowledge regarding sun protection, and inadvertent intake of phototoxic drugs.[14]

Polymorphic light eruption, Parthenium dermatitis with photoaggravation, inadvertent use of photosensitizing drugs and nutritional deficiencies are major concerns in India.

Polymorphous Light Eruption

Polymorphous light eruption (PMLE) is the most common endogenous photodermatosis affecting men and women of all ages. It commonly occurs in fair-skinned individuals with Fitzpatrick skin types I–IV. In an Indian study conducted by Sharma and Basnet, 96% of patients were of skin types IV–VI, out of which 63% were females.[15]

Polymorphous light eruption generally occurs one or two days post exposure to sunlight depending on patient sensitivity and on exposure conditions.[16] The cutaneous lesions may take various forms: typically, they consist of erythematous papules (Fig. 4), lichen nitidus-like papules (small skin-colored pin-point grouped and discrete papules) (Fig. 5), plaques and vesicles. The lesions are often accompanied with pruritus and appear on the sun-exposed areas of the skin. These are mainly located on the V area of chest, extensors of forearms, sides of neck, upper back, lower abdomen and legs but, in the most severe cases, can extend further and often affect the face.

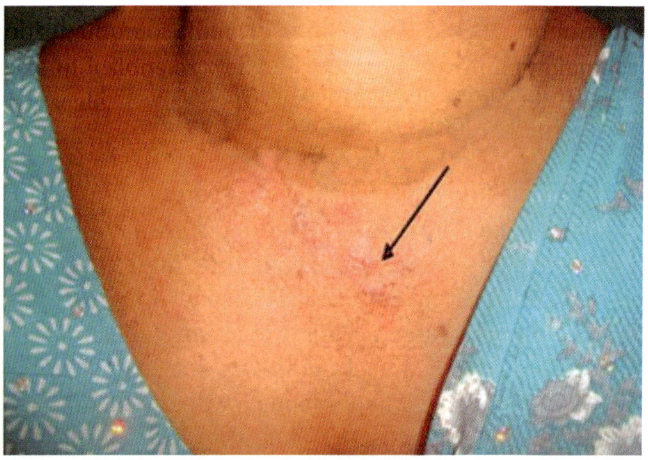

Figure 4: A 35-year-old lady with polymorphous light eruption (PMLE) showing erythematous papules over V area of neck
Courtesy: Dr Sathish Pai, Manipal, India

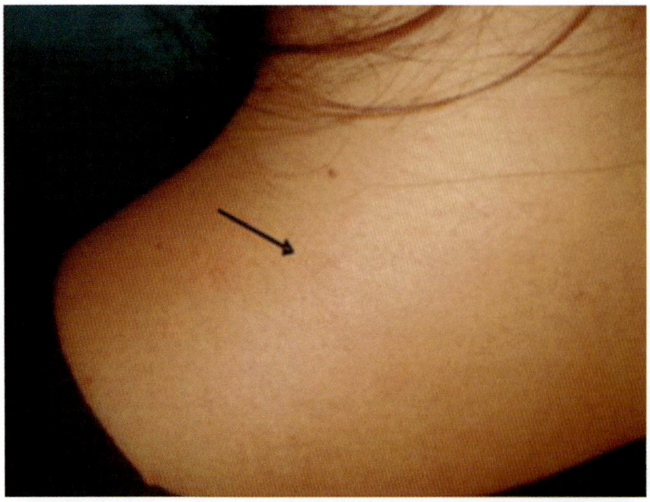

Figure 5: Polymorphous light eruption (PMLE) patient with lichen nitidus-like papules over upper back
Courtesy: Dr Sathish Pai, Manipal, India

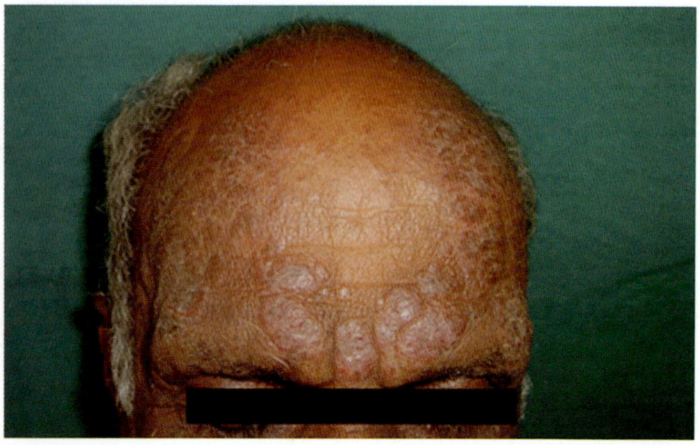

Figure 6: A 65-year-old man with chronic actinic dermatitis (CAD) showing lichenified papules and plaques over forehead
Courtesy: Dr Sathish Pai, Manipal, India

The face is normally spared in most adult patients due to hardening effect, a phenomenon where the sensitivity to light decreases with repeated sun-exposure.

The precise cause of PMLE is not known, despite evidence of immune nature. The action spectrum, however, remains unclear. The solar wavelengths involved in triggering PMLE may include the entire UV spectrum, but it is commonly viewed that PMLE is mainly caused by UVA rays.[17]

The treatment consists of avoidance of sun exposure, use of protective clothing and regular application of sunscreens with high sun-protecting factors against UVB's and UVA's. Since UVA rays are present throughout the day, UV protection should be brought all day long. Rash and itching can be controlled with topical steroids.

Chronic Actinic Dermatitis

Chronic actinic dermatitis (CAD) is a common eczematous photodermatosis due to delayed type hypersensitivity (DTH) reaction against an endogenous, cutaneous, photo-induced allergen, leading to a comparable clinical picture as allergic contact dermatitis. It is characterized by pruritic papules and plaques with lichenification (Fig. 6). Commonly involved sites are the face, V area of the neck, neck (nape and sides), dorsum of the hands and bald areas of the scalp. Areas, such as the upper eyelids, skin creases, sub-chin area and retroauricular regions are usually spared. CAD most frequently affects elderly, of an unusual occurrence below 50 years. In India, patients with CAD exhibit contact sensitivity to *Parthenium hysterophorus*. The action spectrum includes UVB, UVA and rarely visible wavelengths. Treatment consists of strict photoprotection, avoidance of contact allergens, if any, topical steroids, calcineurin inhibitors and systemic immunosuppressive agents.

Solar Urticaria

Solar urticaria is an uncommon condition in which sun exposure leads to urticaria. This is a rare immunoglobulin E (IgE) mediated photodermatosis characterized by transient cutaneous eruption of wheals evoked by exposure to UVR or visible light. Patients present a sensation of tingling over the exposed areas within 5–10 minutes post sun exposure, shortly followed by erythema and wheals. Prophylactic measures are important with appropriate clothing and sunscreen use.

Drug-induced Photodermatoses: Phototoxic and Photoallergic Reaction

In India, drug reactions have become very common. The lack of advice regarding avoidance of sunlight and inappropriate dosing can lead to various drug-induced phototoxic reactions.

A phototoxic reaction is a direct nonimmunologic damage to the skin resulting from a drug or chemical interacting with UV or visible light. The common drugs causing phototoxic reaction are antimicrobials-

Table 1: Comparison of phototoxic and photoallergic reactions[13]		
Feature	*Phototoxic Reaction*	*Photoallergic Reaction*
Incidence	High	Low
Amount of agent required	Large	Small
Onset of reaction	Minutes to hours	24–72 hours
Distribution	Sun-exposed skin only	Sun-exposed skin; may spread to unexposed areas
More than one exposure to agent required	No	Yes
Clinical characteristics	Resembles exaggerated sunburn or blisters	Dermatitis
Immunologically mediated	No	Yes; Type IV

quinolones, tetracyclines, sulfonamides, nonsteroidal anti-inflammatory drugs, retinoids, furocoumarins.

A photoallergic reaction results from an immune response to a product generated by the interaction of the drug/chemical and sun radiation, called photoproduct (Table 1).

Both types of reactions induce clinical lesions confined in the light exposed part of the body. Prophylactic measures are essential minimizing exposure and avoiding the suspected chemical/drug.

Short-term Effects of UV Rays: Erythema and Pigmentation

In this section, we discuss the erythemal and tanning effects of UVA and UVB rays as they are observed visually and measured using instruments recording colorimetric parameters (CIE 1976 L*a*b* color space).[18] L* denotes the lightness (or Luminance) of the skin, ranging from 0 (black) to 100 (white), a* the red component and b* the yellow/blue component of the skin.

Erythema

Erythema is the major and most familiar clinical sign of a sunburn reaction associated with UVR overexposure. It is an acute skin inflammatory reaction associated with redness that results from excessive exposure to UV rays. Erythema is readily visible and can be easily measured using noninvasive methods. Its development can be monitored over time. It is used as an endpoint for many photobiological studies.

The erythemal reaction induced by UV rays depends upon the wavelength range. The ability to induce erythema considerably declines with increasing wavelength. UVB, particularly at 307 nm, is the most effective waveband for eliciting erythema in human skin. UVA rays are 1000-fold less potent in triggering skin erythema. Figure 7 shows the relative action spectrum of erythema at 24 hours post exposure, according to the CIE-1987 standard.[19]

Although the final reaction is an increase in redness of the skin, the time course and the dose response of erythema to UVB and UVA wavebands are different. UVB-induced erythema is a delayed response reaching a peak at 6–24 hours accompanied by pruritus and pain.[20] This erythema fades over a day or longer according to UV dose and skin type.[21] In skin type I, it may last longer compared to skin type III or IV.[22] UVA-induced erythema

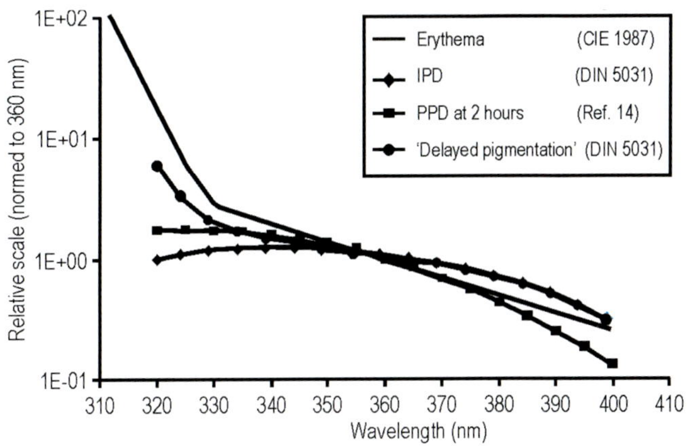

Figure 7: UV-exposed skin, the effects of a variety of clinical response spectra: erythema, IPD, PPD and delayed pigmentation (new pigment formation)
©L'Oréal Research and Innovation
Abbreviations: IPD, immediate pigment darkening; PPD, persistent pigment darkening.

contributes to at about 15% of the total sun-induced erythema.[23] Actinic UVA erythema fades partly within 2 hours. However, when skin type I is exposed to high UVA dose, persistent erythema is observed from 2 hours to 24 hours post exposure. Immediate and persistent UVA erythema is easily inducible with relatively low UVA dose (10–30 J/cm^2) on very fair skin (skin type I). Conversely, high UVA doses (>30 J/cm^2) are necessary to induce erythema on darker skin (skin types III and IV). In this case, UVA erythemal response is mixed with persistent pigment darkening (PPD).[24,25] The time course of UVA-induced erythema is similar to that of PPD reaction.[26] For both reactions the presence of oxygen is required whereas UVB-induced erythema is oxygen independent[25] suggesting that UVA- and UVB-induced erythema involve different chromophores.

The minimal erythema dose (MED) is defined as the lowest dose inducing minimally perceptible or detectable erythema on the UV-exposed site 24 hours post exposure. This biological value obviously varies from one subject to another depending on skin phototype as well as skin color typing and body area. Constitutional pigmentation is well described in the L* vs b* colorimetric plane.[27] MED increases with higher skin type.[28] Since most Indians have Fitzpatrick skin phototypes III–V,[29] they obviously have a higher MED than Caucasian skins. Similarly, people involved in outdoor occupations have a higher MED as compared to people with indoor occupations.

Later changes include hyperkeratosis (increased scaling), acanthosis (epidermal thickening), disorganization and misalignment of keratinocytes, dermal vascular ectasia, and mononuclear perivascular infiltration.

Pigmentation

Skin pigmenting response following exposure to sunlight involves an immediate tanning reaction and delayed production of new melanins. The tanning response of human skin depends on UVR wavelength.

UVA-induced changes in color begin with an immediate darkening of the skin due to photo-oxidation of preexisting melanin; the immediate pigment darkening (IPD).[23] In skin types III and IV, this pigmentation may appear within a short single exposure to UVA (dose less than 6 J/cm^2).[30] This phenomenon is transient and fades within 2 hours post exposure. Following exposure to UVA doses above about 10 J/cm^2, a stable residual pigmentation is observed after the transient part of IPD has faded out. This pigmentation called persistent pigment darkening (PPD) remains detectable for a few days or weeks, depending on the UVA dose received, particularly in skin with phototypes III or IV.[30] The UVA dose required to induce a minimal PPD is 10–15 J/cm^2 and represents a little bit less than the amount received during 1 hour exposure to quasi-zenithal sun. Figure 7 shows the relative action spectra of IPD[31] as observed immediately following exposure and PPD as observed 2 hours post exposure.[30]

Neomelanization or delayed pigmentation is characterized by a visible brown pigmentation in UV-exposed skin reflecting an increase in epidermal melanin content due to stimulation of melanogenesis. Delayed tanning becomes visible within 3 days post exposure. An acute erythemal dose of UVB or multiple suberythemal UVB doses are necessary to induce delayed pigmentation. No pigmentation develops following UVB exposure without a preceding inflammation response. Both UVA and UVB can cause delayed tanning, but UVA is less effective. Whereas the time courses of UVA and UVB erythema markedly differ from each other, the time courses of UVA and UVB delayed tanning, though induced with far different doses of UV energy, are similar. The action spectrum of delayed tanning at 7 days post exposure is broadly similar to that of erythema (Fig. 7).[31] However, melanization produced by cumulative UVA exposures appears to be much longer lasting (several months or even a year) than that acquired with UVB exposures. Reason accounting for such difference is not fully understood but has been suggested to be related to the more basal location of UVA-induced pigment. UVB-induced melanization disappears within one month with the course of epidermal turnover.[32]

In some cases, UV-pigmentation can lead to irregular pigmentation and hyperpigmented areas. In particular melasma, postinflammatory pigmentation and actinic lentigines are associated with exposure to UV rays.[33]

Long-term Effects: Photoaging and Photocarcinogenesis

Photoaging

Chronic insults to the skin by UV rays result in a phototrauma called photoaging or dermatoheliosis. This is of importance with regard to our perception of the age of an individual, most often based on examination of unprotected body sites, face and hands. Photoaged skin is characterized by numerous clinical signs, fine and coarse wrinkling, laxity, leathery appearance, mottled pigmentation reflected by lentigines, fragility, impaired wound healing and telangiectasia. Figure 8 clearly illustrate this impact of chronic sun-exposure upon Indian skin.

Generally, photoaging is associated with changes in skin microrelief and loss of elastic properties. Histologic and ultrastructural studies have revealed that the major alterations in photoaged skin are found in the connective tissue (dermis).[34-36]

The respective role of UVB and UVA wavelengths in the process of photoaging is not fully understood. However, animal models chronically exposed to UV have brought out that exposure to both UVB or UVA for several weeks resulted in wrinkle formation and solar elastosis.[37] In humans, repeated exposures to suberythemal doses of UVA induced alterations within the dermal compartment which were correlated with early damage occurring during photoaging.[38] Gordon et al. showed a case of unilateral dermatoheliosis in a 69-year-old man who had driven a delivery truck for 28 years, strongly suggesting the role of UVA in generating skin alterations related to photoaging[39] since only UVA rays can cross the window glass.

Skin sensitivity to photoaging alterations, such as dermal damage, solar elastosis, and wrinkling also depends on constitutive pigmentation, the lighter skins being more prone to. It has also been suggested that in Asians the major early symptoms of skin photoaging are pigmentary changes, such as solar lentigo, rather than wrinkling.

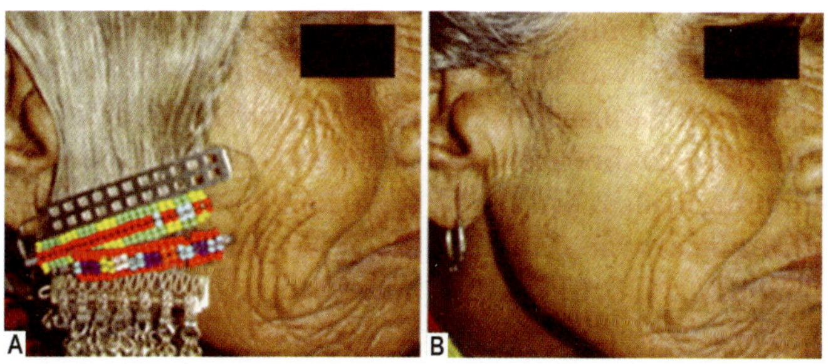

Figures 8: A 70-year-old Indian woman. **A**, Sun-exposed skin. **B**, Sun-protected skin
Courtesy: Dr Arun Inamadar, Bijapur, Karnataka, India

However, a Korean study showed that in the Korean population, wrinkling was a major feature of photoaging together with dyspigmentation and that a statistically significant association was found between both clinical signs and their severity.[40] Durai et al.[41] conducted a study in Puducherry, India, on 500 consecutive elderly individuals attending their Dermatology out-patient department, to evaluate the severity of photoaging in this population (skin types IV and V). Photoaging changes were less common than chronological aging changes in the studied population though prolonged sun exposure was shown a risk factor for photoaging. This study confirmed that, in India, the most important cutaneous changes suggestive of photoaging was dyspigmentation. Interestingly, it also showed that chronological changes were more frequent in females than males, while photoaging was more frequent in males, likely due to occupational exposure to sun.

Photocarcinogenesis

There is strong evidence supporting the direct role of sunlight exposure in the development of skin cancers, especially nonmelanoma skin cancers (NMSC), i.e. squamous cell carcinoma (SCC) and basal cell carcinoma (BCC).[42] These cancers more frequently occur on the head, neck, arms and hands, i.e. the skin areas most frequently exposed to UV. In these body sites, actinic keratoses (AK), which are precancerous lesions are also frequent. About 5–20% of these lesions progress toward SCC. Lightly pigmented individuals (skin type I or II) are more prone to NMSC than those with deeply pigmented skin.[43] Unlike NMSC, the direct association with UV exposure is still under investigation for cutaneous malignant melanoma. It seems that severe sunburn episodes during childhood may have a causal effect in the development of melanoma on sun-exposed areas. A recent Australian study tends to prove that melanoma may be preventable by a regular sunscreen use in adults.[44]

Conventional wisdom is that the incidence of all varieties of skin cancers is lower among Indians due to the protective effects of melanin. Indeed, in most people with type IV or V skin, the incidence of basal cell cancer, squamous cell cancer, and malignant melanoma is very low as compared to patients with lighter skin.[45] BCC is the most common skin cancer worldwide, but various studies from India have reported SCC as the most prevalent skin malignancy.[46,47]

An Indian review showed that there are indirect indications that NMSCs may be on the rise in India.[48]

BIOLOGICAL ASPECTS OF UV-INDUCED SKIN DAMAGE

As discussed above, acute and repeated sun exposure trigger short- and long-term deleterious clinical effects. Tremendous progress has been made in identifying the underlying molecular and cellular events and the respective role of UVB and UVA rays (Table 2).

Molecular Effects

The major chromophores absorbing UVB wavelengths are nucleic acids, and especially cellular DNA. The latter is a very important target since its alterations can impact the whole genome integrity and may affect many cellular functions as well. Predominant lesions resulting from UVB photon absorption occur at pyrimidine bases which become covalently linked and distort the DNA helix. The most frequent UV-induced DNA lesions are cyclobutane-pyrimidine dimers (CPDs) and pyrimidine 6-4 pyrimidone photo-products (6-4 PP) (Fig. 9).

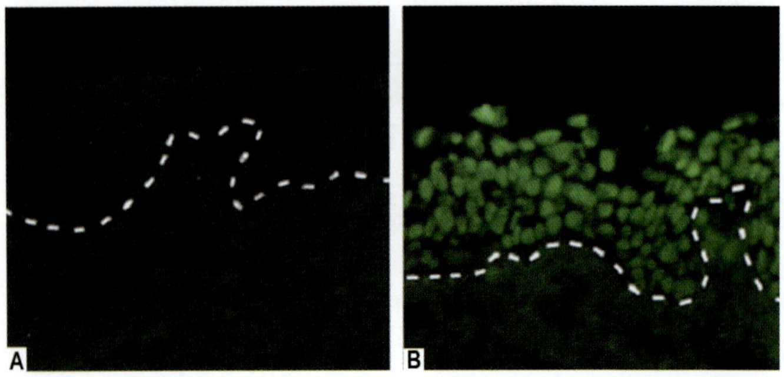

Figure 9: DNA lesions, cyclobutane-pyrimidine dimers (CPDs), immediately produced following UVB exposure of normal human skin. **A,** Non-exposed skin. **B,** UVB-exposed skin ©L'Oréal Research and Innovation

Both DNA lesions are mutagenic and need being repaired to maintain genomic integrity and avoid mutagenesis. The specific repair mechanism of these lesions is called nucleotide excision repair (NER),[49] which proceeds through successive enzymatic steps: recognition of the DNA distortion; DNA unwinding around lesion; stabilization of the multiproteic complex; incision of the lesion; and replicative gap filling. The dramatic consequences of defective repair of UV-induced DNA lesions are demonstrated in patients affected by the genetic disease xeroderma pigmentosum (XP), characterized by mutations in genes involved in NER process, resulting in a high predisposition to develop epidermal skin tumors during childhood, in sun-exposed body sites.[50]

Experimental data show a relationship between the minimal UV dose inducing DNA lesions and skin color/ethnic origin, i.e. lower in light skin and higher in

Table 2: Major biological effects of ultraviolet (UV) light on skin and their clinical consequences

	Mediators	*Short-term Effects*	*Long-term Effects*
DNA damage	Pyrimidine dimers Pyrimidine-pyrimidone Cell death/apoptosis	Sunburn reaction Pigmentation	Cancer Immunosuppression
Free radical generation	ROS	IPD	Cancer Immunosuppression Photoaging
Immunosuppression	LC depletion Cytokines (TNF-α IL-1, IL-10) Urocanic acid isomerization	Susceptibility to infection	Chronic inflammatory diseases Cancer
Inflammation	Inflammation's mediators Cytokines Neuropeptides	Sunburn, erythema, pain, itching	Photoaging Cancer
Alterations of dermal structure	Metalloproteinases Proteases		Photoaging

Abbreviations: ROS, reactive oxygen species; IPD, immediate pigment darkening; LC, Langerhans cells; TNF, tumor necrosis factor; IL, interleukin dark skin.[51] Although the action spectra for CPDs and 6-4 PPs formation peak within the UVB range,[52] recent studies seem to indicate that UVA wavelengths may also be responsible for such DNA lesions.[53] However, the mechanisms underlying their formation are not fully understood. A recent paper clearly demonstrated the ability of long wave UVA's to induce CPDs in human skin.[54] It also emphasized that the latter were preferably localized within the basal layer of the epidermis, including epidermal stem cells as well as the proliferative pool of keratinocytes. This strongly suggests the potential role of long UVA in photocarcinogenesis.

Yet the major DNA damage induced by UVA rays is indirect and results from the generation of reactive oxygen species (ROS). The most abundant UVA-induced DNA lesion is 8-hydroxy-2' deoxyguanine (8-OhdG), also mutagenic if not repaired.[55]

As a consequence of these multiple mechanisms, exposure to full UV spectrum induces a wide range of DNA lesions especially within the epidermal keratinocytes.[56]

Apart from the link between DNA lesions and photocarcinogenesis, it has also been shown that thymidine dinucleotides (pTpT) are involved in the stimulation of melanogenesis and thus participate in the tanning response.[57]

Cellular Effects

Consequences of DNA Damage

One outcome of DNA damage in the cell is the stabilization and accumulation of p53 protein, the product of *p53* tumor suppressor gene (Fig. 10).

P53 plays a major role in protecting genome integrity of the cell, through cell cycle regulation and arrest in G1 phase[58] allowing the cell to repair DNA lesions. However, p53 protein is also involved in apoptosis induction whereby the cell is compelled to enter a process eventually leading to cell death when it is overly damaged resulting in too high risk for impaired DNA to be inadequately repaired. The apoptotic keratinocytes usually observed after an acute UV exposure are called sunburn cells (SBC). These could be clearly detected at 24 hours post exposure and show a specific morphological appearance on histological section, with an eosinophylic cytoplasm, a condensed picnotic nucleus, a round shape and a suprabasal location (Fig. 10).[59] Mutations in the

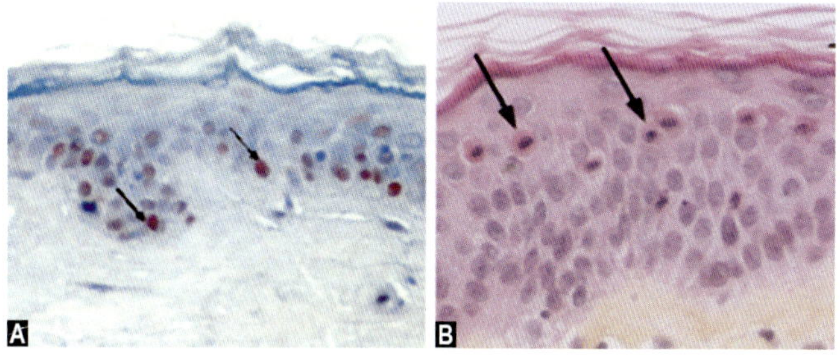

Figure 10: Biological markers associated with sunburn reaction in normal human skin. **A,** p53 (24 h). **B,** Sunburn cells (24 h) ©L'Oréal Research and Innovation

p53 gene leading to its dysfunction facilitate tumor development and more than 50% of skin carcinomas are associated with mutations in *p53* gene.[60] The assessment of p53 mutations *in vivo* and in human skin model *in vitro* revealed that both UVB and UVA wavelength domains could be responsible for p53 mutations, even after few exposures to low doses.[61]

Other cellular events have been linked to UV-induced DNA damage including regulation of gene expression, such as the proto-oncogenes *c-fos* and *c-jun*.

More recently, p53 protein has also been shown to trigger melanogenesis, demonstrating a role in the control of UV-induced pigmentation.[62]

Extracellular Matrix Proteins

Many extracellular matrix proteins as well as matrix proteases have been shown to be involved in UV-induced skin response. Through connective dermal tissue remodeling, they participate in photoaging-related alterations, such as solar elastosis, but also to tumor development by creating a permissive matrix environment.

From a histological point of view, photoaged skin is mostly characterized by a disorganization of the dermal structure.[63] As a result of linearization of the dermal epidermal junction, dermal papillae decrease. In photoaged skin, this superficial dermal area is called the Grenz zone. Underneath the Grenz zone, the structure and organization of the dermis are completely modified with the appearance of so-called solar elastosis pattern. It consists of aggregates of elastotic material, made up of abnormal elastic fibers (Fig. 11), and other extracellular matrix proteins, such as fibronectin which replaces the

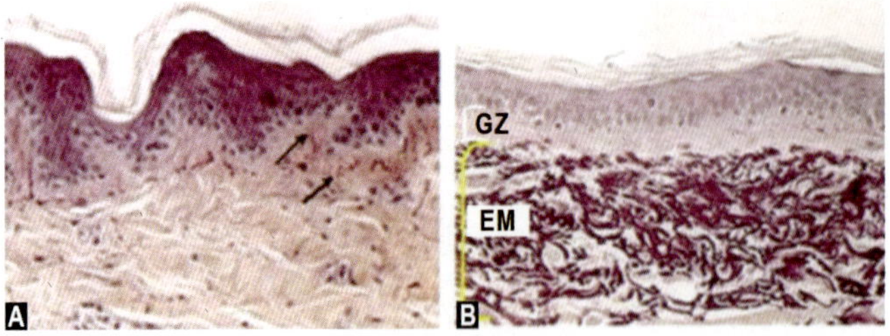

Figure 11: Photoaging of the superficial dermal area. **A,** Young skin 25 years. **B,** Photoaged skin 76 years
©L'Oreal Research and Innovation
Abbreviations: GZ, Grenz zone; EM, elastotic material.

normal matrix essentially composed of collagen.[64] The accumulation of elastotic material depends upon the extent of sun exposure.

Elastic tissue: From a structural point of view, elastic fibers in photoaged skin are degenerated with a swollen appearance. Elastin gene has been shown induced at the transcriptional level by both UVB and UVA exposures resulting in an increase in mRNA levels in dermal fibroblasts of photoaged skin.[65] The microfibrils associated with elastic fibers are composed of fibrillin 1, which has been shown to be downregulated in photoaging.[66] Lysozyme, which is involved in elastolysis process, shows a higher staining in photoaged dermis with deposits on elastotic material. Lysozyme deposition is also increased in human skin after repeated UV exposures. This increase may be related to abnormal turnover and accumulation of elastic tissue in solar elastosis.[67]

Collagens: The staining for collagen in photoaged skin shows sparse labeling compared to dense appearance in normal skin, revealing a decrease in the total amount of collagen content.[64,68] Precursors for type I and type III collagens (procollagens) are reduced in photoaged skin.[69] This decrease seems to be related to the degree of severity of clinical signs. The whole process of collagen I synthesis is altered in photoaged skin resulting in lower levels of mRNA and proteins.[70] Experimental UV exposures induced a dose-dependent reduction of type I procollagen protein.[71] This downregulation is also observed after exposure to UVA only. Type III collagen, another major collagen of the dermal connective tissue, also decreases with photoaging and following UV exposure.[71] Photoaged skin also shows a decrease in Type VII collagen, the major component of anchoring fibrils, responsible for cohesion between the basement epidermal membrane and the underlying dermal structure.[72]

Glycosaminoglycans and proteoglycans: The content of glycosaminoglycans and proteoglycans (PGs) is altered in sun-exposed dermis. Versican, a large chondroitin sulfate PG associated with elastic fibers was shown increased in photoaged skin.[73] The level of versican mRNA is also increased in cultures of dermal fibroblasts from photoaged skin. In contrast another PG decorin, associated with collagen fibers is found decreased.[73]

Matrix-metalloproteinases: Many studies have shown that matrix-metalloproteinases (MMPs), proteases responsible for breakage and degradation of extracellular matrix components, are among the major biological markers of skin response to UV exposure and are key regulators of collagen reduction and disorganization of dermal structure during photoaging.[74] MMP-1 or interstitial collagenase is able to cleave type I collagen fibers and is upregulated by both UVB and UVA.[75-77] The level of MMP-1 mRNA and the amount of MMP-1 protein within the dermis of photoaged skin is increased.[70]

The increase in MMP-1 following UV exposure was studied in reconstructed skin model to better understand the role of keratinocyte and fibroblast in MMP-1 induction.[78] Under UVA exposure, MMP-1 production was directly induced in dermal fibroblasts. Removal of epidermis immediately after UVA exposure did not alter this induction. These results confirmed other data on UVA-induced MMP-1 in cultured fibroblasts.[76,79] In contrast, UVB-induced MMP-1 production required the presence of epidermis. The use of both monolayered cultured keratinocytes and fibroblasts, as well as reconstructed skin demonstrated that UVB-induced MMP-1 resulted from a paracrine mechanism involving the release of epidermal soluble factors, such as cytokines IL-1 α and IL-6.[78]

The expression of gelatinase, MMP2 and MMP9 is also induced by UV exposure.[80] Altogether, these results have suggested a theory for solar elastosis development, based on cumulative damage induced by repeated exposure to low doses of sunlight and imperfect repair leading to "dermal solar scars".[81]

Immune System

Ultraviolet exposure of the human skin induces local and systemic immunosuppression. Various studies have shown that both UVA and UVB are immunosuppressive.[82,83] The action spectrum for immunosuppression has been recently published.[84]

The pathways leading to downregulation are complex, starting from the absorption of UV photons by chromophores in the skin and ending with local and systemic changes in immune mediators, the generation of T and B regulatory cells and inhibition of effectors and memory T cell activation.[85] The process is thought to involve Langerhans cells, the epidermal dendritic cells that play a crucial role in antigen presentation.[86] The role of several cytokines induced by UV exposure, such as TNF-alpha, IL-1 and IL-10 has also been demonstrated to be related to immunosuppression.[87] It has been recently reported that UVB rays could induce apoptosis of T lymphocytes in the inflammatory skin; therefore, narrow band and broad band UVB rays have been widely used for the clinical treatment of many immune-related skin diseases.

Oxidative Stress

As previously mentioned, the major molecular effects of UVA wavelengths result from induced oxidative stress leading to the production of ROS.[88] However, UVB wavelengths could also be responsible for oxidative stress. Photo-oxidative damage has been implicated in several biological deleterious consequences of sun exposure, especially in photoaging but also photocarcinogenesis. ROS production following exposure to UVA or UVB entails absorption of photons by endogenous photosensitizers. Among them, trans-urocanic acid has been shown being directly connected with photoaging.[89] Both UVB and UVA are responsible for lipid peroxidation associated with alterations of cellular membranes.[90,91] In these phenomena, iron which is immediately released following UVA exposure plays a central role. Activation of heme oxygenase (HO-1) gene expression is the major stress response observed in fibroblasts following UVA exposure.[92] This has been closely related to increased levels of cellular ferritin.[93] Dermal fibroblasts seemed to be more sensitive to oxidative stress than epidermal keratinocytes.[94] A recent study investigated the impact of oxidative stress induced by daily UV exposure in a reconstructed skin model.[95] Gene expression of 24 markers involved in oxidative cell response was assessed in fibroblasts and keratinocytes in parallel. The results confirmed a high sensitivity of dermal fibroblasts to oxidative stress.

Protein oxidation has been identified as another deleterious consequence of UV-induced oxidative stress related to photoaging process.[96] The same team also identified the related repair enzyme.[97]

Oxidative stress induced by UVA may also be responsible for mutations in mitochondrial DNA.[98] These mutations, namely the "common deletion" have also been found in the fibroblasts of photoaged skin. They lead to a reduced mitochondrial functionality and a decrease in cellular energy, a classical feature of general aging process.

Finally, ROS production by UV rays is responsible for the activation of several signal transduction pathways leading to MMPs induction and various alterations of extracellular matrix.[99]

Other cell actors involved in the global cellular response to UV are cytokines or growth factors. They often participate to the cascade of signaling, leading to activation of other markers, such as those related to extracellular matrix. For example, it was shown that interleukin-6 participated in the induction of MMP-1.[78,79]

PREVENTION OF ULTRAVIOLET-INDUCED DAMAGE BY SUNSCREENS

Development of Sunscreens

As a result of increased knowledge about UV-induced skin damage and especially UVA effects, public education programs have been developed, including the use of proper sunscreen products.

With advanced technology, many new UV filters have been made available in the last two decades and particularly new UVA filters with improved efficacy and safety.

An appropriate sunscreen product should provide effective protection against both UVB and UVA rays, must be stable to heat and to UVR (photostable), and should be cost-effective and user-friendly to encourage frequent applications and provide reliable protection. To protect against both UVB and UVA, it must contain a combination of filters (either organic or inorganic) within a complex vehicle matrix. Sunscreens can act either by absorption, or reflection or diffusion of UV rays.[100,101]

Table 3: Main UVB and UVA filters with their maximum wavelength

Name	*Maximum Wavelength Absorbed*
UVB filters:	305 nm
Homosalate	307 nm
Phenyl benzimidazole sulfonic acid	
Ensulizole	302 nm
Octocrylene	310 nm
Ethylhexyl methoxycinnamate	
Octinoxate	306 nm
Ethylhexyl salicylate	
Octisalate	
UVA filters:	355 nm
Butyl methoxydibenzoylmethane (Avobenzone)	345 nm
Terephthalylidene dicamphor sulfonic acid (Mexoryl® SX)	
UVB/UVA filters:	287 nm
Benzophenone -3	
Oxybenzone	303 nm, 344 nm
Drometrizole trisiloxane (Mexoryl® XL)	
Methylene bis-benzotriazolyl	305 nm, 360 nm
tetramethylbutylphenol (Tinosorb® M)	310 nm, 343 nm
Bis-ethylhexyloxyphenol	
methoxyphenyl triazine	290 ~ 300 nm
(Tinosorb® S)	
Titanium dioxide	360 ~ 370 nm
Zinc oxide	

Table 3 summarizes the main existing UVB and UVA filters.

Butyl-methoxydibenzoylmethane (BMDM or Avobenzone), with an absorption peak at 355 nm, is the most common long UVA filter. However, it is photo-unstable, i.e. losing its protective potency when exposed to UVR. It is possible to photostabilize Avobenzone by combining it with Octocrylene, a UVB filter or some other ingredients. The most common UVB filter, octyl methoxy cinnamate is also photo-unstable. It is therefore of prime importance to take into account the issue of photo-unstability when assessing the protection factors.

Terephthalylidene dicamphor sulfonic acid (TDSA) or Mexoryl® SX, a broad photostable UVA filter is approved in Europe, Australia and Asia. Three NDA for formulations containing Mexoryl® SX were approved by the FDA in the USA, in 2006. Numerous studies have shown the high efficiency of this filter in preventing DNA damage,[102] photoaging,[103] UV-induced pigmentation,[104] UV-induced immunosuppression[105] and photodermatoses, such as PMLE[106] and solar urticaria.[107]

Drometrizole trisiloxane (DTS) or Mexoryl® XL is the first photostable broad UV filter that affords high protection against both UVA and UVB, introduced on the European market rope in 1998. Mexoryl® XL has two absorption peaks, one in the UVB range at 303 nm and the other one in the UVA range at 344 nm.

Methylene bis-benzotriazolyl tetramethylbutylphenol (MBBT) or Tinosorb® M is a photostable UVA filter that also absorbs in the UVB range. It is available as organic particles, dispersed in the water phase.

Bis-ethylhexyloxyphenol methoxyphenyl triazine (BEMT) or Tinosorb® S is a broad spectrum UV filter, photostable and oil soluble.

Due to the FDA regulations, there are few efficient UVA filters available in the USA. On the contrary, the number of UVA filters approved in Europe and Asia is high. Combination of UVB and UVA filters allows sunscreen products highly efficient against both UVB and UVA to be marketed. Nano-sized titanium dioxide can be used to enhance efficacy against erythema especially by synergetic effect with UVB filters, affording SPF up to 50+.

Synergetic effect between lipophilic and hydrophilic filters is also used in sunscreen formulations to reduce the total amount of UV filters. As an example, Mexoryl® SX (hydrophilic) and Mexoryl® XL (lipophilic) are very often combined. Higher SPF and UVA protection level can be reached thanks to these synergetic effects even if the filter amount is lower. A combination of TDSA and DTS was also shown beneficial in various studies.

Combination of TDSA, DTS, Avobenzone, Octocrylene and titanium dioxide providing a very high SPF 50+ and a very high level of UVA protection [UVA protection factor (UVAPF) higher than 25] completely inhibited photoprovocation-induced lesion in 100% of tested patients with lupus erythematosus whereas only 45% of patients were protected by product having the same SPF but that did not contain the two UVA filters TDSA and DTS.[108] In another study, 16 patients suffering from PMLE were exposed to sun for 6 days with this combination of UV filters applied to half body whereas a product of the same SPF but of a lower UVA protection level was applied to the other half body. Only four subjects developed PMLE where the potent broad spectrum product was applied, whereas 15 out of 16 patients who applied the product with lower UVA-PF developed PMLE.[109]

Finally, an ideal sunscreen product should offer different characteristics. Obviously, it should be safe, stable to heat and photostable, it should offer a well-balanced protection against the UVB and UVA rays to protect against short-term and long-term effects of the sun.

Evaluation of the Efficacy of Sunscreen Products

Determination of Sun Protection Factor

The efficacy of a sunscreen is primarily assessed by its sun protection factor (SPF).[108] The SPF is a ratio calculated from the UV dose required to induce a minimum erythemal response with and without sun product applied to the skin of human volunteers, using UV radiation from an artificial source.

The ISO SPF Test Method is a laboratory method that utilizes a xenon arc lamp solar simulator (or equivalent) of defined and known output. Incremental series of delayed erythemal responses are induced on a number of small sub-sites of the skin of selected human subjects. An area of each subject's skin is exposed to UV light without any protection and another (different) area is exposed after applying a test sun protection product. The delayed erythemal responses are visually assessed for redness intensity 16–24 hours post-UVR exposure, by the judgment of a trained evaluator.

By definition, the SPF determines the protection against erythema and is calculated from the following equation:[110]

$$\text{SPF} = \frac{\text{Minimal erythema dose on skin protected by sunscreen product (MEDp)}}{\text{Minimal erythema dose on unprotected skin (MEDu)}}$$

Since SPF assesses the protection against erythema, which is mainly induced by UVB wavelengths, it does not provide information upon UVA photoprotection level. Indeed, UVA contributes only to a small percentage of the skin erythemal response. Therefore, SPF does not reflect the efficacy of protection against all biological endpoints induced by the entire solar UV spectrum.[111]

Determination of UVA Protection Level

There is no worldwide consensus on how to measure and label the level of protection against UVA. The PPD method was the first one being developed for determining UVAPF since PPD is induced by UVA rays and not by UVB.[112] The Japan Cosmetic Industry Association (JCIA) has adopted the PPD method as the official method for assessment of UVA efficacy of sunscreen products since January 1996.[113] Korea and China have also adopted this method in 2001 and 2007, respectively.[114,115] PPD method is officially recommended by the European Commission since September, 2006.[116]

The UVAPF is determined similarly to the SPF on human volunteers, with the following differences: volunteers of a phototype able to develop immediate pigmentation (phototypes II, III and IV), a UVA source being used instead of a complete solar simulated radiation (SSR), and PPD as endpoint instead of erythema. The higher the UVAPF value, the stronger the UVA protection. The consistency of the results has shown that the *in vivo* PPD method is reproducible and reliable.[117] In 2011, the ISO 24442 standard *in vivo* determination of sunscreen UVA protection was published based on the JCIA method.[118] Another important point in the evaluation of the protection against UV rays is the challenge of product photostability during the test not to overestimate UVA protection level of products which are photo unstable. *In vivo* SPF and *in vivo* UVAPF test methods involving UV exposure take into account the photostability, therefore the results are not overestimated.

$$\text{UVA PF}_{\text{PPD}} = \frac{\text{MPPDp dose on sunscreen protected skin (MPPDp)}}{\text{MPPDu dose of unprotected (MPPDu)}}$$

The UVAPF can be also determined using an *in vitro* method.[119] This method has been validated against the *in vivo* PPD method. The transmission through the sunscreen applied to a polymethyl methacrylate (PMMA) plate substrate was cross-multiplied by the UVA source emission spectrum and the PPD action spectrum.

Another approach is the measurement of the absorbance broadness (also called the critical wavelength method).[120] The UV proofing property of the sunscreen agent can be described by its absorption curve which offers two important parameters: height and width. The height of the curve represents the efficiency of sunscreen agent to absorb the UV wavelengths, which can be reflected by the SPF and the UVAPF of sunscreen product. The width of the curve represents the range of UV wavelengths where the sunscreen agent absorbs, that is to say, whether it has a wide range of absorption. The absorption curve of most sunscreen agents has a common feature, i.e. absorption value is high at the shorter wavelengths, such as 290 nm and decreases gradually with increasing wavelength. The critical wavelength refers to the wavelength (λc) beyond 290 nm where (λc), the area under the absorption curve accounts for 90% of the total area of the entire absorption spectrum (290–400 nm). This method relies on the shape of the UV absorption spectrum and not on its amplitude. Consequently it does not evaluate the level of UVA protection: it only ensures that products absorb at least partly in the long UVA waveband.

In 2006, a minimum requirement for UVA efficacy of sunscreens was chosen in Europe:[116] a UVAPF reaching at least 1/3rd of the SPF of the product is now required, which is equivalent to a ratio SPF/UVAPF equal to or lower than 3. This criterion has also be adopted in 2012 by Australia, the Mercosur countries (viz. Argentina, Brazil, Paraguay and Uruguay), Mexico, South Africa and recently proposed by Health Canada. This value has been chosen based on the calculations presented in Table 4, linking real UV exposure to related visible biological phenomena. In humans, a UVA dose of 15 J/cm^2 can induce several biological signs of acute or chronic damage, implying that this dose should not be attained. Indeed, a UVA dose of 15 J/cm^2 which is reached in about 45 minutes of sun exposure, is able to induce the PPD phenomenon which corresponds to melanin oxidation. This PPD is induced very easily on dark skin (III, IV, V).

Since most Indians have Fitzpatrick skin phototypes IV–V, these calculations suggest that the SPF/UVAPF ratio of a sunscreen should be less than 3 in India too. It is also important to note that UVA damage can occur after acute or repeated UVA exposure below 15 J/cm^2.

Relevance of Well-balanced Sunscreens to Protect Human Skin from Both UVA and UVB Damage

A recent Indian study performed in a high altitude, very dry sun-exposed environment (Ladakh) confirmed that skin disorders due to UV rays can be very important even in darker phototypes.[121] In particular, they showed no significant differences between lowlanders, Ladakhis and tourists in the incidence of UVR-related acute conditions (sunburn, PMLE). Melasma and chronic telangiectasia of the face were very common among Ladakhis—considering that this incidence might be largely underestimated since the study only included those who consulted for dermatological advice. Prevention of all UV-induced skin damage is thus important to consider.

Prevention of Hyperpigmentary Disorders Induced by UV Exposure

As described above, sun exposure induces both UVA and UVB pigmentation phenomena. The use of suncare or daily protection products can thus prevent hyperpigmentation.

Considering the strong association between UV exposure and some hyperpigmentary disorders (solar lentigo, melasma, postinflammatory hyperpigmentation), sun protection is crucial for the prevention of such disorders. Unfortunately, clinical studies showing the benefits of photoprotection in such disorders are scarce, especially on darker skin. One study performed in Morocco demonstrated the effectiveness of a well-balanced sunscreen in the prevention of melasma in pregnant women.[122] One hundred and eighty-five patients

Table 4: Calculation of MED/MPPD ratio depending on skin phototypes, considering a zenithal sun exposure and a MPPD of 15 J/cm^2

Fitzpatrick Skin Phototypes	*Time to Achieve 1 MED*	*UVA Dose Received during 1 MED Time*	*Equivalent of UVA MPPD during 1 MED Time*	*Ratio MED/MPPD*
I/II	15 min	5 J/cm^2	1/3 MPPD	3
III	30 min	10 J/cm^2	2/3 MPPD	1.5
IV	45 min	15 J/cm^2	1 MPPD	1

Abbreviations: MED, minimal erythemal dose; UVA, ultraviolet A; MPPD, minimal persistent pigment dose with skin type from II to V applied this product and only five cases of melasma (3%) were noted which was much lower than the 53% previously observed in an usual condition study (same investigators, same geographical area and same time frame). It is also worth noting that at 6 months, a clinical improvement was observed in 8 out of 12 volunteers who were already affected by melasma at the inclusion visit.

The benefit of a well-balanced photoprotection in preventing hyperpigmentation has been studied in provocative test studies.

Well-balanced photoprotection was shown to prevent hyperpigmentation in Asian skin (phototypes III to V). In one study, six different sunscreen products containing UVA + UVB filters with different SPF/UVAPF ratios were applied to volunteers' skin prior to exposure to solar radiation mimicking standard daily UVR.[123] The *in vivo* protection against UVB- and UVA-induced pigmentation was assessed by determining the pigmentation protection factor (PPF). Results showed that products having a well-balanced UVB and UVA protection [SPF/UVAPF (PPD) ≤3] afforded higher protection against pigmentation (Table 5). For the same level of SPF, products having the highest UVAPF had the highest PPF, and products having a SPF/UVAPF ratio below 3 showed more effective than those with a ratio above 3.

These results were confirmed on Indian skin with sunscreen products of lower SPF; two different sunscreens with a same SPF 15 but different level of UVA protection were tested on nine healthy Indian volunteers exposed to increasing dose of daily UVR.[124] Protection level against UVB- and UVA-induced pigmentation was

Table 5: Summary of SPF, UVAPF, PPF, SPF/UVAPF ratio of six sunscreen products tested on Asian skin

Products	*SPF*	*UVAPF*	*SPF/UVAPF ratio*	*PPF*
A	18	8	2.4	17.2
B	19	4	4.8	11.7
C	30	15	2	18.9
D	30	9	3.3	9
E	50	21	2.4	58.9
F	50	13	3.8	22.3

Abbreviations: SPF, sun protection factor; UVAPF, UVA protection factor; PPF, pigmentation protection factor

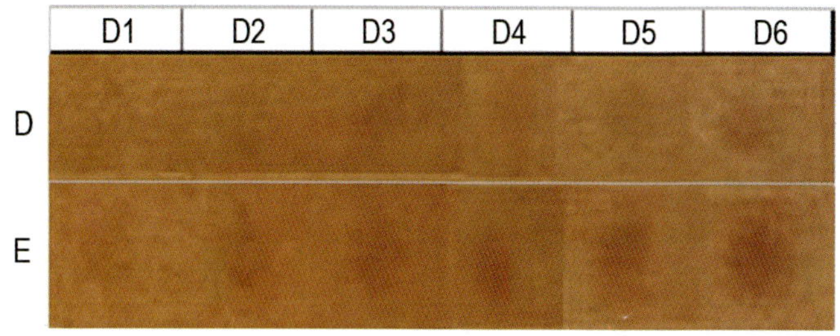

Figure 12: Visual differences of UV-induced pigmentation for product D (well balanced SPF/UVAPF ratio = 1) and product E (SPF/UVAPF ratio= 5, i.e. low UVA protection) 7 days post exposure to increasing daily UV doses (D1 to D6)
©L'Oréal Research and Innovation

assessed by measuring the variation of colorimetric parameters, such as L*a*b* 7 days post UV exposure. Results showed that product with a well-balanced UVB/UVA protection provided a better protection against skin darkening and overall pigmentation than product with a low UVA protection (Fig. 12). This demonstrated that a well-balanced UVB/UVA protection is more efficient in protecting the skin against daily UV-induced pigmentation.

Prevention of Photoaging

Clinical signs of photoaging are the consequence of chronic sun exposure. Even if less reported, photoaging occurs in Indian skin.[41,121] Both UVA and UVB participate in the generation of photodamaged skin during sun exposure. *In vitro* and *in vivo* studies have now demonstrated that UVA rays contribute significantly to long-term dermal structure deterioration and clinical signs of photoaging.[59,77,94,103,125,126]

Ultraviolet A waveband of sunlight can penetrate deep into skin and cumulative exposure to UVA largely explain skin photoaging. Seite et al.[125] found that repeated exposure of healthy volunteers' skin to UVA at suberythemal dose induced changes in elasticity, water content, pigmentation, and histological parameters, and that all these photoaging-related alterations could be blocked by sunscreen product with high UVA protective effect. Seite et al. investigated in depth the effect of UVA rays on a series of metabolic markers, such as ferritin, elastin, tenascin, lysosome and various cells in the dermis, and found a similar protective effect, a significant inhibition of UVA-induced damage with sunscreen products having a high UVA protection level.[103] More recently, the demonstration was performed at the molecular level.[127] The latter study showed that topical application of a daily moisturizer with broad-spectrum sunscreen prevented UVA-induced transcriptional expression of genes that are directly linked to skin aging (i.e. MMP-1) and also reflect the skin's antioxidative stress defense response [i.e. catalase (CAT), superoxide dismutase (SOD), glutathione peroxidase (GPx)]. Furthermore, this study demonstrated that the protection against UV-induced skin damage provided by products with different SPF but with the same UVAPF, was similar; emphasizing the importance of high UVA protection to maintain unaltered essential biologic functions. This data indicates that the use of a daily moisturizer containing broad-spectrum sunscreen with a well-balanced SPF/UVA-PF ratio on a regular basis is highly beneficial to human skin.

Three-dimensional (3D) organotypic models have been developed to identify and understand the early biological events induced by UV light *in vitro*, and thus to evaluate the efficiency of sunscreens to prevent those biological events. The wavelength specific biological damage induced in both epidermis and dermal equivalent allows the photoprotection afforded by various sunscreen formulations to be assessed with regard to damage induced by UVB, UVA, SSR or daily UV radiation (DUVR) exposure.[128-131] The importance of UVB-UVA transmission profile in photoprotection was then evaluated. Products that absorb both UVB and UVA rays were shown to provide better protection toward photoaging markers than those absorbing mostly in the UVB range.[128]

An *in vitro* study using a skin reconstructed model was conducted to assess the protection afforded by two different sunscreens under standard DUVR exposure conditions.[129] The two sunscreens had the same SPF factor value but different profile of UVA-PF (ratio SPF/UVA-PF (PPD) < 3 for sunscreen A and > 3 for sunscreen B). The results showed that compared to sunscreen B, sunscreen A with a well-balanced photoprotection gave a better protection from daily UVR with regard to photoaging-related biomarkers, i.e. fibroblast alterations and MMP-1 release (Fig. 13). Thus, for a given SPF value, efficient photoprotection requires a significant UVA absorption potency.

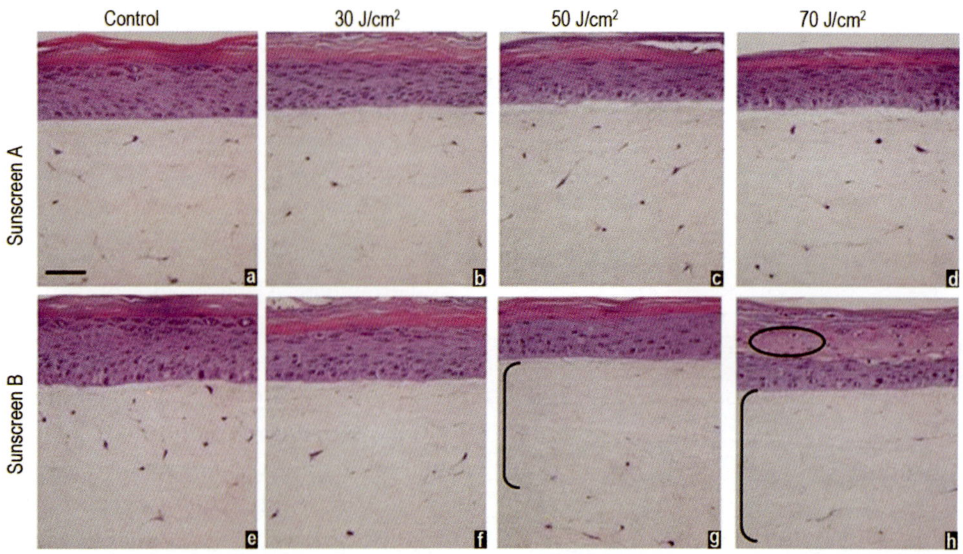

Figure 13: Evaluation of protection by sunscreens A and B in reconstructed skin exposed to increasing doses of daily UV radiation (DUVR). Sunscreens A and B had same SPF15 but different SPF/UVA-PF ratio, less than and more than 3, respectively. Products were applied onto samples before exposure to DUVR (0, 30, 50 or 70 J/cm^2). *Note:* a good protection where product A was applied compared to alterations in samples protected with product B. Scale bar: 50μm. Oval: alterations in the epidermis. Brackets: the depth of dermal alterations (Hematoxylin-eosin-saffron staining, ×200 magnification)
©L'Oréal Research and Innovation

In order to characterize the protection afforded by a well-balanced sunscreen (SPF: 67.5 ± 6.2 and UVA-PF (PPD method): 31.1 ± 6.4) at the molecular level, a semiglobal gene expression analysis was performed.[131] 244 genes in keratinocytes and 227 in fibroblasts were analyzed separately in the reconstructed skin after UVA exposure with or without prior application of the sunscreen. In both skin compartments, UVA radiation modulated the expression of several genes involved in extracellular matrix, oxidative stress response, heat shock response, cell growth, inflammation and epidermal differentiation. Prior application of sunscreen abrogated these effects or reduced them significantly. This revealed a very high photoprotective activity of the sunscreen that could be evidenced using an unsupervised clustering analysis or a gene by gene comparison approach. This data indicated that a well-balanced sunscreen was able to prevent from UVA-induced gene responses.

Efficacy against DNA Damage

The epidemiological data available suggests that sun UV rays were the major environmental factor for the onset of skin tumor. DNA damage can lead to mutations and genetic instability that can facilitate skin cancer development. As previously described, UVB directly impact DNA whereas genotoxicity of UVA mainly depends on indirect mechanisms involving ROS generation.

DNA damage activates the p53 tumor suppressor gene. Thus, the expression of p53 protein following UV exposure provides a sensitive biological endpoint for the evaluation of sunscreen efficacy against damage that may lead to skin cancer. Following this observation, the level of protection against p53 accumulation provided by two sunscreen products having the same SPF25 but different UVAPF was compared in human volunteers in outdoor sun exposure conditions.[132] One test product contained a potent UVA filtering combination (Mexoryl SX, Mexoryl XL, Avobenzone) of a UVA-PF of 14, measured by the PPD method, whereas UVA-PF of the other product was 6. The volunteers self-applied the products in a realistic amount (0.8 mg/cm^2). They were exposed for 6 days to sun with an increasing UV dose from 6 MED to 10 MED. Although the two tested sunscreens provided a similar level of protection against erythema, sunscreen with a well-balanced UV protection SPF/UVAPF less than 3 showed a far higher protective potency against p53 accumulation.

Protection of the Immune System

The immunosuppressant effect of UV is now well documented. UV exposure of human skin induces both local and systemic immunosuppression. As shown by Kelly et al. this immunosuppressive effect does exist in darker skin (phototypes III/IV) at a higher dose compared to lighter skins (phototypes I/II).[133]

Various studies have shown that both UVA and UVB are immunosuppressive.[83,105,134,135] The process is thought to involve Langerhans cells (LC), the epidermal dendritic cells that are pivotal in antigen presentation.

The protective effect of sunscreens on UV-induced immunosuppression has been demonstrated. In particular, the importance of an effective protection against UVA has been stressed. The protective potential of two sunscreens having the same SPF 25 but widely different regarding the level of UVA protection (UVA-PF 14 vs. 6) as determined by the PPD method, has been compared *in vivo* in outdoor conditions[111] consisting in six exposure sessions from 6 MED to 10 MED with an average amount of 0.8 mg/cm^2 of sunscreen applied by the volunteers before each exposure. Results showed that both sunscreens only partially prevented the reduction of LC density and morphological alteration induced by repeated SSR exposure. However, a significantly lower level of LC damage was seen in the skin area protected by sunscreen with higher UVA-PF. This again demonstrates the need for an efficient, balanced protection with a SPF/UVAPF (PPD) ratio less than 3 to prevent impairment of immune competent cells.

The delayed-type hypersensitivity (DTH) response to recall antigens was also studied to evaluate the protective role of sunscreens against immunosuppression induced by UV exposure. Acute and repeated exposures to UVA induced a significant decrease in the DTH responses. The efficacy of sunscreens with different levels of UVA protection has been evaluated under both SSR and outdoor real-life exposure conditions.[105] The results confirm the importance of well-balanced photoprotection using the SPF/UVAPF ratio less than or equal to 3 criterion. When comparing products with same SPF, the product with the higher UVAPF and with SPF/UVAPF ratio less than or equal to 3 always afforded a significant higher protection against photoimmunosuppression than the product with a lower UVAPF (SPF/UVAPF >3).

Protection against Photodermatoses

Photosensitivity, an abnormal reaction to sunlight, is a general term including phototoxicity, photoallergy and photodermatoses. The wavelengths causing these skin abnormal reactions to sunlight lie principally in the UVA range.

Rational use of sunscreen product is an important measure to prevent or treat many photosensitive skin diseases. In particular, the preventive efficacy of sunscreen products on PMLE has been demonstrated.[136] An outdoor study was performed on 10 females prone to PMLE to compare, under natural sunlight realistic conditions of exposure and product applications, the efficacy of two sunscreen products with same SPF 50+ but different UVA protection level, UVA-PF 28 vs.17 and thus different SPF/UVAPF ratios 2.1 and 3.5, respectively. Each product was applied per half body (right or left according to randomization). Only 3 delayed and less intense eruptions were observed on the half-body treated with the sunscreen SPF 50+ with the high UVA-PF 28 whereas 9 cases of PMLE appeared on the half-body treated with the SPF 50+ UVAPF17.

The sunscreen with the highest UVA protection level (UVA-PF 28) SPF/UVAPF 2.1 allowed a better PMLE prevention than the sunscreen with lower UVA protection (UVA-PF 17), SPF/UVAPF 3.5.

SUN PROTECTION STRATEGIES

Photoprotection can be achieved in three different ways. First is behavioral change, e.g. avoiding sun exposure between 9 am and 3 pm, trying to seek shade when outdoors. Second is wearing appropriate clothing, e.g. garment with high ultraviolet protection factor (UPF), and thirdly use of appropriate sunscreen.

Behavioral Changes

The intensity of sunlight varies from place to place. The amount of sun rays received by a person can be altered by certain changes in behavior. The issue at stake is UV avoidance. The various ways of reducing direct sun exposure are:

- Minimizing sun exposure during its peak, when UV rays are maximum, i.e. between 9 am and 3 pm
- Try to seek shade. The amount of UV rays reduced by shade is about 50%.[137] Trees with dense leaves provide protection against UVB rays.[138]

Patients should be aware of reflected light from sand, snow, glass and metal. These can reflect up to 85% of UVB.[139] It should be noted that:

- Water is not a shield from sun exposure. UVB can penetrate up to a depth of 60 cm
- Window glass effectively absorbs UVB rays
- Plastic blinds blocks UV rays and visible light below 470 nm and can be used in the management of patients with severe photodermatoses.

Clothing as a Photoprotective Measure

Use of proper clothing forms an integral part of photoprotection. The photoprotective property of the clothing can be measured by an *in vitro* method method known as the UPF of the garment or clothing. A spectrophotometer is used to assess the UPF. It is defined as the ratio of average effective UV irradiance to the average effective UV irradiance transmitted through the garment. It tells us how much longer a person can remain under the sun with the garments on. Based on the UPF, garments are categorized into three types, e.g. those with good protection (UPF 15–24, blocks 93.3–95.9% of UV rays), very good protection (UPF 25–39, blocks 96–97.4% UV rays) and excellent protection (UPF 40–50, blocks 97.5%–99% of UV rays). Several factors affect the UV protective property of the clothing, its weaving being the most important. Tightly woven clothing gives the maximum protection. The simplest way to test clothing is to hold it against light. Absence of light, observed from the other side, the clothing is likely to give good protection against sunlight. Other factors affecting the UPF are color (dark colored is better), weight (heavier the better), stretch (easily stretchable less protective), wetness (wetness reduces UPF by 50%), fitting (loosely fitting garments give better protection), washing (washing increases the UPF) and material[140] (polyester is the best, then wool, silk and nylon and the least protective are cotton and rayon. Use of physical barriers is the key for prevention of photodermatoses, photoaging and pigmentation. The recommendation is to cover as much skin as possible using long sleeved shirts, full length trousers, full collars, and wide brimmed hat and UV protective glasses to protect the eyes.

Sunscreens

The final preventive measure is the use of an appropriate sunscreen. An ideal sunscreen should protect the skin from both UVB and UVA rays. It should be nonoily, noncomedogenic, photostable, water resistant and cosmetically acceptable.

To be effective, a sunscreen should be applied properly. Ideally, sunscreen should be re-applied every 2 hours or even more frequently depending on sun exposure and the level of photoprotection used and immediately after contact with water. The recommended amount is 2 mg/cm^2.

An even uniform layer should be applied and it should not be rubbed into the skin. Rubbing sunscreen vigorously into the skin decreases its photoprotective value.[141] The amount of sunscreen to be applied can be measured by the teaspoon rule[142] or crown tin lid[143] method. In the teaspoon rule, a little more than half teaspoon (3 mL) is required for each arm, face and neck. A little more than a teaspoon (6 mL) is needed for each leg, chest and back. The crown tin lid of an aerated bottle provides a consistent measure for dispensing a sunscreen. Half full of the lid is required for the face and neck and one full lid for each upper limb, and 2 full lids for the back.

CONCLUSION

Indian people having in majority a moderately to highly pigmented skin, conventional wisdom is that Indians are not concerned about the sun damaging effects although exposed to high doses of solar UV all along the year. Nevertheless, Indians presented some typical sun-induced damage: photodermatoses, hyperpigmentation, photoaging and to a lesser extent photocarcinogenesis. Furthermore, with regard to the increase of life expectancy and emergence of new lifestyles, it is very important for dermatologists to be aware of all the damaging effects of sun and the importance of sun protection.

It is now proved that both UVB and UVA play a major role in the detrimental effects of solar rays on skin. An efficient well-balanced photoprotection combining UVB and UVA absorption seems more and more crucial because of the increasing knowledge related to the harmful effects of UVA. This chapter clearly demonstrates the importance of UVA protection and that the SPF value does not appear sufficient *per se to* evaluate the protecting effects of a sunscreen against all biological end-points induced by the entire solar UV spectrum. All the above studies show the importance of a well-balanced photoprotection with a ratio SPF/UVAPF (PPD) less than or equal to 3 to prevent most of the damage induced by UV exposure. A well-balanced sunscreen appears an effective protection against hyperpigmentary disorders, photoaging, DNA damage, alterations of the skin immune system and the onset of photodermatoses. In particular, hyperpigmentary disorders being major issues in India, it is very important to emphasize the role of prevention and the use of adapted sun protection behavior and sunscreens with well-balanced filtration systems.

REFERENCES

1. Diffey BL. What is light? Photodermatol Photoimmunol Photomed. 2002;18:68-74.
2. Jablonski NG, Chaplin G. Colloquium Paper: Human skin pigmentation as an adaptation to UV radiation. Proc Natl Acad Sci USA. 2010;11:8962-8.
3. Balasaraswathy P, Kumar U, Srinivas CR, et al. UVA and UVB in sunlight, optimal utilization of UV rays in sunlight for phototherapy. Indian J Dermatol Venereol Leprol. 2002;68:198-201.
4. Frederick JE, Lubin D. Possible long-term changes in biologically active ultraviolet radiation reaching the ground. Photochem Photobiol. 1988;47:571-8.
5. Frederick JE, Snell EH, Haywood EK. Solar ultraviolet radiation at the earth's surface. Photochem Photobiol. 1989;50:443-50.
6. Lubin D, Jensen EH. Effects of clouds and stratospheric ozone depletion on ultraviolet radiation trends. Nature. 1995;377:710-3.
7. Christiaens FJ, Chardon A, Fourtanier A, et al. Standard ultraviolet daylight for nonextreme exposure conditions. Photochem Photobiol. 2005;81:874-8.
8. Ma J, Guicherit R. Effects of stratospheric ozone depletion and tropospheric pollution on UVB radiation in the troposphere. Photochem Photobiol. 1997;66:346-55.
9. Loughlin PE, Box MA. Investigating biological response in the UVB as a function of ozone variation using perturbation theory. J Photochem Photobiol B. 1998;43:73-85.
10. Krzyscin JW. Total ozone influence on the surface UVB radiation in the late spring-summer 1963-1997: An analysis of multiple timescales. J Geophys Res. 2000;105:4993-5000.
11. Frederick JE, Qu Z, Booth CR. Ultraviolet radiation at sites on the antarctic coast. Photochem Photobiol. 1998;68:183-90.
12. Vernez D, Milon A, Vuilleumier L, et al. Anatomical exposure patterns of skin to sunlight: relative contributions of direct, diffuse and reflected ultraviolet radiation. Br J Dermatol. 2012;167:383-90.
13. Sharma VK, Sahni K, Wadhwani AR. Photodermatoses in pigmented skin. Photochem Photobiol Sci. 2013;12:65-77.
14. Srinivas CR, Sekar CS, Jayashree R. Photodermatoses in India. Indian J Dermatol Venereol Leprol. 2012;78:S1-8.
15. Sharma L, Basnet A. A clinicoepidemiological study of polymorphic light eruption. Indian J Dermatol Venereol Leprol. 2008;74:15-7.

16. Palmer RA, Van De Pas CB, Campalani E, et al. A simple method to assess severity of polymorphic light eruption. Br J Dermatol. 2004;151:645-52.
17. Ortel B, Tanew A, Wolff K, et al. Polymorphous light eruption: Action spectrum and photoprotection. J Am Acad Dermatol. 1986;14: 748-53.
18. Commission Internationale De l'Eclairage: Colorimetry, 2nd Edition. Publication CIE N; 1986. pp. 15-2.
19. Mc Kinlay AF, Diffey BL. A reference action spectrum for ultraviolet induced erythema in human skin. CIE J. 1987;6:17-22.
20. Farr PM, Diffey BL. The erythemal response of human skin to ultraviolet radiation. Br J Dermatol. 1985;113:65-76.
21. Fitzpatrick TB. The validity and practicality of sun-reactive skin types I through VI. Arch Dermatol. 1988;124:869-71.
22. Kollias N, Malallah Y, Al-Ajmi H, et al. Erythema and melanogenesis action spectra in heavily pigmented individuals as compared to fair-skinned caucasians. Photodermatol Photoimmunol Photomed. 1996;12:183-8.
23. Kaidbey K, Kligman A. The acute effects of long-wave ultraviolet radiation on human skin. J Invest Dermatol. 1978;72:253-6.
24. Chardon A, Moyal D. Immediate and delayed pigmentary responses to solar UVA radiation (320-400 nm). In: Ortonne JP, Ballotti R, (Eds). Mechanisms of Suntanning. London: Martin Dunitz Ltd; 2002; pp. 315-25.
25. Auletta M, Gange RW, Tan OT, et al. Effect of cutaneous hypoxia upon erythema and pigment responses to UVA, UVB, and PUVA (8-MOP + UVA) In human skin. J Invest Dermatol. 1986;86:649-52.
26. Moyal D, Fourtanier A. Acute and chronic effects of uv on skin: what are they and how to study them? In: Rigel DS, Weiss RA, Lim HW, Dover JS, (Eds). Photoaging. New York: Marcel Dekker, Inc; 2004. pp. 15-32.
27. Chardon A, Crétois I, Hourseau C. Skin colour typology and suntanning pathways. Int J Cosm Sci. 1991;13:191-208.
28. Harrison GI, Young AR. Ultraviolet radiation-induced erythema in human skin. Methods 2002;28:14-9.
29. Mehta RV, Shenoi SD, Balachandran C, et al. Minimal erythema dose (MED) to solar simulated irradiation in normal Indian skin. Indian J Dermatol Venereol Leprol. 2004;70:277-9.
30. Chardon A, Moyal D, Hourseau C. Persistent pigment darkening response as a method for evaluation of UVA protection assays. In: N Lowe, N Shaat and M Pathak, (Eds). Sunscreens: Development, Evaluation and Regulatory Aspects, 2nd Edition. New York: Marcel Dekker Inc; 1997. pp.559-82.
31. Deutsche Norm: Strahlungsphysik im optischen Bereich und Lichttechnik - Teil 10: Photobiologisch wirksame Strahlung, Grösen, Kurzziechen und Wirkungsspektrum. DIN 5031-10. 1996.
32. Halprin KM. Epidermal "Turnover Time". A Re-Examination. Br J Dermatol. 1972;86:14-9.
33. Khanna N, Rasool S. Facial Melanoses: Indian Perspective. Indian J Dermatol Venereol Leprol. 2011;77:552-63.
34. Tsoureli-Nikita E, Watson RE, Griffiths CE. Photoageing: The darker side of the sun. Photochem Photobiol Sci. 2006;5:160-4.
35. Griffiths CE. The clinical identification and quantification of photodamage. Br J Dermatol 1992;127:37-42.
36. Smith JG, Davidson EA, Sams WM, et al. Alterations in human dermal connective tissue with age and chronic sun damage. J Invest Dermatol. 1962;39:347-50.
37. Kligman LH, Akin FJ, Kligman AM. The contributions of UVA and UVB to connective tissue damage in hairless mice. J Invest Dermatol. 1985;84:272-6.
38. Seite S, Moyal D, Richard S, et al. Effects of repeated suberythemal doses of UVA in human skin. In: Rougier A, Schaefer H, (Eds). Protection of the Skin against Ultraviolet Radiations. Paris, France: John Libbey Eurotext; 1998. pp. 159-66.
39. Gordon JRS, Brieva JC. Images in clinical medicine. Unilateral Dermatoheliosis. N Engl J Med. 2012;366:e25.
40. Chung JH. Photoaging in Asians. Photodermatol Photoimmunol Photomed. 2003;19:109-21.
41. Durai PC, Thappa DM, Kumari R, et al. Aging in elderly: Chronological versus photoaging. Indian J Dermatol. 2012;57: 343-52.
42. Black HS, De Gruijl FR, Forbes PD, et al. Photocarcinogenesis: An Overview. J Photochem Photobiol B. 1997;40:29-47.
43. Halder RM, Bridgeman-Shah S. Skin cancer in African Americans. Cancer. 1995;75:667-73.
44. Green AC, Williams GM, Logan V, et al. Reduced melanoma after regular sunscreen use: randomized trial follow-up. J Clin Oncol. 2011;29:257-63.
45. Verma SB. Dermatology for the elderly: An indian perspective. Clin Dermatol. 2011;29:91-6.
46. National Cancer Registry Programme. Indian Council of Medical Research. Consolidated Report of the Population Based Cancer Registries. 1990-96.
47. Adinarayan M, Krishnamurthy SP. Clinicopathological cancer. Indian J Dermatol. 2011;56:670-2.
48. Panda S. Nonmelanoma skin cancer in India: current scenario. Indian J Dermatol. 2010;55:373-8.
49. De Boer J, Hoeijmakers JH. Nucleotide excision repair and human syndromes. Carcinogenesis. 2000;21:453-60.
50. Magnaldo T, Sarasin A. Xeroderma Pigmentosum: From symptoms and genetics to gene-based skin therapy. Cells Tissues Organs. 2004;177:189-98.
51. Del Bino S, Sok J, Bessac E, et al. Relationship Between skin response to ultraviolet exposure and skin color type. Pigment Cell Res. 2006;19:606-14.
52. Setlow RB. Action spectra: skin. In: Gasparro FG, (Ed). Sunscreen Photobiology: Molecular, Cellular and Physiological Aspects. Berlin: Springer-Verlag; 1997. pp. 1-8.
53. Rochette PJ, Therrien JP, Drouin R, et al. UVA-induced cyclobutane pyrimidine dimers form predominantly at thymine-thymine dipyrimidines and correlate with the mutation spectrum in rodent cells. Nucleic Acids Res. 2003;31:2786-94.
54. Tewari A, Sarkany RP, Young AR. UVA1 induces cyclobutane pyrimidine dimers but not 6-4 photoproducts in human skin in vivo. J Invest Dermatol. 2012;132:394-400.
55. Kozmin S, Slezak G, Reynaud-Angelin A, et al. UVA Radiation is highly mutagenic in cells that are unable to repair 7,8-dihydro-8-oxoguanine in saccharomyces cerevisiae. Proc Natl Acad Sci USA. 2005;102:13538-43.
56. Song EJ, Gordon-Thomson C, Cole L, et al. 1α,25-Dihydroxyvitamin D(3) reduces several types of UV-induced DNA damage and contributes to photoprotection. J Steroid Biochem Mol Biol. 2013;136:131-8.
57. Gilchrest BA, Eller MS. DNA Photodamage stimulates melanogenesis and other photoprotective responses. J Investig Dermatol Symp Proc. 1999;4:35-40.
58. Campbell C, Quinn AG, Angus B, et al. Wavelength Specific patterns of p53 induction in human skin following exposure to UV radiation. Cancer Res. 1993;53:2697-9.

59. Bernerd F, Asselineau D. Successive alteration and recovery of epidermal differentiation and morphogenesis after specific UVB-Damages in skin reconstructed in vitro. Dev Biol. 1997;183:123-38.
60. Nataraj AJ, Trent JC, Ananthaswamy HN. P53 gene mutations and photocarcinogenesis. Photochem Photobiol. 1995;62:218-30.
61. Huang XX, Bernerd F, Halliday GM. Ultraviolet a within sunlight induces mutations in the epidermal basal layer of engineered human skin. Am J Pathol. 2009;174:1534-43.
62. Cui R, Widlund HR, Feige E, et al Central role of p53 in the suntan response and pathologic hyperpigmentation. Cell. 2007;128: 853-64.
63. Gilchrest BA. Dermatoheliosis (Sun-Induced Aging). In: Gilchrest BA, (Ed). Skin and Aging Process. Boca Raton, FL: CRC Press; 1989. pp. 97-116
64. Chen VL, Fleischmajer R, Schwartz E, et al. Immunochemistry of elastotic material in sun-damaged skin. J Invest Dermatol. 1986;87:334-7.
65. Bernstein EF, Brown DB, Urbach F, et al. Ultraviolet radiation activates the human elastin promoter in transgenic mice: a novel in vivo and in vitro model of cutaneous photoaging. J Invest Dermatol. 1995;105:269-73.
66. Watson RE, Griffiths CE, Craven NM, et al. Fibrillin-Rich microfibrils are reduced in photoaged skin. Distribution at the dermal-epidermal junction. J Invest Dermatol. 1999;112:782-7.
67. Seite S, Zucchi H, Septier D, et al. Elastin changes during chronological and photo-ageing: the important role of lysozyme. J Eur Acad Dermatol Venereol. 2006;20:980-7.
68. Oikarinen A, Karvonen J, Uitto J, et al. Connective tissue alterations in skin exposed to natural and therapeutic UV-radiation. Photodermatol. 1985;2:15-26.
69. Talwar HS, Griffiths CE, Fisher GJ, et al. Reduced type I and type III procollagens in photodamaged adult human skin. J Invest Dermatol. 1995;105:285-90.
70. Chung JH, Seo JY, Choi HR, et al. Modulation of skin collagen metabolism in aged and photoaged human skin in vivo. J Invest Dermatol. 2001;117:1218-24.
71. Fisher GJ, Datta S, Wang Z, et al. C-Jun-dependent inhibition of cutaneous procollagen transcription following ultraviolet irradiation is reversed by all-trans retinoic acid. J Clin Invest. 2000;106:663-70.
72. Craven NM, Watson RE, Jones CJ, et al. Clinical features of photodamaged human skin are associated with a reduction in collagen VII. Br J Dermatol. 1997;137:344-50.
73. Bernstein EF, Fisher LW, Li K, et al. Differential expression of the versican and decorin genes in photoaged and sun-protected skin. comparison by immunohistochemical and northern analyses. Lab Invest. 1995;72:662-9.
74. Fisher GJ, Datta SC, Talwar HS, et al. Molecular basis of sun-induced premature skin ageing and retinoid antagonism. Nature. 1996;379:335-9.
75. Brenneisen P, Sies H, Scharffetter-Kochanek K. Ultraviolet-B irradiation and matrix metalloproteinases: from induction via signaling to initial events. Ann N Y Acad Sci. 2002;973:31-43.
76. Scharffetter K, Wlaschek M, Hogg A, et al. UVA irradiation induces collagenase in human dermal fibroblasts in vitro and in vivo. Arch Dermatol Res. 1991;283:506-11.
77. Fagot D, Asselineau D, Bernerd F. Matrix metalloproteinase-1 production observed after solar-simulated radiation exposure is assumed by dermal fibroblasts but involves a paracrine activation through epidermal keratinocytes. Photochem Photobiol. 2004;79:499-505.
78. Fagot D, Asselineau D, Bernerd F. Direct role of human dermal fibroblasts and indirect participation of epidermal keratinocytes in MMP-1 production after UVB irradiation. Arch Dermatol Res. 2002;293:576-83.
79. Wlaschek M, Bolsen K, Herrmann G, et al. UVA-induced autocrine stimulation of fibroblast-derived-collagenase by IL-6: a possible mechanism in dermal photodamage? J Invest Dermatol. 1993;101:164-8.
80. Koivukangas V, Kallioinen M, Autio-Harmainen H, et al. UV irradiation induces the expression of gelatinases in human skin in vivo. Acta Derm Venereol. 1994;74:279-82.
81. Fisher GJ, Wang ZQ, Datta SC, et al. Pathophysiology of premature skin aging induced by ultraviolet light. N Engl J Med. 1997;337: 1419-28.
82. Cooper KD, Oberhelman L, Hamilton TA, et al. UV Exposure reduces immunization rates and promotes tolerance to epicutaneous antigens in humans: relationship to dose, CD1a-DR+ epidermal macrophage induction, and langerhans cell depletion. Proc Natl Acad Sci USA. 1992;89:8497-501.
83. Kuchel JM, Barnetson RS, Halliday GM. Ultraviolet A augments solar-simulated ultraviolet radiation-induced local suppression of recall responses in humans. J Invest Dermatol. 2002;118:1032-7.
84. Damian DL, Matthews YJ, Phan TA, et al. An action spectrum for ultraviolet radiation-induced immunosuppression in humans. Br J Dermatol. 2011;164:657-9.
85. Norval M, Halliday GM. The consequences of UV-induced immunosuppression for human health. Photochem Photobiol. 2011;87:965-77.
86. Seite S, Zucchi H, Moyal D, et al. Alterations in human epidermal langerhans cells by ultraviolet radiation: quantitative and morphological study. Br J Dermatol. 2003;148:291-9.
87. Barr RM, Walker SL, Tsang W, et al. Suppressed alloantigen presentation, increased TNF-Alpha, IL-1, IL-1Ra, IL-10, and modulation of TNF-R in UV-irradiated human skin. J Invest Dermatol. 1999;112:692-8.
88. Scharffetter-Kochanek K, Wlaschek M, Brenneisen P, et al. UV-Induced reactive oxygen species in photocarcinogenesis and photoaging. Biol Chem. 1997;378:1247-57.
89. Hanson KM, Simon JD. Epidermal trans-urocanic acid and the UVA-induced photoaging of the skin. Proc Natl Acad Sci USA. 1998;95:10576-8.
90. Morliere P, Moysan A, Santus R, et al. UVA-induced lipid peroxidation in cultured human fibroblasts. Biochim Biophys Acta. 1991;1084:261-8.
91. Brenneisen P, Wenk J, Klotz LO, et al. Central role of ferrous/ferric iron in the ultraviolet B irradiation-mediated signaling pathway leading to increased interstitial collagenase (Matrix-Degrading Metalloprotease (MMP)-1) And Stromelysin-1 (MMP-3) mRNA levels in cultured human dermal fibroblasts. J Biol Chem. 1998;273:5279-87.
92. Applegate LA, Noel A, Vile G, et al. Two genes contribute to different extents to the heme oxygenase enzyme activity measured in cultured human skin fibroblasts and keratinocytes: implications for protection against oxidant stress. Photochem Photobiol. 1995;61:285-91.
93. Vile GF, Tyrrell RM. Oxidative stress resulting from ultraviolet a

irradiation of human skin fibroblasts leads to a heme oxygenase-dependent increase in ferritin. J Biol Chem. 1993;268:14678-81.
94. Bernerd F, Asselineau D. UVA exposure of human skin reconstructed in vitro induces apoptosis of dermal fibroblasts: subsequent connective tissue repair and implications in photoaging. Cell Death Differ. 1998;5:792-802.
95. Marionnet C, Pierrard C, Lejeune F, et al. Different oxidative stress response in keratinocytes and fibroblasts of reconstructed skin exposed to non extreme daily-ultraviolet radiation. Plos One 2010;5:E12059.
96. Sander CS, Chang H, Salzmann S, et al. Photoaging is associated with protein oxidation in human skin in vivo. J Invest Dermatol. 2002;118:618-25.
97. Ogawa F, Sander CS, Hansel A, et al. The repair enzyme peptide methionine-s-sulfoxide reductase is expressed in human epidermis and upregulated by UVA radiation. J Invest Dermatol. 2006;126:1128-34.
98. Berneburg M, Grether-Beck S, Kurten V, et al. Singlet oxygen mediates the UVA-induced generation of the photoaging-associated mitochondrial common deletion. J Biol Chem. 1999;274:15345-9.
99. Wlaschek M, Tantcheva-Poor I, Naderi L, et al. Solar UV irradiation and dermal photoaging. J Photochem Photobiol B. 2001;63:41-51.
100. Forestier S. Rationale for sunscreen development. J Am Acad Dermatol. 2008;58:S133-8.
101. Moyal D. The Development of efficient sunscreens. Indian J Dermatol Venereol Leprol. 2012;78 (Suppl 1):S31-4.
102. Young AR, Sheehan JM, Chadwick CA, et al. Protection by ultraviolet A and B sunscreens against in situ dipyrimidine photolesions in human epidermis is comparable to protection against sunburn. The Society for Invest Dermatol. 2000;115:37-41.
103. Seite S, Moyal D, Richard S, et al. Mexoryl® SX: a broad absorption UVA filter protects human skin from the effects of repeated suberythemal doses of UVA. J Photochem Photobiol B. 1998; 4469-76.
104. Moyal D. Prevention of ultraviolet-induced skin pigmentation. Photodermatol Photoimmunol Photomed. 2004;20:243-7.
105. Moyal D, Fourtanier A. Broad-spectrum sunscreens provide better protection from the suppression of the elicitation phase of delayed-type hypersensitivity response in humans. J Invest Dermatol. 2001;117:1186-92.
106. Moyal D. Polymorphous light eruption: its reproduction and prevention by sunscreens. In: Lowe N, (Ed). Sunscreens development, evaluation and regulatory aspects. New York: Marcel Dekker Inc; 1997. pp. 611-7.
107. Nocera T, Peyron JL, Moyal D, et al. Protection of solar urticaria using a broad-spectrum sunscreen and determination of a solar urticaria protection factor. Nouv Dermatol. 1998;17:01-4.
108. Stege H, Budde MA, Grether-Beck S, et al. Evaluation of the capacity of sunscreens to photoprotect lupus erythematosus patients by employing the photoprovocation test. Eur J Dermatol. 2002;12: VII-VIX.
109. Moyal D, Binet O, Richard A. Prevention of polymorphism light eruption by a new broad-spectrum sunscreen. 57th annual meeting of the American Academy of Dermatology. New-Orleans. 1999.
110. ISO 24444 ISO Sun Protection Factor (SPF) Test Method. Geneva. 2010.
111. Fourtanier A, Bernerd F, Bouillon C, et al. Protection of skin biological targets by different types of sunscreens. Photodermatol Photoimmunol Photomed. 2005;21:1-11.
112. Moyal D, Chardon A, Kollias N. Determination of UVA protection factors using the persistent pigment darkening (PPD) as the endpoint. (Part 1). Calibration of the method. Photodermatol Photoimmunol Photomed. 2000;16:245-9.
113. JCIA. Measurements standard for UVA protection efficacy. Japan Cosmetic Industry Association (Tokyo Japan). 1996.
114. Korean FDA. Korean measurement standards for UV protection efficacy. 2004.
115. MOH, China. Hygenic standard for cosmetics. UVA protection factor (PFA) test method of cosmetic sunscreens. 2007.
116. European Commission Recommendation. On the efficacy of sunscreen products and the claims made relating thereto. Official J Eur Union. 2006;265:39-43.
117. Moyal D, Pissavini M, Boyer F, et al. In vivo persistent pigment darkening method: proposal for a new standard product for UVA protection factor determination. Int J Cosm Sci. 2007;29:443-9.
118. ISO 24442. In vivo determination of sunscreen UVA protection. 2011.
119. ISO 24443. Determination of sunscreen UVA photoprotection in vitro. 2012.
120. Diffey BL. A method for broad-spectrum classification of sunscreens. Int J Cosm Sci. 1994;16:47-52.
121. Singh G, Chatterjee M, Grewal R, et al. Incidence and care of environmental dermatoses in the high-altitude region of Ladakh, India. Indian J Dermatol. 2013;58:107-12.
122. Lakhdar H, Zouhair K, Khadir K, et al. Evaluation of the effectiveness of a broad-spectrum sunscreen in the prevention of chloasma in pregnant women. J Eur Acad Dermatol Venereol. 2007;21:738-42.
123. Fourtanier A, Moyal D, Seite S. UVA filters in sun protection products: regulatory and biological aspects. Photochem Photobiol Sci. 2012;11:81-9.
124. Moyal D, Battie C, Tricaud C. Prevention of skin pigmentation in darker skin: experimental evidence in India. Poster International Congress of Dermatology, New Delhi, India, 2013.
125. Seite S, Moyal D, Richard S, et al. Effect of repeated suberythemal doses of UVA in human skin. Eur J Dermatol. 1997;7:204-9.
126. Ou-Yang H, Stamatas G, Saliou C, et al. A chemiluminescence study of UVA-induced oxidative stress in human skin in vivo. J Invest Dermatol. 2004;122:1020-9.
127. Seité S, Reinhold K, Jaenicke T, et al. Broad-spectrum moisturizer effectively prevents molecular reactions to UVA radiation. Cutis. 2012;90:321-6.
128. Bernerd F, Vioux C, Lejeune F, et al. The sun protection factor (SPF) inadequately defines broad-spectrum photoprotection: demonstration using skin reconstructed in vitro exposed to UVA, UVB or UV-solar simulated radiation. Eur J Dermatol. 2003;13:1-8.
129. Lejeune F, Christiaens F, Bernerd F. Evaluation of sunscreen products using a reconstructed skin model exposed to simulated daily ultraviolet radiation: relevance of filtration profile and SPF value for daily photoprotection. Photodermatol Photoimmunol Photomed. 2008;24:249-55.
130. Bernerd F, Vioux C, Asselineau D. Evaluation of the protective effect of sunscreens on in vitro reconstructed human skin exposed to UVB or UVA irradiation. Photochem Photobiol. 2000;71:314-20.
131. Marionnet C, Grether-Beck S, Seité S, et al. A broad-spectrum sunscreen prevents UVA radiation-induced gene expression in reconstructed skin in vitro and in human skin in vivo. Exp Dermatol. 2011;20:477-82.
132. Fourtanier A, Bernerd F, Bouillon C, et al. Protection of skin

biological targets by different types of sunscreens. Photodermatol Photoimmunol Photomed. 2005;21:1-11.

133. Kelly DA, Young AR, Mcgregor JM, et al. Sensitivity to sunburn is associated with susceptibility to ultraviolet radiation-induced suppression of cutaneous cell-mediated immunity. J Exp Med. 2000;191:561-6.
134. Damian DL, Barnetson RS, Halliday GM. Low-dose UVA and UVB have different time courses for suppression of contact hypersensitivity to a recall antigen in humans. J Invest Dermatol. 1999;112:939-44.
135. Levee GJ, Oberhelman L, Anderson T, et al. UVA II exposure of human skin results in decreased immunization capacity, increased induction of tolerance and a unique pattern of epidermal antigen presenting cell alteration. Photochem Photobiol. 1997;65:622-9.
136. Fourtanier A, Moyal D, Seité S. Sunscreens containing the broad-spectrum UVA absorber, Mexoryl® SX, prevent the cutaneous detrimental effects of UV exposure: a review of clinical study results. Photodermatol Photoimmunol Photomed. 2008;24:164-74.
137. Moseley H. Photoprotection. In: Ferguson J, Doverjs, (Eds). Photodermatology. Manson Publishers Ltd; London: 2006. p. 22.
138. Carolyn B, Lyde R, Bergstresser PR. Ultraviolet protection from sun avoidance. Dermatol Ther. 1997;4:72-8.
139. Kullavanijaya P, Lim HW. Photoprotection. J Am Acad Dermatol. 2005;52:937-58.
140. Crews PC, Kachman S, Beyer AG. Influence on UVB transmission of undyed woven fabric. Textile Chern Colorist. 1993;31:17-26.
141. Haywood R. Relevance of sunscreen application method, visible light, and sunlight intensity to free radical protection: A study of ex vivo skin. Photochem Photobiol. 2006;82:1123-31.
142. Schneider J. The teaspoon rule of applying sunscreen. Arch Dermatol. 2002;138:838-9.
143. Castanedo-Cazares JO, Lepe V, Torres-Alvarez B, et al. A simple measure for applying sunscreen while on holidays. Dermatology Online J. 2003;9:23.

Chapter 8

Stratum Corneum, Dry Skin, Xerosis and Moisturizers

Mark Donovan, *L'Oréal Research and Innovation, Aulnay-sous-Bois, France*
Reena Rai, *PSG Institute of Medical Science and Research, Coimbatore, India*
Muthuvel Kumaresan, *PSG Institute of Medical Science and Research, Coimbatore, India*

WATERTIGHT SKIN

A key step in evolution of life on earth was the development of a functional exogenous barrier which allowed vertebrates to leave the oceans and live on dry land. The ultimate barrier is that of human skin which has beautifully evolved to be an effective and impermeable protective shield allowing us to tolerate and live in all sorts of climatic and environmental conditions. Human skin is composed of three tissue compartments: (1) the epidermis, (2) the dermis and (3) the hypodermis (Fig. 1). The upper tissue is the epidermis and one of its main functions is to form the stratum corneum; the cornified layer which is body's front line barrier to the external environment. The stratum corneum (Fig. 2) consists of highly specialized anucleated cells known as corneocytes and intercellular arrays of organized lipids. This structure, which has long been considered biologically inert, is in fact very much alive from a biochemical point of view and it plays a key role in the homeostasis of the skin functional barrier.

KEY FEATURES OF THE STRATUM CORNEUM[1-7]

The Keratinocyte Cycle

The corneocyte starts its life as a keratinocyte stem cell in the lower layers of the epidermis—the stratum basale. Over the course of 28 days, the young keratinocyte migrates towards the surface while undergoing several morphological and physiological changes. During the first few days of this lunar cycle, keratinocytes proliferate rapidly in the basal layer. They become regularly arranged, adhering to neighboring cells via specialized protein bridges known as desmosomes and to the basement membrane, the dermal-epidermal junction, through hemidesmosomes. A certain percentage of these keratinocytes become the so-called transit-amplifying cells and start to differentiate, change shape and migrate upwards to the stratum spinosum which is also called the prickle cell layer due to the histological observation of spine-like structures between neighboring keratinocytes. Here, the keratinocytes take on a polyhedral shape and start to synthesize new keratin proteins, K1 and K10, which are characteristic of differentiating keratinocytes. These keratins are organized into large filamentous bundles through which keratinocytes adhere to desmosomes. As the cells migrate towards the upper layers they become increasingly larger in size, start to flatten and acquire new organelles—lamellar granules also known as Odland bodies. In the granular layer, the stratum granulosum, keratinocytes enter the latter

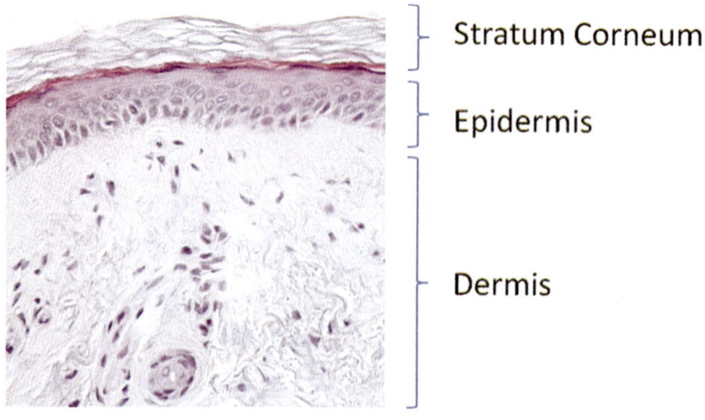

Figure 1: Histology section of skin showing the three different compartments: (1) the dermis, (2) epidermis and (3) the outer cornified layer the stratum corneum
©L'Oréal Research and Innovation

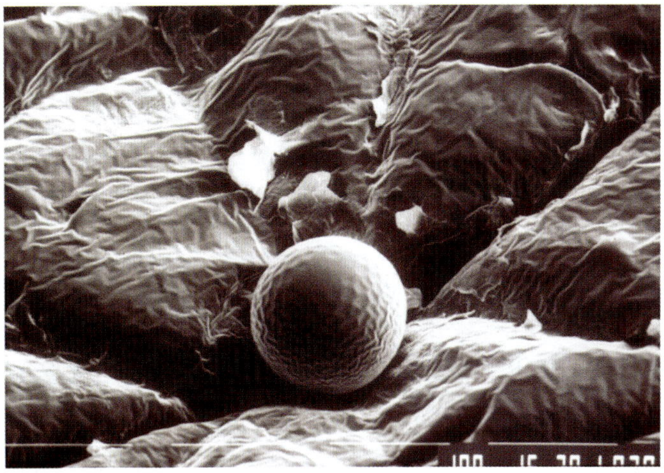

Figure 2: Electron micrograph of the skin surface—the stratum corneum showing the arrangement of corneocytes that provide our watertight barrier to the external environment
©L'Oréal Research and Innovation

stages of differentiation before reaching the uppermost layer of the epidermis. Here, the morphology of keratinocytes dramatically changes as it undergoes an apoptotic form of cell death including the destruction of cellular organelles and of the nucleus in addition to deoxyribonucleic acid (DNA) fragmentation. In the granular layer, keratinocytes are characterized by the presence of keratohyalin granules which are primarily composed of keratin intermediate filaments, profilaggrin and loricrin. These proteins play an instrumental role in the composition of the ultimate cell stage, corneocyte and its envelope. In the stratum granulosum, many membrane bound lamellar granules are present in the cytoplasm of keratinocytes which contain in abundance the lipids, glycoproteins and glycolipids that will serve as the precursors to found the architecture of the stratum corneum barrier. The keratinocyte now enters the uppermost layer of the epidermis, the stratum corneum after terminally differentiating into a corneocyte, a polygonal flat cell, which is 30–50 μm in diameter, far different from the one originating in the basal layer 14 days before. Indeed, it will be another 14 days before the corneocyte reaches the surface where it is shed into the surrounding environment through a process known as desquamation (Fig. 3). In the stratum corneum, corneocytes form a dual compartment with tightly

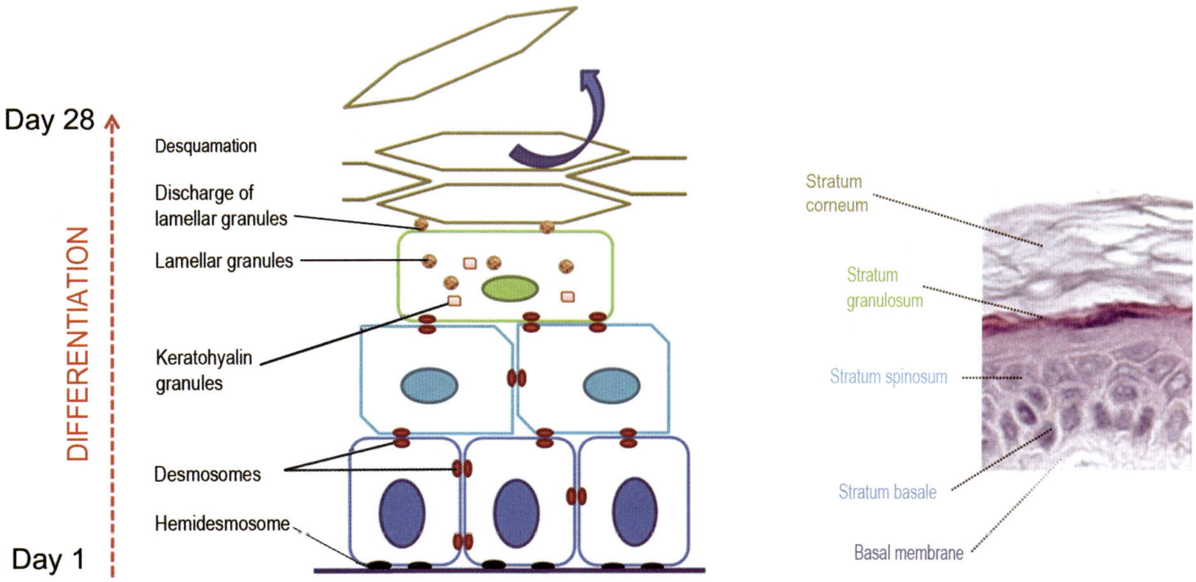

Figure 3: Graphic showing the different layers of epidermis from the basal membrane to the stratum corneum. The lifecycle of a keratinocyte is approximately 28 days. Starting as an undifferentiated cell in the basal membrane until it is finally shed from the surface as a corneocyte through the process of desquamation
©L'Oréal Research and Innovation

packed cells and an extracellular lamellar lipid matrix. This functions as a dense barrier providing mechanical protection to the skin and preventing excessive transcutaneous water loss while permitting permeation of soluble substances from the environment.

Structural Organization of the Stratum Corneum[8-9]

Initial perspective of the stratum corneum was based on histological images which depicted it as multilayered tissue with a "basket weave" appearance. Higher resolution electron microscope images, however, show that the barrier is quite a compact and highly organized structure composed of several layers of corneocytes with densely packed keratins and a loricrin-rich envelope surrounded by a continuous extracellular lipid matrix. A brick and mortar model is often used to describe the organization of the stratum corneum as a dual compartment system where the corneocytes are the bricks and the lipids the mortar or cement (Fig. 4).

One of the chief components of the stratum corneum are the corneocytes, flat polyhedral shaped, anucleated cells, primarily composed of intermediate filament networks. These are mainly made up of keratins and another protein, filaggrin. Keratins and filaggrin constitute as much as 80% of the proteins found in the stratum corneum. Filaggrin is initially expressed in the stratum granulosum as profilaggrin, a large histidine-rich and highly cationic phosphoprotein with large 37 kDa repeating domains. During the early stages of terminal differentiation, profilaggrin is processed into the mature form of the protein, filaggrin, which organizes the keratins into highly ordered and condensed arrays of filaments in the corneocytes of the lower stratum corneum. In this region, which is often referred to as the stratum compactum, the filamentous network in corneocytes is quite dense and plays a key role in collapsing the corneocytes into a flatter and compact shape—a characteristic feature which contributes to the mechanical properties of the stratum corneum.

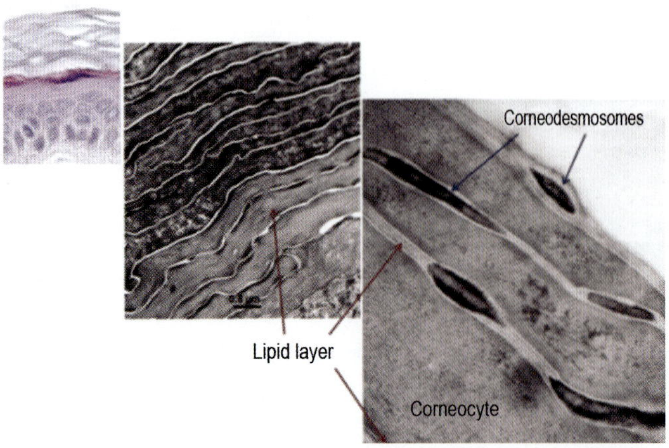

Figure 4: Electron micrograph of stratum corneum showing the arrangement of corneocytes and lipid layers. Each corneocyte is tethered to a neighboring Corneocytes via bridges called corneodesmosomes (dark structure on image on the right) *Courtesy:* AM Minondo, L'Oréal Research and Innovation

Each corneocyte is surrounded by a protein shell known as the cornified cell envelope which replaces the keratinocyte plasma membrane during cornification. It is approximately 10–15 nm thick, composed of an intricate network of highly cross-linked proteins including envoplakin, periplakin, involucrin, loricrin and small proline-rich proteins. The major protein of the cornified envelope is loricrin, an insoluble 38 kDa protein with a high content in serine and glycine amino acids. It accounts for as much as 70–85% of the cell envelope protein mass where it functions as the key structural reinforcement protein. The adhesion between loricrin and the other components of the cornified envelope and corneocyte cytoskeleton is reinforced by protein cross-linking, isopeptide bonds, catalyzed by specialized enzymes known as transglutaminases. As many as three of these enzymes, transglutaminases type 1, 3 and 5 are thought to be involved in the cross-linking of cornified envelope proteins. Their function is essential to the building of a functional stratum corneum barrier. This is evident in skin diseases which are characterized by very dry and flaky skin conditions due to loss of function mutations in the gene encoding transglutaminase 1. The whole construction of the cornified envelope is genetically orchestrated in a highly organized and controlled fashion. The proteins involved in this process are expressed one after another in time reflecting the arrangement of genes on chromosome one—known as the differentiation complex. Even transglutaminases appear to act in a timely fashion with transglutaminases 3 and 5 catalyzing in turn the formation of isopeptide bonds between the earlier expressed proteins in the complex while transglutaminase 1 cross-links the later expressed proteins, such as loricrin to the emerging envelope scaffold and keratins of the corneocyte cytoskeleton.

At the macroscopic level, two types of cornified envelope exist: (1) fragile envelopes which are irregularly shaped with a crumpled surface and which are predominantly found in the lower layers of the stratum corneum and (2) rigid envelopes which are polygonal in shape, showing a smooth flat surface, and of which about 80% are found in the superficial layers of the stratum corneum (Fig. 5). Corneocytes with rigid envelopes are considered to be mature. The ratio of rigid to fragile corneocytes can vary from one body site to another with more exposed sites, such as the face and the back of the hand displaying a higher percentage of fragile envelopes in the superficial layers. This observation suggests that external environmental factors, such as ultraviolet (UV) and humidity can influence the maturation of the cornified envelope.

In the epidermis the adhesion of keratinocytes is facilitated by junctions known as desmosomes. In the stratum corneum, corneodesmosomes are the adhesive bridges between neighboring corneocytes. These are large macromolecular complexes made up of several glycoproteins. The main ones are desmoglein and desmocollin, large cadherin like proteins which span the lipid enriched *sheets* between corneocytes and adhere to keratin filaments via a conglomerate of proteins—plakoglobins, desmoplakins and plakophilins. The whole complex is reinforced by cross-linking catalyzed by transglutaminases. Corneodesmosome composition is very similar to that of epidermal desmosomes but they are not identical. The difference is that corneodesmosomes contain an additional protein which is unique to the stratum corneum—corneodesmosin. This protein is secreted by lamellar bodies into the extracellular space in the upper levels of the stratum granulosum where it is associated with the desmosomal protein complex that converts desmosomes into their cornified layer cousins known as the corneodesmosomes. It is thought that corneodesmosin strengthens the structure of these complexes and protects them against proteolytic degradation in the stratum corneum. In fact, it is the controlled proteolysis of corneodesmosin itself which is a pivotal first step in the desquamation process, the exfoliation of corneocytes from the surface of the skin (Fig. 3).

Electron micrographs of the stratum corneum show an electron lucent layer, approximately 10 nm thick, that has been observed between the cornified envelope and the sheets of extracellular lipids. This is the cornified lipid envelope whose membrane-like structure is composed of omega-hydroxyceramides. These lipids possess very

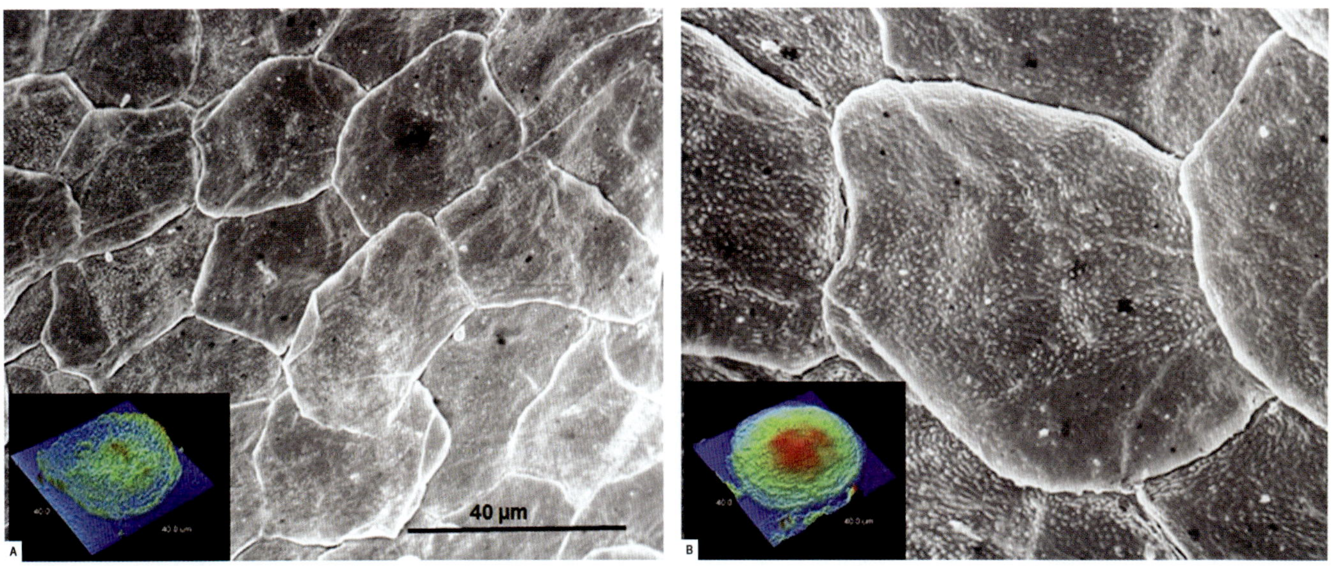

Figure 5: Scanning electron micrograph and atomic force microscopy (inserts) of corneocytes. **A,** Immature and **B,** Mature
Courtesy: Dr G Luengo, L'Oréal Research and Innovation

long chain fatty acids which are covalently bound to the cornified envelope via involucrin through ester links thought to be catalyzed by transglutaminases.

The extracellular spaces between corneocytes in the stratum corneum are filled with lipids—the so-called mortar between the bricks in the stratum corneum model described in the literature. This lipid matrix essentially consists of ceramides, cholesterol and fatty acids. All of the free fatty acids and those linked to ceramides are nonbranched structures and this characteristic allows the construction of a continuous and ordered tightly packed lipid layer. The loss of phospholipids is characteristic of the final step of keratinization. Since very few or no phospholipids are found in these lipid layers, in contrast to the plasma membranes found in the living epidermis, the stratum corneum lipid bilayers are less fluid and considerably less permeable than other biological membranes.

The precursors to the stratum corneum lipids are either synthesized or acquired in the stratum granulosum and stored in vesicles known as lamellar granules or Odland bodies. During the final stages of epidermal differentiation, lamellar granules, which account for approximately 10% of the cytosol in the stratum granulosum, fuse with the plasma membrane of keratinocytes releasing stacks of lipid lamellae into the surrounding extracellular matrix. The lipids are then processed into their mature forms by specialized enzymes which are also stored and secreted by lamellar granules. Phospholipids are metabolized by acid hydrolases while glucosylceramides are converted into ceramides by the enzyme β-glucocerebrosidase. Once the lipids are modified, they are arranged in ordered stacks of lamellar sheets. Ceramides and cholesterol form the lamellar phase of the lipid sheets while fatty acids play an important role in their lateral packing. The whole structure is held together and tethered to neighboring lipid sheets by a lipid that is unique to cornified epithelium—acyl glucosylated ceramide. This lipid contains a very long chain of essential fatty acid—linoleic acid. The length of the chain allows this specialized lipid to span the lipid bilayers and it inserts into neighboring sheets using the linoleate tail as a molecular rivet. The lipids exist either in a solid crystalline state or in a gel or liquid crystalline state. The lipids in the lower levels of the stratum corneum are mostly in a solid crystalline state and are tightly packed in an orthorhombic pattern resulting in an excellent barrier. In the upper layers, there is a transition to a more fluid gel state and the lipids are packed hexagonally resulting in a weaker barrier. Skin which is deficient in essential fatty acid has poor barrier function and increased transepidermal water loss (TEWL). The synthesis of lipid matrix, which accounts for approximately 20% of the stratum corneum volume, takes place continuously under physiological conditions. These intercellular lipids are crucial in the keratinization process and skin humidity.

Desquamation

Corneocyte exfoliation from the surface of the skin is the final step in the life cycle of a keratinocyte taking place some 28 days after its first migratory steps from the basal layer of the epidermis. In normal and healthy skin this process is essentially invisible as one layer of the stratum corneum is shed into the surrounding environment every day. However, if desquamation is impaired, such as in dry skin conditions, the corneocytes tend to clump and detach as clusters producing a visible rough skin texture.

Corneocyte desquamation is orchestrated by specific hydrolytic enzymes that progressively degrade the corneodesmosomal links between neighboring cells. In the upper layers of the stratum corneum, hydrolysis of cholesterol sulfate results in a more fluid lipid bilayer allowing proteolytic enzymes access to the corneodesmosomes. These are progressively degraded according to a time sequence of events involving a battery of glycosidases and serine/cysteine/aspartic proteases. The first step in the degradation process is believed to be removal of external glycans from corneodesmosomal proteins through the action of glycosidases. This opens the way to the concerted action of proteases, mainly the stratum corneum chymotryptic and tryptic enzymes (also known as kallikrein 7 and kallikrein 5, respectively), to degrade corneodesmosin, desmocollin and desmoglein—the key components of corneodesmosomes. Other proteases such as cathepsins L-2, D and E are all known to be involved in the desquamation process. The activity of all these proteases is strictly regulated by corresponding endogenous protease inhibitors which act to silence their corresponding protease. The whole process is dependent on physiological parameters such as pH and water content which are essential to invisible desquamation.

The Physiology of the Stratum Corneum

Many of the enzymes involved in the desquamation process and other key functions of the stratum corneum are pH dependent. A pH gradient exists across normal stratum corneum where pH level of 4.5–5 is commonly found in the outer layers up to around pH 7 in the deeper layers. The optimal pH for the activity of the stratum corneum chymotryptic and tryptic enzymes is 7 while a more acidic environment—pH 5—favors stratum corneum cysteine protease and cathepsin activity. The lipid processing enzymes involved in the lipid layer homeostasis are also pH dependent. Both lipid hydrolases, beta-glucocerebrosidase and acidic sphingomyelinase share acidic pH for optimal activity while other lipid enzymes such as steroid sulfatase preferably operate in a more neutral pH environment. The pH of the stratum corneum can also influence the way lipids are ordered in the bilayers with a more fluid pattern at the acidic pH found at the surface of the stratum corneum. In pathological conditions, such as dermatitis, the pH gradient is abolished with an increase in pH level to neutral in the upper layers of the stratum corneum. This results in inappropriate changes in activity of the key hydrolytic enzymes with disruptive consequences for desquamation and lipid organization. The importance of a pH gradient across the stratum corneum is also underlined by the fact that skin exposure to substances with an alkaline pH is known to deteriorate the performance of the barrier. Thus, the treatment of skin conditions, such as psoriasis, where the pH is neutral in the upper layers of the stratum corneum, with an acidic formulation might prove beneficial. The pH, therefore, is essential to the integrity and the cohesion of the stratum corneum. It also plays a vital role in another function of the stratum corneum, antimicrobial defense. Normal flora, such as the propionibacteria, flourishes best at acidic pH while pathogenic strains such as *Staphylococcus aureus* prefer a more neutral pH. Thus, it would be important to maintain an acidic environment in the upper layers of the stratum corneum to minimize infection by pathogenic bacteria. This is particularly true in newborns who have an increased risk of skin infection and with the onset of atopic skin condition, particularly during the first three months of life where the pH of the upper levels of the stratum corneum is neutral.

While it is clear that a pH gradient exists across the stratum corneum, the molecular basis for its generation and maintenance is less clear. It has been proposed that the free fatty acids produced through phospholipase activity are instrumental to the acidification of the barrier while the natural moisturizing factor urocanic acid may also be involved in the process.

The bivalent cation calcium is another important physiological factor in the homeostasis and maintenance of stratum corneum barrier function. In normal skin, a calcium gradient exists across the epidermis with the highest level of calcium ion found in the stratum granulosum and very low levels in the basal layer of the epidermis and in the outer layers of the stratum corneum. It is well known that calcium is a very important cofactor for epidermal differentiation and the correct function of transglutaminases which as described above, are crucial in the formation and maturation of the cornified envelope. Several of the enzymes involved in lipid synthesis such as glycosylceramide synthase are calcium dependent. Likewise, many of the cornified envelope proteins and filaggrin bind calcium suggesting that this ion plays an important role in their function and structural organization. The calcium gradient present in normal skin is disturbed in both psoriasis and atopic dermatitis (AD). In the latter disease, there is a notable increase in calcium level in the stratum corneum and stratum granulosum compared to the spinous and basal epidermal layers resulting in a steeper than normal gradient across the epidermis. Since calcium regulates enzymes that are key factors in the homeostasis of the epidermis and the stratum corneum, such disruption of the calcium gradient would have significant consequences for normal barrier function. It has been suggested that skin reacts to such changes by increasing the level of a specialized protein, the calmodulin skin like protein (CLSP) to mop up excess calcium and thereby restoring a normal gradient. In skin wounds, CLSP levels are particularly high along the wound edge. Once the wound has closed up and barrier function is restored, CLSP levels return to normal. Thus, CLSP acts as a biosensor of calcium and plays a pivotal role in restoring the barrier by reestablishing the normal calcium gradient through the modulation of calcium binding protein function. In acute AD, where the barrier function and calcium gradient are disturbed, there is a significant increase in CLSP levels. Thus, in this disease the protein could have an important role in regulating calcium gradient in the upper layers of the epidermis.

Functions of the Stratum Corneum

The stratum corneum has been long considered as a dead layer of cornified cells with a principal function as a barrier against TEWL and external aggressions. However, the use of modern research tools in molecular biology, such as proteomics, have demonstrated that the stratum corneum is far from being just a dead conglomerate of corneocytes but in fact, a tissue which is biologically very much alive with a plethora of important biochemical functions.

The stratum corneum acts as an important biological sensor for our skin endowed with the capacity to adapt rapidly to changes in the external environment. For example after prolonged exposure to a humid environment (greater than 80% relative humidity) the barrier function of the stratum corneum decreased. In contrast, following sustained exposure to low humidity level (less than 20% relative humidity), the barrier function is enhanced. Rapid changes between extreme hydration conditions results in decreased barrier function but, in time, the stratum will adapt to its new environment. The ideal relative humidity to maintain an optimally functional stratum corneum barrier is between 40% and 60%.

Skin barrier function can be impaired by single or prolonged exposure to irritant substances. The stratum corneum responds to such external stimuli by releasing a number of signaling molecules known as cytokines into the intercellular spaces. How these molecules are stored in the stratum corneum has yet to be fully elucidated, but once released, they migrate towards the epidermis to stimulate appropriate biological responses to restore normal barrier function. In recent years, thanks primarily to the application of proteomics, there has been an exponential increase in the identification of new bioactive molecules that reside in the stratum corneum. This has been very much the case in the discovery of the proteins and peptides that constitute cutaneous antimicrobial defense. It is an impressive arsenal of antimicrobial peptides, toll-like receptors, chemokines and proteases that make up the first line of defense in the skin's innate immune system. Keratinocytes express several families of antimicrobial peptides, β-defensins, cathelicidins and ribonucleases. RNase 7, a member of the latter family, is the most abundant antimicrobial peptide found in the stratum corneum and it possesses a very broad spectrum of antibacterial and antifungal activity. The importance of these antimicrobial peptides is underscored in skin diseases and wound healing. In AD, low levels of antimicrobial peptides are present in disease-affected, lesional skin resulting in a potentially high prevalence of *S. aureus* at these sites. By contrast, high levels of another antimicrobial peptide, psoriasin, and RNase 7 minimize the number of infections in psoriasis. High levels of antimicrobial peptides are also found in healing wounds decreasing once the wound has closed up.

The stratum corneum also has a role to play in photoprotection, particularly in darker colored skins. The main component that protects skin from UV-induced damage is the naturally occurring skin pigment, melanin. It is produced by melanocytes in the basal epidermis and packaged into melanosomes which are transferred to keratinocytes whereby the pigment is dispersed throughout the epidermis. In Caucasian and light skins, melanosomes are typically degraded in the spinosum layers of the epidermis. In darker skin types, however, melanosomes, which are larger in size and contain different melanin type with high photostability, persist unaltered in the upper layers of epidermis and their slow degradation results in the presence of melanin granules in the stratum corneum. Black skin is also known to contain a greater number of corneocyte layers in the stratum corneum than Caucasian skin thus providing a more cohesive and compact structure. It is possible that the stratum corneum has adapted in darker skins to act both as a natural filter of sunlight and scavenger of free radicals produced by reactive oxygen species (ROS). Urocanic acid, which is a component of natural moisturizing factor natural moisturizing factors (NMF) (see next section), is another potential natural UV-filter in the stratum corneum. The trans isoform of urocanic acid is a good absorber of UV radiation in the UVB range. However, on UV exposure it is converted to its cis-isomer, which induces immunosuppression in the skin. It is unclear whether the amount of trans-urocanic acid is sufficient to afford appreciable protection to skin against UV radiation but its presence in normal healthy stratum corneum suggests that this tissue contributes to some extent to natural defense against the harmful rays of the sun, except in light skin.

Hydration and Barrier Function[10-11]

One of the major functions of the stratum corneum is to act as a barrier to restrict the loss of water. It is such an effective barrier that even a small molecule such as water is not readily lost from the surface of normal skin. Generally, the stratum corneum barrier does not allow the passive penetration of molecules with a mass greater than 500 daltons. The stratum corneum water content, which can be as much as 25–30% in healthy skin, is very important for the stratum corneum to properly fulfill its barrier function. It is essential for optimal activity of enzymes involved in the maturation and desquamation of corneocytes since increased TEWL impairs their function resulting in dry skin. Mother nature has, therefore, devised several biological mechanisms in the stratum corneum to retain water. The stratum corneum lipids are packed and organized in lamellar sheets in a gel like fashion to provide a tight and semi permeable barrier to water. The dove and tail organization of corneocytes and their insoluble protein and lipid envelopes ensure that water must follow a tortuous route to reach the external world. The stratum corneum also produces hygroscopic molecules known as NMFs to aid water retention. The NMFs consist of amino acids, lactic acid and sugars. This mix has high water retention capacity and acts as a natural surface humectant. The major source of NMF amino acids comes from filaggrin which is hydrolyzed in the outer layers of the stratum corneum into free histidine, glutamine and arginine. These are subsequently deaminated into derivatives, pyrrolidone carboxylic acid and urocanic acid, which represent a major part of the functional osmotic material in the stratum corneum. The sugar content is likely to derive from the glycosaminoglycan, hyaluronan. This very large and highly anionic polysaccharide plays a major role in the hydration and lubrication of tissues in the human body. More than half the total body mass of hyaluronan is found in the skin. It is instrumental in both hydration and regulation of cell behavior in dermis and epidermis. Glycerol is often used as a prime moisturizer in cosmetic compositions tailored to treat dry skin. However, the skin actually produces its own glycerol to enhance the hydration of the stratum corneum. It is believed that endogenous glycerol originates from the hydrolysis of triglycerides in the sebaceous glands and its transport to the surface is facilitated by specialized membrane water channels known as aquaporins. The transport of another NMF component, urea to the surface of the skin is also believed to involve aquaporins.

Site Differences[12]

There are significant differences in the characteristics of the stratum corneum according to body location. The stratum corneum of facial skin is considerably thinner than that of the palms or of the sole of the foot. In the latter regions it is an extremely thick and tough tissue, while remaining soft and relatively smooth in normal conditions, adapted to withstand constant mechanical stress and friction. Unsurprisingly, these areas have a significantly greater number of corneocyte layers than facial areas.

Elsewhere, the stratum corneum of normal healthy skin is a smooth and soft membrane often no more than 30 μm thick. On the forehead and scalp, the stratum corneum is as much as two times more permeable than on other body sites such as trunk and limbs. Furthermore, on sites with a higher density of hair follicles like the face, scalp or upper back, allergens and irritants are more likely to penetrate the skin via pores or sweat ducts and thereby cause inflammatory responses. Thus, it would be important that any cosmetic product be tested on a small area of a subject's skin in order to assess its allergen or irritant potential before general application.

Transepidermal water loss also varies according to body site. TEWL measured on facial skin is much higher than on the scalp, forearm, upper arm, trunk and lower extremities. The nape and elbow areas unexpectedly show high TEWL values as do palmo-plantar regions despite their thick stratum corneum.

Typically, turnover takes about two weeks but on the face the process is believed to occur within a week. This is reflected in the phenotype of corneocytes isolated from facial sites which are much smaller in size than those from arms, legs or trunk. There is also a much higher rate of fragile cornified envelopes in the upper layers of facial stratum corneum as compared to other body sites and this is likely due to the higher stratum corneum turnover in this region. Plantar skin also shows a very high level of fragile corneocytes, as high as 90% compared to the reported 20% in the stratum corneum of the forearm. Such a high ratio of immature cornified envelopes is also characteristic of lesional skin of hyper proliferative skin disorders such as psoriasis and AD.

Ethnic Differences[13-20]

Data on racial differences in stratum corneum structure are rather conflicting. Many of the studies reported in the literature involve small patient populations and less-than-optimal study designs. Consequently, definitive conclusions cannot be drawn, and further research is warranted.

An early study by Weigand et al. investigated the cell layers and density of the stratum corneum in black and fair-skinned subjects through recording the number of tape strips necessary to completely remove the stratum corneum, microscopic observation, and measuring the air density in the stratum corneum. There was a greater variability in the amount of tape strips required to remove the stratum corneum in black subjects as compared to fair-skinned subjects, but this variability was not correlated with pigmentation. Microscopic visualization also demonstrated ethnic differences in the stratum corneum. Black subjects demonstrated greater air density in the stratum corneum; however, buoyant densities were similar between the two ethnic skin types. Because the average stratum corneum thickness was found similar between the two ethnic groups, it was concluded that black stratum corneum was more compact than white stratum corneum, perhaps reflecting greater intercellular cohesion.

Reed et al. compared the skin structure of subjects with skin types V and VI to those with lightly pigmented skin types II and III. The darkly pigmented subjects required more tape strippings to disrupt the epidermal barrier. The authors drew two conclusions from these data. First, darkly pigmented skin probably had more cornified cell layers, and therefore was more compact than lightly pigmented skin. Second, dark skin was thought to have superior epidermal barrier function. These data are of particularly interesting because the differences in cell layers and barrier protection were demonstrated to be related to the skin hue and skin phototype and not to ethnic type.

La Ruche and Cesarini, in a review of other authors' research, concluded that stratum corneum compactness and lipid content were greater in black skin as compared to white skin. Again, their conclusions were based on studies involving small patient populations.

Corcuff et al. examined corneocyte surface area, mean surface area and spontaneous desquamation in African-Americans, White Americans and Asians of Chinese extraction (18–25 subjects per group). There was no difference in corneocyte surface area between all three ethnic groups, and no difference in spontaneous corneocyte desquamation between the Chinese and white skin groups. However, spontaneous desquamation was increased in the black group compared with the white and Asian groups. These data appear contradictory to Weigand's findings. If black skin requires more tape strippings to remove the stratum corneum, then we would expect spontaneous desquamation to be less, not greater in black skin.

Johnson reported that black skin showed a trend toward possessing a thicker stratum corneum compared with white skin. However, other studies do not confirm such findings. Studies using various methods failed to demonstrate differences in stratum corneum thickness between black skin (of Africans, Australoids and African-Americans) and white skin (of Europeans and Americans).

Finally, other studies have suggested that there is a greater lipid content in black versus white stratum corneum. This could account for the greater density of black stratum corneum, a conclusion supported by Weigand et al. showing that when lipids were removed from stratum corneum samples extracted from both skin types, the specimens were of equal weight.

Neonatal Skin[21-22]

The development of the stratum corneum starts with the stratification of the epidermis in the uterus during the first trimester of pregnancy. At 32–34 weeks of gestation, the barrier becomes fully mature and is ready for the transition from the aqueous environment of the uterus to a dry external one. During the third trimester, fetal skin becomes coated by a biofilm called vernix caseosa which apparently is unique to humans. It is composed of corneocytes and a rich mix of lipids including ceramides, cholesterol, triglycerides, wax, sterol esters, squalene and phospholipids. It also contains a unique long chain ceramide containing branched fatty acids. Since these corneocytes are devoid of corneodesmosomal components and the lipids lack lamellar architecture, vernix caseosa is more fluid and permeable than the stratum corneum. It is also rich in antimicrobial peptides and contains as much as 80% water. Thus, vernix caseosa acts as a moisturizer as well as an antimicrobial biofilm and facilitates the adaptation of a newborn's stratum corneum to the external environment in the first hours and days after birth. Once this protective film is shed, the stratum corneum of the infant starts to adapt to its new environment. At birth, corneocyte morphology in the stratum corneum is similar throughout the body but during the first few weeks the barrier morphologically changes so that it provide the functional needs of each body site. Nonetheless, during the first year of life, the concentration of NMFs is significantly lower than that in adult skin and TEWL values remain high. The exception is the face and scalp where ample sebum excretion maintains adequate hydration of the stratum corneum. However, this hydrated condition of the face starts to decrease after a few months due to a decrease in sebum and surface lipids and thus the skin of infants often becomes dry in the long and cold winter months. Such a seasonal trend can occur every winter until a child reaches the age of puberty when sebaceous glands start to produce sebum in sufficient amounts to keep skin moisturized.

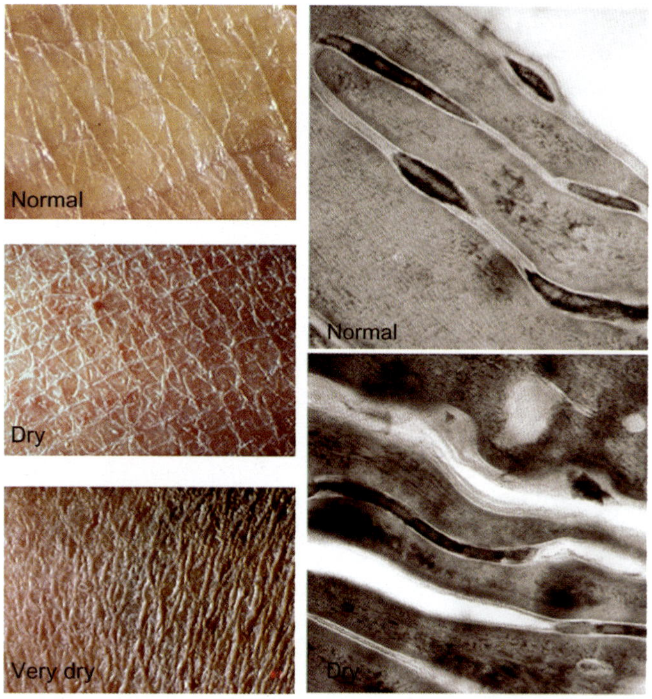

Figure 6: Images of the surface of normal, dry and very dry skin as observed by video microscopy. On right, transmission electron microscopic imaging of stratum corneum from normal and dry skin—in the latter, note the disorder in the lipid layers and the diffuse arrangement of corneodesmosomes
©L'Oréal Research and Innovation

STRATUM CORNEUM AND SKIN DISEASES[23-24]

Several well-known skin diseases are associated with defects in the stratum corneum barrier and affected patients often show a very dry and flaky skin phenotype (Figs 6 to 8).

Lamellar ichthyosis, which is characterized by a dramatically dry and scaly skin (Fig. 9) is caused by mutations in the gene for transglutaminase 1. The much reduced activity of this enzyme results in abnormal cornified envelope and organization of the lipid lamellae leading to significant alterations in barrier function and subsequent increase in TEWL. Bathing suit ichthyosis, a clinical form of congenital ichthyosis, is also characterized by pronounced scaling but only in areas covered by the bathing suit. This condition is not only due to reduced activity of transglutaminase 1 but also of transglutaminase 3 and cathepsin D, the aspartic protease which has an important role in desquamation process. Interestingly, the phenotype of this disease appears to be triggered by an increase in temperature under the bathing suit suggesting that this form of the disease is temperature sensitive. A scaly skin phenotype is also characteristic of another inherited disease, Vohwinkel's syndrome. Here, mutations in the gene for loricrin, the major cornified envelope protein, result in an attenuated barrier. Netherton syndrome, which is caused by mutations in the *SPINK5* gene encoding for an inhibitor (which is known as *LEKTI*) of the desquamation proteases kallikreins 5 and 7 is characterized by a thin stratum corneum, lack of cohesion between corneocytes and impaired barrier function. A less common form of this type of dermatological condition affecting barrier function is X-linked ichthyosis. This is an X-linked recessive disease producing fine scaly skin in males and originating from mutations in the steroid sulfatase gene which results in increased levels of cholesterol sulfate in the stratum corneum.

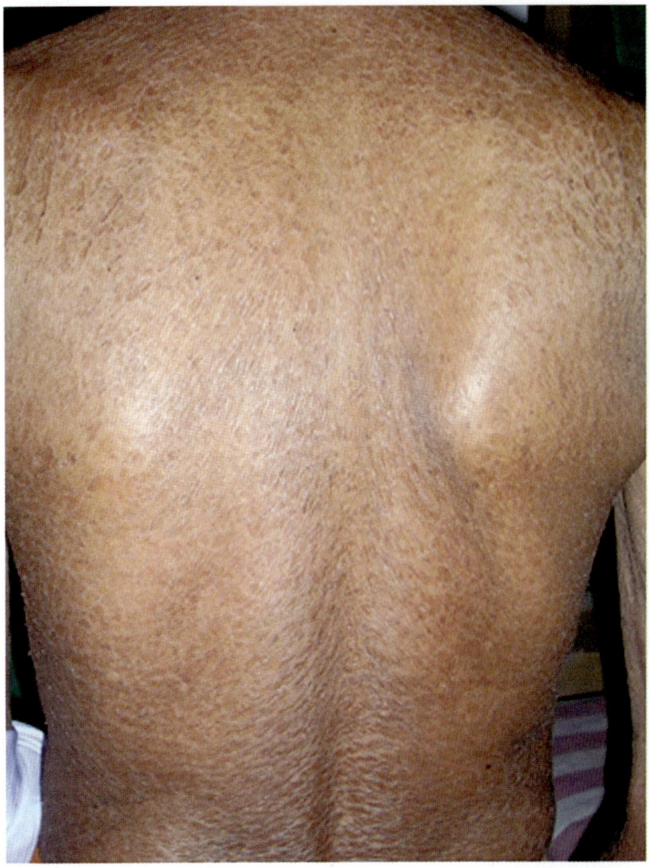

Figure 7: Xerosis of the back
Courtesy: Dr Reena Rai and Dr Muthuvel Kumaresan, Coimbatore, India

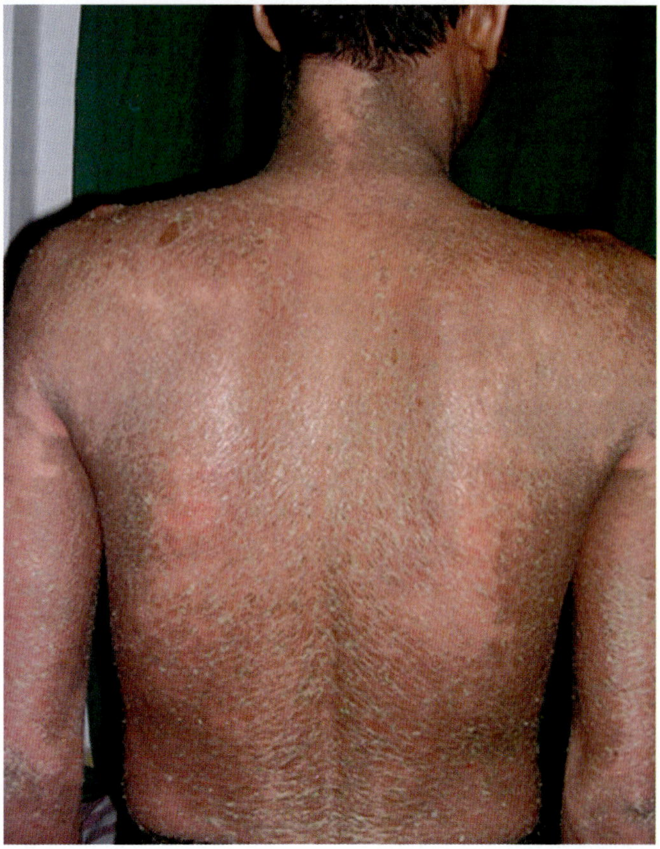

Figure 9: Large pigmented scales in a patient with lamellar icthyosis
Courtesy: Dr Reena Rai and Dr Muthuvel Kumaresan, Coimbatore, India

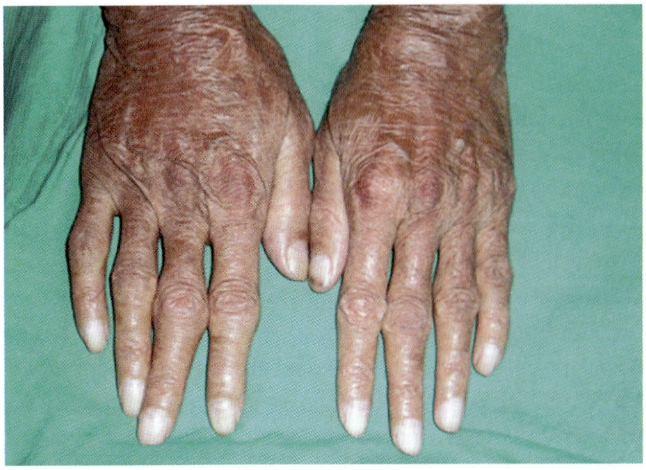

Figure 8: Large pigmented scales in the hands
Courtesy: Dr Reena Rai and Dr Muthuvel Kumaresan, Coimbatore, India

Disrupted barrier function is symptomatic of several other skin diseases. The most potentially severe is probably Gaucher's disease. Babies born with this disease have decreased levels of beta-glucocerebrosidase, a key enzyme in ceramide processing, and thus they have abnormal barrier function. A smaller number of these patients who have severe deficiencies of the enzyme develop a collodian membrane instead of a proper stratum corneum and often die during the neonatal period.

Recent research has shown that two of the most common heritable skin conditions, ichthyosis vulgaris (IV) and AD are due to loss of function mutations in the profilaggrin gene. IV, which occurs in one in 250 individuals, is characterized by abnormal or absent keratohyalin granules as well as a stratum granulosum devoid of filaggrin. The consequence is a disrupted barrier resulting in a dry and scaly skin. Deficiency in filaggrin is also a factor in as many as 50% of the patients with AD. It is becoming increasingly evident that the development of a defective stratum barrier is an early primary event in the genesis of AD leading to subsequent inflammatory events. Indeed, several scientific reports have described other key molecular changes that play a critical role in barrier dysfunction in AD such as elevated pH, altered proteolytic activity, altered levels of anti-microbial peptides, abnormal desquamation, impaired lamellar body function and decreased ceramide synthesis. All of these molecular and cellular changes conspire to form a defective stratum corneum barrier allowing easier access of allergens which initiate the inflammatory processes associated with AD. Thus, it is believed that therapies aimed at restoring normal barrier function could prove to be an excellent strategy to treat AD symptoms or even as measures to prevent the onset of the disease itself. The epidermis has an excellent capacity to rapidly restore stratum corneum barrier to its right condition. It has been shown that when the three keys stratum corneum lipids: (1) cholesterol, (2) fatty acids and (3) ceramides—are supplied in equal measure and they enhance the restoration of normal barrier function. Thus, compositions with optimized mixtures of these physiological lipids may prove efficient in the treatment of clinical dry skin conditions.

MOISTURIZERS[25-26]

A moisturizer is an agent designed to make the stratum corneum soft and more pliant by increasing hydration of dry skin resulting in smoother, more supple and healthier looking skin. There are four main classes of moisturizers: (1) occlusive agents, (2) humectants, (3) emollients and (4) rejuvenators. The moisturizing treatment involves a four-step process:

- Repairing the skin barrier
- Increasing water content
- Reducing TEWL
- Restoring water barrier function of lipids.

Occlusive Agents

Occlusive ingredients reduce TEWL by forming a hydrophobic layer on the surface of the skin providing an exogenous barrier to water loss. They prevent water evaporation from the skin and hence can be particularly effective when applied to already dampened skin. They are the most common type of moisturizers used in cosmetic formulations and are well tolerated among individuals. There is a wide range of agents with occlusive properties. Petrolatum, the occlusive prototype is most commonly used in skin care products, after water. Petrolatum helps restore the stratum corneum barrier by penetrating into its upper layers and initiating the production of intercellular lipids, including free sterols, sphingolipids and free fatty acids. Dimethicone is the second most common occlusive ingredient used in moisturizers today. Like petrolatum, it is hypoallergenic and noncomedogenic, and non-acnegenic. Limitations of occlusive agents are odor, potential allergenicity and greasy feel associated with most of them.

Humectants

Humectants increase the water content of skin by enhancing water retention from the dermis into the epidermis. All humectants have a hydroxyl group which attracts water. Humectants include hydroxy acids, propylene glycol, sorbitol, propylene glycol and urea. The most common humectant used in moisturizers is glycerol or glycerin. This hydroscopic compound is the most effective humectant and can also activate transglutaminase activity in the stratum corneum, accelerating the maturation of corneocytes and reducing scaling in xerotic skin. Glycerol also has some unique characteristics including its ability to produce moisturizing effects in the skin long after it is no longer present. Overall, when combined with occlusive agents, glycerol has the ability to produce significant moisturizing effects in the skin. Urea and alpha-hydroxy acids (AHA's), in addition to their humectant properties, are keratolytic. Urea is a humectant in lower concentrations (10%), but in higher concentrations (20–30%), it is mildly keratolytic through disrupting hydrogen bonds. AHA's, such as lactic acid or glycolic acid, appear to increase cohesion of the stratum corneum cells, thereby reducing roughness and scaling.

Emollients

Emollients smooth skin by filling spaces between skin flakes with droplets of oil, and are not usually occlusive unless applied heavily. When combined with an emulsifier, they may help hold oil and water in the stratum corneum. Examples of emollients include mineral oil, lanolin, fatty acids, cholesterol, squalene and structural lipids. Emollients vary according to their oil (lipid) to water ratio. In lotions, the lipid content is low whereas it is high in ointments (medium in creams). Emollients with high lipid content are greasier and stickier—they also make the skin shinier.

Rejuvenators

This class of moisturizers is intended to replenish essential proteins in skin. Collagen, keratin and elastin are skin proteins often found in rejuvenators. Since these proteins are relatively large, a considerable limitation to rejuvenators is their difficulty in penetrating the stratum corneum. Although rejuvenators may not be able to successfully replenish proteins in the dermis, they can have a role similar to emollients and improve skin appearance by creating a film that aesthetically smoothes the skin and stretches out and fills in fine lines.

CONCLUSION

The stratum corneum has been viewed, for some considerable time in textbooks, as a dead tissue, with the sole function of providing an excellent barrier to the diffusion of external and internal substances. However, research over the last twenty years or so has shown that the stratum corneum is not just an inert human shield but instead quite an active tissue from a metabolic point of view. It turns out to be very much alive, participating in a multitude of biological and biochemical functions essential to skin homeostasis. More recently, the stratum corneum barrier has been implicated in the pathogenesis of several atopies and diseases involving dry skin conditions. Thus, the stratum corneum presents a realistic therapeutic and accessible target for the medical and cosmetic treatment of xerosis and genetic disorders such as AD.

REFERENCES

1. Candi E, Schmidt, R, Melino G. The cornified envelope: a model of cell death in the skin. Nat Rev Mol Cell Biol. 2005;6:328-40.
2. Elias PM and Feingold KR eds. Skin Barrier. 1st ed. Informa Healthcare: New York, USA; 2006.
3. Elias P. Stratum Corneum Defensive Functions: An Integrated View. J Invest Dermatol. 2005;125:183-200.
4. Haake A, Scott GA, Holbrook KA. Structure and function of the skin: overview of the epidermis and dermis. In: Freinkel RK, Woodley DT, editors. The biology of the Skin. Parthenon Publishing: New York, USA; 2001.
5. Harding CR, Long S, Richardson J, Rogers J, Zhang Z, et al. The cornified cell envelope: an important marker of stratum corneum maturation in healthy and dry skin. Int J Cosmet Sci. 2003;25:157-67.
6. Marks R, Lévêque JL, Voegeli R. The essential Stratum Corneum. Martin Dunitz Ltd.: London, UK; 2002.
7. Masion K. Barrier function of the skin: "La raison d'être" of the epidermis. J Invest Dermatol. 2003;121:231-41.
8. Norlén L, Al-Amoudi A. Stratum Corneum Keratin Structure, Function and Formation: The Cubic Rod-Packing and Membrane Templating Model. J Invest Dermatol. 2004;123:715-32.
9. McGrath JA, Uitto J. The filaggrin story: novel insights into skin barrier function and disease. Trends Mol Med. 2008;14:20-7.
10. Rawlings AV and Leyden JJ. Skin Mosturization. 2nd ed. Informa Healthcare: New York, USA; 2009.
11. Rawlings AV, Matts PJ. Stratum corneum moisturization at the molecular level: an update in relation to the dry skin cycle. J Invest Dermatol. 2005;124:1099-110.
12. Tagami H. Location-related differences in structure and function of the stratum corneum with special emphasis on those of the facial skin. Int J Cosmet Sci. 2008;30:413-34.
13. Weigand DA, Haygood C, Gaylor JR. Cell layers and density of Negro and Caucasian stratum corneum. J Invest Dermatol. 1974;62:563-8
14. Reed JT, Ghadially R, Elias PM. Skin type, but neither race nor gender, influence epidermal permeability barrier function. Arch Dermatol. 1995;131:1134-8.
15. La Ruche G, Cesarini JP. Histology and physiology of black skin. Ann Dermatol Venereol. 1992;119:567-74.
16. Corcuff P, Lotte C, Rougier A, Maibach HI. Racial differences in corneocytes. A comparison between black, white and oriental skin. Acta Derm Venereol. 1991;71:146-8.
17. Johnson LC, Corah NL: Racial differences in skin resistance. Science. 1960;139:766-7.
18. Rawlings AV. Ethnic skin types: are there differences in skin structure and function? Int J Cosmet Sci. 2006;28:79-93.
19. Taylor SC. Skin of color: Biology, structure, function, and implications for dermatologic disease. J Am Acad Dermatol. 2002; 46:S41-S62.
20. Man MQ, Xin SJ, Song SP, Cho SY, Zhang XJ, et al. Variation of skin surface pH, sebum content and stratum corneum hydration with age and gender in a large Chinese population. Skin Pharmacol Physiol. 2009;22:190-9.
21. Hoath SB, Pickens WL, Visscher MO. The biology of vernix caseosa. Int J Cosmet Sci. 2006;28:319-333.
22. Nikolovski J, Stamatas GN, Kollias N, Wiegand BC. Barrier function and water-holding and transport properties of infant stratum corneum are different from adult and continue to develop through the first year of life. J Invest Dermatol. 2008;128:1728-36.
23. Cork MJ, Danby SG, Vasilopoulos Y, Hadgraft J, Lane ME, et al. Epidermal barrier dysfunction in atopic dermatitis. J Invest Dermatol. 2009;129:1892-908.
24. Schmuth M, Gruber R, Elias PM, Williams ML. Ichthyosis Update: Towards a function-driven model of pathogenesis of the disorders of cornification and the role of corneocyte proteins in these disorders. Adv Dermatol. 2007;23:231-56.
25. Loden M. The clinical benefit of moisturizers. J Eur Acad Dermatol Venereol. 2005;19:672-88
26. Nolan K, Marmur E. Moisturizers: reality and the skin benefits. Dermatol Ther. 2012;25:229-33.

Chapter 9

Sensitive Skin

Roland Jourdain, *L'Oréal Research and Innovation, Aulnay-sous-bois, France*
Frédéric Amaral, *L'Oréal Research and Innovation, Aulnay-sous-bois, France*
Arun C Inamadar, *SBMP Medical College, BLDE University, Bijapur, India*
Kiran Godse, *D.Y. Patil Medical College and Hospital, Nerul, Navi Mumbai, India*

INTRODUCTION

Sensitive skin is an extremely common topic among cosmetics consumers and professionals, although this syndrome lacks a clear consensual definition. Subjects with sensitive skin complain about more or less severe discomfort sensations after topical applications or when confronted with certain environmental factors. Very often, these subjective complaints especially occuring on the face do not express clinical signs. Epidemiological surveys have shown that this syndrome is very common worldwide and concerns all ethnicities. Some experimental results have evidenced of its clinical reality. Although common and matters of many publications, sensitive skin remains a very challenging issue. This self-declared condition without evident clinical traits is hard to diagnose and quantify, little being known about its pathophysiology. These different points explain how difficult the challenge is for the dermatologist to well manage individuals with sensitive skin and for cosmetic industry to develop suitable products. This chapter aims at reviewing the comprehensive facts established on that syndrome and the challenges to be overcome by scientific and dermatological communities on such complex skin condition.

GENERAL DEFINITION

Well described by Thiers in 1962,[1] sensitive skin is currently a highly common condition for cosmetics consumers and professionals. No one knows who first used the term "sensitive skin" to describe persons who have disagreeable reactions to drugs, cosmetics and toiletries that are in fact well tolerated by most consumers.[2] Sensitive skin was the subject of a comprehensive textbook edited in 2006 by Berardesca, Fluhr and Maibach[3] and of a number of papers written worldwide. Despite such abundant publications, finding a consensual definition of sensitive skin is a hard task. For example, the definition varies with chapters in the previous quoted textbook. It seems likely easier to describe what sensitive skin is and/or what it is not rather than define it with words. Sensitive skin subjects have been recently described as people complaining of severe sensations of discomfort such as burning, stinging or itching after application of cosmetics or toiletries, such as sunscreens and soaps without any clinical stigmata of scaling, induration and/or erythema that would be expected in known inflammatory or allergic processes.[4] Beyond these purely subjective symptoms, some authors include in the scope of sensitive skin some visible signs such as erythema and scaling.[5,6] Some others consider physical environmental factors such as ultraviolet (UV) light, heat, cold and wind as triggering factors as relevant as cosmetics or toiletries.[5-7] Others simply consider them as a possible source of worsening of that skin condition[8] or as a useless source of increased complexity.[2] The common theme of all definitions recently published is the discomfort reported by sensitive skin subjects. As previously seen, controversies still exist on whether sensitive skin is confined to reactions to cosmetics and whether visible findings such as erythema and scaling are an integral part of the syndrome.[9] The complexity of the debates and the difficulty in comparing the published findings also arise from the terminology used to nominate sensitive skin. Different synonyms have been used for sensitive: reactive, hyper-reactive, intolerant or irritable. Other terms perhaps more accurate for this self-perceived entity have been proposed, such as subjective, neurosensory, chemosensory or psychophysical irritation[2] making all these different definitions/denominations a great source of misunderstanding between authors. For instance, the use of "irritable" or "irritation" might suggest that sensitive skin is similar to irritant contact dermatitis. Sensitive skin syndrome deserves to be clearly defined albeit, for the time being, such a definition is elusive since the frontiers of sensitive are fuzzy.

CLINICAL FEATURES

The content of this paragraph and of some following greatly depends upon the definition accepted for sensitive skin. For instance, taking erythema as a visible manifestation and climatic factors as causes is meaningless if we consider relevant the definition limited to cosmetics and to purely invisible subjective signs. In the absence of a consensus to date, we chose to consider a larger view of sensitive skin by including in its scope both visible signs and triggering factors other than cosmetics.

Symptoms

Sensitive skin is characterized by subjective, sensorial signs, such as stinging, burning and itching sensations on a seemingly normal looking skin. Other possible sensations are tightness and dryness. Signs of sensitive skin are not continuous but often triggered by various factors often of chemical nature (drugs, cosmetics, toiletries). Generally, the symptoms that may be severe and painful, appear quickly after the skin stimulation and disappear in a few minutes. Sensitive skin merely concerns the face because of its dense nervous network and its great exposure to triggering factors whatever their nature (cosmetics or physical factors). Indeed, the face is the main target for cosmetic routines and is constantly exposed to the various assaults from the environment. Nevertheless, not limited to the face, sensitive skin symptoms can also arise on other locations, such as hands or the scalp.[10,11] Albeit these unpleasant cutaneous signs tend to quickly disappear, this condition can impair the quality of life.[7]

Visible signs, such as erythema or flaking are far from being systematically present. For example, Groot reported that subjective irritation without any visible signs represented 50% of the adverse reactions to cosmetics.[12] Indeed, a detailed study assessing irritancy of soaps showed that panelists reported feeling of dryness several washing cycles before observable signs of dryness.[13] It is unknown whether this result obtained with the feeling of dryness would be strictly identical to discomfort sensations, such as stinging, burning or itching. If such is the case, this would indicate the necessity to fully focus upon subjective sensations more than on visible signs to thoroughly assess the safety of a new formulation. Indeed, invisible signs are perhaps preliminary signs of irritation but they are keys to determine whether the consumer will continue to use the product.

Triggering Factors

There is a consensus among scientists and professionals for considering topical drugs, cosmetics, and toiletries as major triggering factors of sensitive skin symptoms. Uncomfortable skin reactivity to cosmetics was even at the origin of its first description.[1] The concept gained substance in the 1970s with the observation that some individuals using a sunscreen containing a derivative of para-aminobenzoic acid (PABA) complained of stinging reactions despite the fact that this ingredient had shown no evidence of toxicity in previous safety evaluations.[14] Since then, other compounds have been identified as discomfort inducers, such as benzoyl peroxide, tretinoin (all-trans retinoic acid), glycolic acid and some volatile alcohols. In the late 1990s, the class of chemicals most likely troublesome to sensitive skin consumers was that of surfactants.[15] The uncomfortable sensations with no visible signs were fairly common and represented 50% of the adverse reactions to cosmetics and toiletries reported some years ago.[12] This subjective reactivity to cosmetics often makes difficult for people with sensitive skin to use cosmetic products, having even troubles in seeking products that they can possibly use, i.e. not generating discomfort sensations. Such cosmetic intolerance syndrome is generally limited to one or several products easily recognizable by the consumer. This subjective reactivity to cosmetics, however, can extend to an extreme state called status cosmeticus in which the subject gradually becomes completely intolerant to any cosmetic product.[4] Consequently, since aware of such problem, cosmetic manufacturers have tried to develop formulations without ingredients likely prone to induce uncomfortable sensations.[16] Products labeled for sensitive skins have met with a growing success. For instance, by around 2000, these products were purchased by 80% of self-assessed sensitive skin subjects and by 25% of those with nonsensitive skin.[17]

The diversity of triggering factors beyond topical drugs, cosmetics and toiletries was soon described by Johnson and Page.[18] When asking consumers what they believed was triggering their manifestations, a list of more than 20 factors was obtained that could be divided into four categories: intrinsic (age, hormones, heredity), environmental (sun, cold, pollution), product use (soaps, fragrances, cosmetics) and lifestyle (diet, stress). These items have been used to build questionnaires increasingly relevant for collecting data about the possible causes other than chemical. Epidemiological surveys have confirmed the existence of these different factors.[5-7,19,20] Among the other factors, environmental factors seem of great importance. For instance, some surveys have revealed the existence of subgroups of sensitive skin individuals more sensitive to environment than to cosmetics.[14,21] Although the reaction to topically applied products is the more accepted and consensual triggering factor, it is not the more frequent. A recent French survey has showed the incidence of the following triggering factors: cold (66%), stress (61%), sun exposure (51%), soaps (42%), wind (42%), swimming-pool water (40%), variations of temperature (38%), shower water (29%), heat (28%), friction from clothes (28%), cosmetics (28%), menstruation (24%), sweating (23%), pollution (18%), food (15%) and dermatological drugs (11%).[10] In the view of these incidences of skin reactivity to environment, cosmetic industry has tried to enlarge its product lines to also alleviate these sensitive skins by developing soothing ingredients.

Diathesis Factors

Thiers has first suggested that diathesis features could explain this syndrome.[1] Recent epidemiological data have confirmed the link between sensitive skin and some clinical features. In these surveys, the interviewees who declared that they had dry, oily or combination skin also reported a more frequent incidence of sensitive skin than those with normal skin.[5-7] The findings regarding the link with phototype are more divergent. Some authors have reported a link with fair phototype,[6,7] a fact not observed by others.[20] Sensitive skin subjects also more frequently report current skin disorder. A Japanese survey has recently confirmed the link between sensitive skin and an atopic diathesis previously reported in the UK.[6,19] In the UK survey, however, only 49% of the sensitive skin population presented an atopic diathesis. Hence, all sensitive skins should not be considered as atopic skins.

EPIDEMIOLOGY

Since the first epidemiological findings,[2,18] a lot of studies were conducted to establish the prevalence of self-reported sensitive skin in different geographic areas worldwide. Now relevant data are available with regard to Europe, USA, Japan and China although data from India is still lacking. Some findings are also expected soon from Brazil and Russia.[6] These different locations represent variably mature cosmetic markets. The methodologies used until now to question large cohorts of subjects varied: sending of sensitive skin self-assessment questionnaires by mail,[19] phone surveys[6,7,20,22] or face-to-face interviews at home.[5] Their objective often differed. Some concerned only one gender, the majority of these studies considered both genders. Some studies aimed at establishing the prevalence of sensitive skin in a determined and restricted area. For instance, one survey was conducted within a 10-mile radius of High Wycombe (Buckinghamshire, UK)[19] and another in San Francisco Bay (California, USA).[20] Conversely, a recent survey concerned three different Chinese megalopolises (Beijing, Shanghai, Guangzhou) located in very different climatic and latitude regions.[5] Comparably, a recent American study was conducted on about 1000 subjects chosen by the quota method. This representative sample of the American population gathered people from both genders, different ethnic backgrounds, living in varying regions (East, Central, West, Mountain) and areas of residence (urban, suburban, rural).[7] The way to question subjects about their self-reported sensitive skin also varied between the different surveys. For example, in the San Francisco Bay study,[20] subjects were asked to express whether they "strongly agree", "somewhat agree", "somewhat disagree" or "strongly disagree" with the sentence: "I have a sensitive facial skin". In other studies, the responses to the question "Do you have sensitive skin?" were recorded through a 4-point scale: very sensitive, sensitive, slightly sensitive, not sensitive at all[7] or very sensitive, rather sensitive, not very sensitive, not sensitive.[6] Even though modalities are finally gathered during the data analysis to constitute only two groups (sensitive and not sensitive skins), this number of modalities accounts for the continuous nature of this skin disorder. All the questionnaires used for these surveys contain questions relating to the objective and subjective symptoms and the possible triggering factors. But there again, the questionnaires also slightly differ on these topics. As it is hard to estimate the impact of how the subjects are asked, it seems important to deeply harmonize the wording of the questions to make possible pertinent comparisons. It has been recently implemented for a survey in China by using the questionnaire of a previous study in the UK.[5]

Despite the varying methods and the used questionnaires, these different surveys afforded a general view of the sensitive skin prevalence. Although initially believed to be an abnormal reaction to common products occurring in only some consumers, all epidemiological surveys indicated an amazing prevalence of sensitive skin in the industrialized countries.[23] Indeed, Willis et al. reported a sensitive skin incidence of 51% in the women and of 38% in the men among 2,058 persons questioned in the UK.[19] Still in Europe, 38.4% of 4,506 interviewees in eight European countries (Belgium, France, Greece, Germany, Italy, Portugal, Spain and Switzerland) reported having a "sensitive" or "very sensitive" skin. The incidence ranged from 25.8% in Belgium to 53.8% in Italy.[22] In the San Francisco area, the prevalence in four ethnic groups of women (African-American, Asian, Euro-American and Hispanic) was found as 52% without significant difference between the different groups.[20] In a recent study in Japan, the overall incidence was around 54%.[6] Overall, the incidence of sensitive skin in developed countries often concerns more than 50% of the population especially in women. This incidence seems to have increased recently as suggested by a US survey in 2006 on more than 1000 subjects indicating that about one-third of the total population perceived that their skin was getting more sensitive.[24] A recent study performed on 9,154 subjects in China seems to indicate a somewhat different picture, the mean prevalence being 8.6% in men and 15.9% in women. The authors explained this lower incidence by the fact that "sensitive skin" was a new term and known to the Chinese population since recent years only.[5] For example, 9.4% of participants who were prickling after using cosmetics did not consider themselves as having a sensitive skin. This study also highlighted the higher prevalence in women. This almost recurrent finding[7,19,21-23] has been recently challenged by a survey in Japan which failed at significantly differentiating women (56%) from men (52.8%) in terms of sensitive skin incidence.[6] The authors proposed as a possible explanation that the Japanese population is highly aware of that skin condition and that this awareness is not restricted to a given gender. This explanation could also be relevant for an American survey showing no gender difference.[25] This difference of awareness could also explain the higher incidence in younger respondents seen in some studies,[5,6] but not confirmed by others.[7,25] In a Chinese survey, it was observed that the prevalence of sensitive skin gradually decreased with age, from 19.3% in women less than 25 years old to 11.8% in women more than 50 years old, such difference being also found in male population.[5] The authors explained these differences by a possible lower level of awareness of sensitive skin by the older respondents. The differences due to age and gender possibly decrease in concert with increased advertising of sensitive skin products marketed to men and older people. Beyond the information on sensitive skin incidence and its possible link with gender and age, epidemiological surveys are important since affording a list of possible objective and subjective symptoms and of the different triggering factors (topical applications, environmental or cultural factors). They have also been used to assess possible links with skin type, phototype and other skin conditions, and to study all the anatomical skin areas possibly affected (face, hands and scalp).[11,21,26,27] These epidemiological surveys are essential tools to quantify and qualify what sensitive skin is for the consumers and to better understand their expectations in terms of cosmetic products.

PATHOPHYSIOLOGY

The etiology of sensitive skin is poorly known and understood. There is a decrease in the "tolerance threshold" of the skin without any immune or allergic mechanism.[10] The condition is generally thought being mainly linked to heightened neurosensory input and/or diminished barrier. Understanding these factors is helpful in identifying the pathophysiology (Fig. 1) of varied presentations of sensitive skin.[21,23,27]

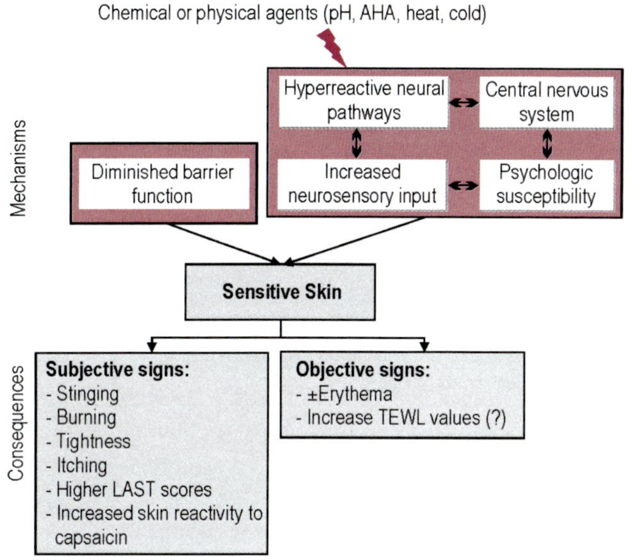

Figure 1: Schematic representation of the pathophysiology of sensitive skin

Abbreviations: AHA, alpha-hydroxy acid; TEWL, transepidermal water loss; LAST, lactic acid stinging test.

Neural Basis

Sensitive skin expresses itself by a variety of discomfort signs (stinging, burning, itching and tingling) associated or not with erythema and scaling.[28] These unpleasant sensations are, at least partly, mediated by unmyelinated C-fibers. These nerve endings are equipped with sensory receptors activated by different chemical or physical agents (pH, capsaicin, heat and cold). Some of these receptors are also present and functional on keratinocytes which play a more and more evidenced role in skin surface perception.[29,30] This repertoire of varied receptors is certainly the physiological support to the great diversity of triggering factors linked to sensitive skin. People with sensitive skin react more strongly to a determined stimulus than people with nonsensitive skin or react to lower stimuli. This property has been taken into account to develop psychophysical tests dedicated to diagnose people with sensitive skin. Some of them detailed later on in this chapter use chemicals able to induce discomfort sensations, such as lactic acid and capsaicin. Capsaicin is a natural agonist of transient receptor potential vanilloid 1 (TRPV1) expressed on keratinocytes and nerve fibers. Subjects with sensitive skin detect lower concentrations of topically applied capsaicin. This observation clearly indicated that the peripheral activation of neuroreceptors such as TRPV1 was linked to sensitive skin condition.[31]

The sensations of pain, which are the hallmark of this condition, also implied possible integration dysfunctions in the central nervous system (CNS). The possible involvement of CNS has been investigated by measuring cerebral responses to lactic acid stinging test. According to their answers to a self-assessment questionnaire, subjects were divided into two balanced groups: severe self-perceived sensitive skin and non-self-perceived sensitive skin. Inclusion criteria involved absence of any dermatological, neurological or vascular condition affecting the face. Event-related functional magnetic resonance imaging (fMRI) was used to measure cerebral activation induced by split-face application of lactic acid and its vehicle (control). In sensitive skin subjects, prefrontal and cingulate activity was significantly higher demonstrating a CNS involvement in sensitive skin physiologic pathway. This study highly contributed to give evidence of the clinical reality of this syndrome.[21,32]

As seen above, there is a clear evidence of implication of the peripheral and central nervous system in that skin condition, although through an unknown mechanism. To date, little is known about a possible alteration or changes in cutaneous nerve endings density, about a possible difference in the repertoire of neuroreceptors in terms of number, distribution or functionality.

Skin Barrier Function

As a high basal transepidermal water loss (TEWL) predicts susceptibility to sodium lauryl sulfate-induced irritation in normal skin,[33] some researchers attempted to understand whether such alteration in barrier function could predict sensitive skin condition, a simple and logical question. A weak barrier should inadequately protect nerve endings and facilitate access of molecules able to induce discomfort sensations. Variable and significant alterations in barrier function in sensitive skin subjects have been observed. A study on 10 sensitive skin women (self-reported sensitive skin and responder to lactic acid stinging test) found a significant TEWL increase on cheekbones as compared to a nonsensitive control group. The other facial areas (forehead, paranasal, lateral cheek, oral commissure and chin) showed an increased TEWL but the difference was not significant.[34] A similar study performed on 26 female volunteers with self-reported sensitive skin showed a trend toward an increased TEWL on the cheek as compared to 26 age-matched nonsensitive women.[35] However, a more recent study on 50 volunteers classified as sensitive skin or not according to their self-assessment did not confirm such finding.[36] In total, how can we understand these conflicting data? Since detailed information about classifying subjects in terms of sensitive skin is sometimes missing, comparison of panels remains a difficult task. For instance, there is no precise reported information about the respective degrees of skin reactivity to environmental factors and to topically applied products, items of great importance. In fact, an alteration of barrier function certainly favors the penetration of molecules toward nerve endings more than physical or environmental parameters, such as temperature and wind. The differences described above are perhaps due to the differences of tested subjects in terms of skin reactivity to factors other than chemical ones.

DIAGNOSIS

The ability to identify sensitive skin is of paramount importance both to dermatologists and to cosmetics companies. In fact, since the sensitive skin population is the target for products dedicated to this skin condition, it is obviously more relevant to test them especially for safety purpose on subjects with clear sensitive skin attributes. The real question is how to well diagnose sensitive skin.[37] The diagnosis of sensitive skin is a challenging and problematic issue, considering the lack of consensual definition and objective assessments for evaluating major symptoms such as stinging, burning and itch and the variability of clinical manifestations. Consequently, diagnosis mostly relies upon the way subjects report to feel sensations[27,38] through questionnaires or during a provocative test such as lactic acid stinging test. Of course, diagnosing sensitive skin should start by a thorough clinical examination to eliminate obvious as well as more subtle atypical dermatoses such as eczema, atopic dermatitis and rosacea which could be mistaken as sensitive skin.[4]

Table 1: A modified survey questionnaire which can be used in an Indian scenario

Nb	*Question*	*Response*
1	How do you describe your skin?	Oily/dry/normal
2	Is your facial skin easily irritated?	Yes/No
3	Have you experienced an adverse reaction to a cosmetic product?	Yes/No
4	Do some cosmetic products make your skin burn or irritated?	Yes/No
5	Do some cosmetic products make your skin itch within 30 minutes?	Yes/No
6	Do some cosmetic products make your skin sting within 30 minutes?	Yes/No
7	Have you suffered an adverse reaction to any cosmetic product in the last 12 months?	Yes/No
8	Have you ever suffered from eczema or dermatitis?	Yes/No
9	Do you regard yourself as having a sensitive scalp?	Yes/No
10	Do you suffer from eczema or dermatitis at this moment?	Yes/No
11	Do some hair products make your scalp itch, sting or smart?	Yes/No
12	Did you suffer from eczema or dermatitis as a child?	Yes/No
13	Have you ever suffered from asthma or hay fever?	Yes/No
14	Do you blush or flush easily?	Yes/No
15	Do you tend to suffer from dandruff?	Yes/No
16	Is your skin sensitive to environmental factors? a. Variation in temperature b. Pollution c. Air conditioning d. Water	 Yes/No Yes/No Yes/No Yes/No
17	Is your skin sensitive to climatic factors? a. Cold b. Heat c. Wind d. Dry air e. Wet air/humid air	 Yes/No Yes/No Yes/No Yes/No Yes/No

Questionnaires

Initially, studies dealing with sensitive skin used open questionnaires to collect as exhaustive as possible information on self-perception of sensitive skin. People were asked to describe what they felt, in what circumstance with their own words. All this information was then gathered to establish questionnaires used as appropriate methods for conducting epidemiological studies on sensitive skin condition worldwide. For example, a modified survey questionnaire which can be used in an Indian scenario is presented in Table 1.

These questionnaires which allow mathematical treatment of collected information are relevant when used to obtain epidemiological data by comparing large groups of subjects. At individual level, self-assessment through a questionnaire, whatever its relevance, is not always a good way for classifying the skin as sensitive or nonsensitive because the meaning of sensitive skin is quite individual for any given subject. Indeed, for the time being, no questionnaire has been validated as a diagnosis tool perfectly relevant by itself. To select people with sensitive skin, it is generally recommended to add to the self-reported sensitive skin statement a positive result to a relevant psychophysical test.

Psychophysical Tests

Psychophysical tests are designed to investigate the heightened neurosensory aspects of the sensitive skin. They rely upon the induction of discomfort sensations similar to those characterizing sensitive skin most often by a chemical applied to the skin. Assessment of the sensation is performed by the subjects themselves. Most common site of test is nasolabial fold, a facial site richly innervated with sensory fibers, followed by cheek and forearm. Seasonal influence can be observed as a more intense stinging response in winter than summer, probably due to the cumulative effect of heightened neurosensory input combined with defective barrier function possibly associated with the winter xerosis.[39]

Lactic Acid Stinging Test

This test, initially proposed in 1977, relies upon the intensity of stinging sensations induced by a lactic acid solution applied to the nasolabial folds. This test can be performed by two different methods.[28,40] In the first method, the subjects first undergo a facial sauna treatment for 5–15 minutes or are conditioned to a state of profuse sweating in an environmental chamber at 110°F and 80% relative humidity. An aqueous 5% lactic acid solution is applied with a cotton swab to the test site later to see the response. In the second method, a 10% aqueous solution of lactic acid at room temperature is rubbed with a cotton swab on the test site. Inert substance, such as saline solution, is applied to the contralateral test site, used as control. Stinging experience is rated on a 4-point scale by patient at 2.5, 5 and 8 minutes post application. Subjects with scores equal to or above 3 are considered as stingers. This very simple test is very popular and largely performed by cosmetic manufacturers for the selection of "stingers". This selected population prone to experience neurosensory problems with topical products is asked to test new products to substantiate claims indicating that they are appropriate for sensitive skin. Although very useful for product safety, the lactic acid stinging test does not fully render the complexity of self-assessed sensitive skin, as illustrated by the discrepancy between acid lactic response and self-perception of sensitive skin.[35] In the year 2000, this difference was taken into account for the recommendation to include "stingers" with a concomitant self-declared sensitive skin as panelists for safety testing.[17] Lactic acid stinging test is based on the reported sensations by the subject in terms of nature and intensity and has thus raised controversies owing to the use of a subjective individual pain scale. Indeed, there is no agreed scale for quantifying the intensity of the sensory response experienced.[9] A new test with capsaicin has been recently proposed to overcome this bias, as expressed below.

Capsaicin Detection Threshold Test

This test was designed to measure the cutaneous neurosensitivity with a greater accuracy because it does not rely on the quantification of the intensity of the response. It is based on the determination of individual detection thresholds of topically applied capsaicin. Five capsaicin concentrations are used in 10% ethanol aqueous solution ($3.16 \times 10^{-5}\%$; $1 \times 10^{-4}\%$; $3.16 \times 10^{-4}\%$; $1 \times 10^{-3}\%$; $3.16 \times 10^{-3}\%$). The method used to attain the detection threshold consists in applying increasing concentrations of capsaicin to the nasolabial folds. The vehicle is simultaneously applied following a split-face, single-blind plan. The test is stopped as soon as the subject reports a specific sensation on the capsaicin side. The test allows the classification of the test population according to six threshold levels corresponding to the sensitive reaction to one of the five capsaicin concentrations and to the absence of sensitivity to the highest concentration. This new test of skin neurosensitivity is easy, quick and truly painless. It appears to be a promising tool for the cosmetic diagnosis of sensitive skin.[31] It was used to explore the controversial issue of ethnic variations in sensitive skin in 144 American women of three ethnicities: Asian, African and Caucasian. Each ethnic group was split into six subgroups according to the threshold levels of sensitivity to capsaicin. Asian women tended to have higher capsaicin detection thresholds than Caucasians, but lower thresholds than Africans. Nevertheless, the differences according to ethnic background appeared minimal.[41]

Noninvasive Biophysical Instruments

Many studies aimed at objectively diagnosing sensitive skin with the various available techniques. It was expected that physiologic changes indicative of sensitive skin could be detected at low levels before clinical visible signs.[15] These different techniques (TEWL, corneometry, skin capacitance, skin hydration, pH) have been applied either at baseline or after provocative test to identify biophysical variations linked to sensitive skin condition. The results obtained after or during provocative tests were slightly more conclusive than those at baseline. Indeed, these techniques are fully pertinent to assess the induced visible signs, such as redness. But, their usefulness is less established to assess the neurosensorial signs including burning, itching and stinging, the major features of sensitive skin. In such a large repertoire of biophysical tools, the most popular test is TEWL measurement. As barrier function impairment tends to exist at baseline on sensitive skin subjects, it is certainly the most appropriate biophysical test.

For the time being, unfortunately, no test allows sensitive skin condition to be perfectly and undoubtedly diagnosed. For that purpose, it would be careful to confirm the information collected through a questionnaire about the self-perceived sensitive skin by a psychophysical test with lactic acid or capsaicin and a baseline TEWL measurement. These difficulties to diagnose sensitive skin are a major problem in identifying a sensitive skin panel.

MANAGEMENT

Since sensitive skin greatly varies in its manifestations and causes, managing sensitive skin appears a real challenge to the dermatologist. A major concern is to identify the triggering factors causing sensitive skin whatever their nature: cosmetic formulations or environmental factors. Management of sensitive skin due to cosmetics involves simple procedures with a step by step elimination, avoidance and introduction of cosmetics.[27] As it is hard to shield individuals from their different environments, managing subjects with sensitive skin to environment will rely more on a treatment approach. Recent developments in the treatment of sensitive skin will be presented in the following paragraph.

There is no simple, ready to follow routine for managing skin sensitivity to cosmetics. For a given subject, identifying the ingredient and/or product responsible for sensitive skin manifestations could be a great task in view of the high number of ingredients present in cosmetics and toiletries. It involves a detailed protocol which should provide logical recommendations for cosmetics usage. A detailed approach to manage subjects with sensitive skin to cosmetics has been proposed. As explained by Draelos, the proposed algorithm is based more on the art of medicine than science. The 14 successive steps encompass an initial 2-week period of discontinuation of any topical application except for synthetic detergent (Syndet) soap, a clinical examination for any underlying dermatosis (e.g. rosacea, psoriasis), a test battery (patch, photopatch, lactic acid stinging test, contact urticaria) and a progressive reintroduction of the cosmetics and skin-care products according to a specific protocol in terms of reintroduction order and modalities of application. Even time-consuming, this systemic and thorough approach is useful in practice for a given individual because it allows the possible ingredients responsible for his/her skin reactivity to cosmetics to be identified and, consequently, pertinent product to be recommended.[27,42] Identification of sensitive skin triggering factors contained in cosmetics has allowed establishing a list of basic recommendations that may help subjects with sensitive skin to cosmetics.[42] The main recommendation principles cover selecting cosmetics for sensitive skin, reducing the total number of cosmetics used per day, strictly following instructions for use and only using cosmetics before expiry date.

FORMULATING PRODUCTS SPECIFICALLY DESIGNED FOR SENSITIVE SKINS

Among the recommendations to subjects presented in the previous paragraph, the most frequent is certainly to use basic formulations with few ingredients to minimize the risk of encountering a problem. Subjects with sensitive skin have also the possibility to use formulations specifically designed for them. The first generation of cosmetics suitable for sensitive skins has been thought to avoid the manifestations of sensitive skin. This preventive approach was merely dedicated to the increasing number of individuals complaining about skin reactivity to cosmetics. It has consisted in suppressing or reducing any ingredient known or suspected to induce discomfort and/or skin barrier impairment such as glycolic acid or propylene glycol. This "ingredient-free" concept for formulating products was not always satisfying. Indeed, in some cases such as glycolic acid for instance, the reduction concerned the ingredient bearing the claimed activity. Moreover, this preventive approach was less adapted to the needs of subjects with sensitive skin to environmental factors. Recently, taking advantage of some advances in the knowledge of the physiological mechanisms involved in sensitive skin condition and their *in vitro* applications, a new approach has emerged proposing formulations dedicated to treat sensitive skin.

In Vitro Sensitive Skin Models

Unmyelinated sensory C-fibers network take charge of nociceptive sensations in the skin and are associated with sensitive skin symptoms. In particular, they can detect various pruritus induced stimuli and then integrate the signal to the CNS.[43] Some molecular receptors have been implicated in this pathway. TRPV1 was the first identified as a key integrator of itch sensation.[44] This nonselective cation channel is the receptor for capsaicin, the pungent ingredient of hot pepper. It is a thermoreceptor activated by temperatures up to 42°C and also by protons. More recently, TRPV3 and TRPA1 have also been identified as nociceptive receptors.[45-47]

When activated by capsaicin, TRPV1 mediates the release of different neuropeptides [substance P (SP) and calcitonin gene-related peptide (CGRP)] and propagates neurogenic inflammation. The substance P will then bind to its receptor expressed by mast cells. It leads to histamine release which activates TRPV1 by intracellular pathway. This pathway forms an itch initiation loop in the skin.

The TRPV1 is also expressed by other skin cells including keratinocytes.[48-51] Some work reported the keratinocytes as initiators and integrators of skin nociception.[29] The mechanisms remain unclear but keratinocytes have been described to be able to release SP.[52]

Considering TRP biological targets, an *in vitro* itch modelization can be performed using transfected cell lines overexpressing TRPV1 and other receptors. The receptor activation is assessed by electrophysiology or calcium influx quantification using fluorescent probes. Calcium mobilization mimics the depolarization of nerve fibers for CNS signal transmission. This screening model has already allowed trans-4-tert-butylcyclohexanol to be identified as a selective antagonist of TRPV1 able to reduce *in vivo* the skin reactivity to capsaicin.[53] Other assays focus on TRPV1 activation cascade by measuring SP and/or CGRP release by dorsal root ganglion neurons alone or in coculture with keratinocytes.[54] Such a model has been successfully used to select an extract of a probiotic strain called *Bifidobacterium longum* as a new approach for treating sensitive skin.[55]

These different *in vitro* models that mimic cutaneous nociception open new ways to alleviate sensitive skin by introducing compounds decreasing neuron reactivity in cosmetic products. In this perspective, the *in vitro* evaluation approach could be very valuable to identify compounds of interest before enhancing clinical trials.

Testing Formulations on Sensitive Skin Panels

Despite the difficulty to build sensitive skin panels,[37] in vivo testing on sensitive skin subjects is valuable in product development to determine the likelihood of adverse consumer reports after product release in the general sensitive skin population.[15] In such a testing procedure, in addition to visible signs (erythema, visible squames, vesicles, papules, etc.), it is of tremendous importance to ask subjects to report any information regarding invisible signs, such as stinging, burning and itching that could be perceived without any visible manifestation. Such a procedure allows compounds or cosmetic formulations potentially causing discomfort or disagreeable sensations to be identified when used by sensitive skin consumers. Consequently, these compounds or formulations should not be marketed as suitable for sensitive skins. The second testing procedure follows the more recent developments of actives aiming at decreasing the signs of sensitive skin induced by topical applications and environmental factors. In that case, it is of great interest to induce discomfort sensations by capsaicin or lactic acid before or after test product application to assess preventive or curative effects toward neurosensorial signs. Such a reduction in induced discomfort sensations will be certainly predictive of an effective management of the neurosensory hyperreactivity which characterizes the sensitive skin condition.

CONCLUSION

Sensitive skin syndrome is a very common phenomenon in any country where epidemiological surveys have been conducted but still lacks a clear and consensual definition. This syndrome is merely expressed through subjective discomfort sensations, such as stinging, burning and itching. These symptoms above all affecting the face are most often caused by exogenous factors, such as heat, cold, fast changes in temperature, wind, pollution and contact with some products not suitable for sensitive skins. Most of the time, these subjective symptoms are not accompanied by visible signs. To date, no testing protocol emerged as the gold standard diagnostic tool able to fully encompass the complexity of this self-diagnosed syndrome. Consequently, diagnosing sensitive skin is a hard and challenging task for the dermatologist. Some recent findings allowed both heightened cutaneous nervous reactivity and increased stratum corneum permeability to be pointed up as possible pathophysiological support of sensitive skin. Cosmetics and toiletries manufacturers have integrated these results for formulating products more designed to treat sensitive skin syndrome than aimed at avoiding its induction.

REFERENCES

1. Thiers H. Peau sensible. In: Thiers H, editor. Les Cosmétiques. 2nd ed. Paris: Masson;1986. pp. 266-8.
2. Kligman AM, Sadiq I, Zhen Y, et al. Experimental studies on the nature of sensitive skin. Skin Res Technol. 2006;12(4): 217-22.
3. Sensitive Skin Syndrome. In: Berardesca E, Fluhr JW, Maibach HI, editors. New York: Taylor & Francis; 2006.
4. Lev-Tov H, Maibach HI. The sensitive skin syndrome. Indian J Dermatol. 2012;57(6):419-23.
5. Xu F, Yan S, Wu M, et al. Self-declared sensitive skin in China: A community-based study in three top metropolises. J Eur Acad Dermatol Venereol. 2013;27(3):370-5.
6. Kamide R, Misery L, Perez-Cullell N, et al. Sensitive skin evaluation in the Japanese population. J Dermatol. 2013;40(3):177-81.
7. Misery L, Sibaud V, Merial-Kieny C, et al. Sensitive skin in the American population: prevalence, clinical data, and role of the dermatologist. Int J Dermatol. 2011;50(8):961-7.
8. Berardesca E, Fluhr JW, Maibach HI. What is sensitive skin? In: Berardesca E, Fluhr JW, Maibach HI, editors. Sensitive Skin Syndrome. New York: Taylor & Francis; 2006. pp.1-6.
9. Slodownik D, Williams J, Lee A, et al. Controversies regarding the sensitive skin syndrome. Expert Rev Dermatol. 2007;2:579-84.
10. Saint-Martory C, Roguedas-Contios AM, Sibaud V, et al. Sensitive skin is not limited to the face. Br J Dermatol. 2008;158(1):130-3.
11. Misery L, Sibaud V, Ambronati M, et al. Sensitive scalp: does this condition exist? An epidemiological study. Contact Dermatitis. 2008;58(4):234-8.
12. Groot AC, Nater JP, Lender R, et al. Adverse effects of cosmetics and toiletries: A retrospective study in general population. Int J Cosmet Sci. 1987;9(6):255-9.
13. Simion FA, Rhein LD, Morrison BM, et al. Self-perceived sensory responses to soap and synthetic detergent bars correlate with clinical signs of irritation. J Am Acad Dermatol. 1995;32(2 Pt 1):205-11.
14. Morizot F, Guinot C, Lpoez S, et al. Sensitive skin: analysis of symptoms, perceived causes and possible mechanisms. Cosmetics & Toiletries. 2000;115:83-9.
15. Draelos ZD. Sensitive skin: perceptions, evaluation and treatment. Am J Contact Dermat.1997;8(2):67-78.
16. Robinson MK. Population differences in skin structure and physiology and the susceptibility to irritant and allergic contact dermatitis: implications for safety testing and risk assessment. Contact Dermatitis. 1999;41(2):65-79.
17. Bowman JP, Floyd AK, Znaniecki A, et al. The use of chemical probes to assess the facial reactivity of women, comparing their self-perception of sensitive skin. J Cosmet Sci. 2000;51:267-73.
18. Johnson AW, Page DJ. Making sense of sensitive skin. Poster 700. Proceedings of the 18th IFSCC Congress 1992, Yokohama, Japan.
19. Willis CM, Shaw S, de Lacharrière O, et al. Sensitive skin: an epidemiological study. Br J Dermatol. 2001;145(2):258-63.
20. Jourdain R, de Lacharrière O, Bastien P, et al. Ethnic variations in self-perceived sensitive skin: epidemiological survey. Contact Dermatitis. 2002;46(3):162-9.
21. de Lacharrière O. Self-perceived sensitive skin. In: Draelos ZD, editors. Cosmetic Dermatology: Products and Procedures. 2010; p. 22-6.
22. Misery L, Boussetta S, Nocera T, et al. Sensitive skin in Europe. J Eur Acad Dermatol Venereol. 2009;23(4):376-81.
23. Berardesca E, Farage MA, Maibach HI. Sensitive skin: an overview. Int J Cosmet Sci. 2013;35(1):2-8.
24. Farage MA. Perceptions of sensitive skin: changes in perceived severity and associations with environmental causes. Contact Dermatitis. 2008;59(4):226-32.
25. Farage MA. How do perceptions of sensitive skin differ at different anatomical sites? An epidemiological study. Clin Exp Dermatol. 2009;34(8):e521-30.

26. Farage MA, Maibach HI. Sensitive skin: closing in on a physiological cause. Contact Dermatitis. 2010;62(3):137-49.
27. Inamadar AC, Palit A. Sensitive skin: an overview. Indian J Dermatol Venereol Leprol. 2013;79(1):9-16.
28. Christensen M, Kligman AM. An improved procedure for conducting lactic acid stinging tests on facial skin. J Soc Cosmet Chem. 1996;47:1-11.
29. Denda M, Nakatani M, Ikeyama K, et al. Epidermal keratinocytes as the forefront of the sensory system. Exp Dermatol. 2007;16(3):157-61.
30. Ständer S, Schneider SW, Weishaupt C, et al. Putative neuronal mechanisms of sensitive skin. Exp Dermatol. 2009;18(5):417-23.
31. Jourdain R, Bastien P, de Lacharrière O, et al. Detection thresholds of capsaicin: a new test to assess facial skin neurosensitivity. J Cosmet Sci. 2005;56(3):153-66.
32. Querleux B, Dauchot K, Jourdain R, et al. Neural basis of sensitive skin: an fMRI study. Skin Res Technol. 2008;14(4):454-61.
33. Agner T. Basal transepidermal water loss, skin thickness, skin blood flow and skin colour in relation to sodium-lauryl-sulfate-induced irritation in normal skin. Contact Dermatitis. 1991;25(2): 108-14.
34. Distante F, Rigano L, D'Agostino R, et al. Intra- and inter-individual differences in sensitive skin. Cosmetics & Toiletries. 2002;117:39-46.
35. Seidenari S, Francomano M, Mantovani L. Baseline biophysical parameters in subjects with sensitive skin. Contact Dermatitis. 1998;38(6):311-5.
36. Cho HJ, Chung BY, Lee HB, et al. Quantitative study of stratum corneum ceramides contents in patients with sensitive skin. J Dermatol. 2012;39(3):295-300.
37. Marriott M, Basketter D, Cooper K, et al. Identification of a sensitive skin panel. In: Berardesca E, Fluhr JW, Maibach HI, editors. Sensitive Skin Syndrome. New York: Taylor & Francis; 2006. pp. 107-19.
38. Yosipovitch G. Evaluating subjective irritation and sensitive skin. Cosmetics and Toiletries. 1999;114:41-2.
39. Leyden JJ. Risk assessment of products used on skin. Am J Contact Dermatitis. 1993;4:158-62.
40. Frosch P, Kligman AM. A method for appraising the stinging capacity of topically applied substances. J Soc Cosmet Chem. 1977;28:197-209.
41. Jourdain R, Maibach HI, Bastien P, et al. Ethnic variations in facial skin neurosensitivity assessed by capsaicin detection thresholds. Contact Dermatitis. 2009;61(6):325-31.
42. Draelos ZD. Treatments for sensitive skin: an update. In: Berardesca E, Fluhr JW, Maibach HI, editors. Sensitive Skin Syndrome. New York: Taylor & Francis; 2006. pp.245-53.
43. Basbaum AI, Bautista DM, Scherrer G, et al. Cellular and molecular mechanisms of pain. Cell. 2009;139(2):267-84.
44. Caterina MJ, Schumacher MA, Tominaga M, et al. The capsaicin receptor: a heat-activated ion channel in the pain pathway. Nature. 1997;389:816-24.
45. Steinhoff M, Bíró T. A TR(I)P to pruritus research: role of TRPV3 in inflammation and itch. J Invest Dermatol. 2009;129(3):531-5.
46. Wilson SR, Gerhold KA, Bifolck-Fisher A, et al. TRPA1 is required for histamine-independent, Mas-related G protein-coupled receptor-mediated itch. Nat Neurosci. 2011;14(5):595-602.
47. Wilson SR, Nelson AM, Batia L, et al. The ion channel TRPA1 is required for chronic itch. J Neurosci. 2013;33(22):9283-94.
48. Denda M, Fuziwara S, Inoue K, et al. Immunoreactivity of VR1 on epidermal keratinocyte of human skin. Biochem Biophys Res Commun. 2001;285(5):1250-2.
49. Ständer S, Moormann C, Schumacher M, et al. Expression of vanilloid receptor subtype 1 in cutaneous sensory nerve fibers, mast cells, and epithelial cells of appendage structures. Exp Dermatol. 2004;13(3):129-39.
50. Bodó E, Kovács I, Telek A, et al. Vanilloid receptor-1 (VR1) is widely expressed on various epithelial and mesenchymal cell types of human skin. J Invest Dermatol. 2004;123(2):410-3.
51. Kim SJ, Lee SA, Yun SJ, et al. Expression of vanilloid receptor 1 in cultured fibroblast. Exp Dermatol. 2006;15(5):362-7.
52. Dieamant Gde C, Velazquez Pereda Mdel C, Eberlin S, et al. Neuroimmunomodulatory compound for sensitive skin care: in vitro and clinical assessment. J Cosmet Dermatol. 2008;7(2): 112-9.
53. Kueper T, Krohn M, Haustedt LO, et al. Inhibition of TRPV1 for the treatment of sensitive skin. Exp Dermatol. 2010;19(11):980-6.
54. Pereira U, Boulais N, Lebonvallet N, et al. Development of an in vitro coculture of primary sensitive pig neurons and keratinocytes for the study of cutaneous neurogenic inflammation. Exp Dermatol. 2010;19(10):931-5.
55. Guéniche A, Bastien P, Ovigne JM, et al. *Bifidobacterium longum* lysate, a new ingredient for reactive skin. Exp Dermatol. 2010;19(8):e1-8.

Chapter 10

Acne and Cosmetic Care

Prashant S Hegde, *L'Oréal Research and Innovation, Bengaluru, India*
Abir Saraswat, *Indushree Skin Clinic, Lucknow, India*
AK Bajaj, *Bajaj Skin Clinic, Allahabad, India*

INTRODUCTION

Acne vulgaris is a most common skin disorder of the pilosebaceous unit.[1] It is generally characterized by seborrhea, comedone formation, inflammatory lesions and increased colonization by *Propionibacterium* spp. *Staphylococcus* spp. and yeasts of the *Malassezia* spp. within the follicular canal.[2]

Animals do not get acne. The latter is specific to humans who tend to view it as a rite of passage.[3] It is stated that 90% of male and female individuals, experience some degree of acne between puberty and 30 years of age. A report in the British Medical Journal in 1989 stated that in a lifetime, a person is more likely to have acne than any other disease.[4] However, the prevalence of acne in India remains unknown due to the paucity of published data. Experience from dermatology clinics in urban areas, where it is easily the most common skin disease, suggests that acne is as common in India as in European Union (EU) and the USA (consensus of the Indian Acne Alliance).[5] With over a billion of inhabitants and a great proportion of young individuals, acneic subjects in India amount to some 200–300 millions. Half of them are expected to have acne severe enough to experience physical and psycho-social morbidity and are, therefore, in need of systematic and rational treatment.

Although very common, this disorder can cause significant emotional distress and physical scarring if untreated. Acne impacts profoundly quality of life (QOL), psychosocial development and career prospects. Underestimating its importance is of serious consequences.[6]

PATHOGENESIS OF ACNE

Acne results from an obstruction and a further inflammation of the sebaceous follicles, a subtype of pilosebaceous units. Sebaceous follicles show dominant sebaceous gland and rudimentary hair. The primary and pathognomonic lesion of acne is the microcomedo, a microscopic lesion invisible to the eye. Some microcomedones evolve into either a noninflammatory comedo (open or closed), or an inflammatory lesion such as papule, pustule, nodule or macule in the most severe cases.

The development of acne is a multifactorial process involving both endogenous and exogenous factors. There are four primary pathogenic factors, which interact in a complex manner to produce acne lesions:[7] (1) increased sebum production by the sebaceous gland, (2) alteration in the keratinization process, (3) follicular colonization by *Propionibacteria* spp. and (4) release of inflammatory mediators into the skin. Other contributing factors include hormonal influences from estrogen and androgens, such as dehydroepiandrosterone sulfate (DHEAS), which increases sebum production in prepubescent children, leading to acne.[8,9] Genetic factors may also play a role in the development of acne:[10-12] a possible association was found between the CYP17-34T/C polymorphism and the development of severe acne in Chinese patients. More recently, Chinese investigators identified two new susceptibility loci at 1q24.2 and 11p11.2 that conferred a higher risk of severe acne.[13]

Seborrhea and Sebaceous Gland Hyperplasia

Excess of sebum secretion, sebaceous gland hypertrophy and hyperplasia are the hallmarks of acne. The sebaceous glands are beginning to enlarge through an androgenic stimulus (DHEA) at about 7–8 years of age, with a net increase in sebum excretion.[14,15] The overall size of the sebaceous follicles increases along with number of lobules per gland.[16]

Acne subjects, male and female, excrete more sebum than normal subjects, and the sebum excretion rate correlates well with the severity of acne.[17-19] The increase in sebum production is mainly due to a difference in the response of the target organ (sebaceous follicle), to an increase in circulating androgens, or both. The target-organ responsiveness is variable and may explain the bilateral asymmetry of acne.[20] *In vitro* studies have shown that sebocytes from different areas of the body respond differently to dihydrotestosterone and testosterone.[21] Sebocytes from the leg do not respond or have a lower response than those from the face and show a dose-dependent proliferation.

Altered Follicular Keratinization

One of the most crucial initial events in the development of acne lesions is hyperkeratinization in the follicular infundibulum and sebaceous duct resulting in micro-comedones.[22] Comedogenesis occurs when abnormally desquamating corneocytes accumulate within the sebaceous follicle and form a keratinous plug.[23] When the latter enlarges below a very small follicular ostium at the skin surface, it becomes visible as a closed comedone (whitehead). An open comedone (blackhead) occurs if the follicular ostium dilates. The small closed comedones are the precursors of inflammatory lesions.[5] The pathogenesis of follicular hyperkeratinization is still unclear. Immunohistochemical studies described an increased proliferation rate of the basal keratinocytes and an abnormal differentiation of the follicular keratinocytes in the follicle wall of microcomedones and comedones.[23-25] Several factors have been suggested to induce this hyperproliferation: sebum composition, response to androgens, etc. For example, these abnormalities may possibly be due to a relative decrease in sebaceous linoleic acid.[26] An androgen controlled defect may also contribute to abnormal proliferation through the 5-α reductase enzyme (type 1) in the infundibulum.[27] Cytokines are also involved in comedogenesis. High levels of biologically active interleukin-1α (IL-1α) have been detected in comedones, believed to be expressed by follicular keratinocytes and triggered by changes in sebum composition and secretion.[28,29] IL-1α may compromise follicular barrier and thus induce inflammation.

Propionibacterium Acnes Follicular Colonization

It is widely accepted that Propionibacteria species (acnes, granulosum, avidum, etc.), are a major factor in the pathogenesis of acne. *P. acnes* is a common skin resident and one of the major component of the microbial flora of the pilosebaceous follicle.[30] In acne, the abnormal accumulation of corneocytes and the excess of sebum in the infrainfundibular portion of the duct becomes a privileged niche to microbial colonization. Most members of this resident flora produce lipases that are responsible for hydrolysis of triglycerides and release of free fatty acids. They also produce other exoenzymes like proteases, hyaluronidases, which may contribute to the inflammatory process and to the rupture of the follicular wall,[31] a key factor that further propagates the inflammatory reaction to neighboring follicles. In addition, *P. acnes* is being linked to toll-like receptors (TLR), a transmembrane protein with a cytoplasmic portion homologous to IL-1 receptor. *P. acnes* binds to and activates TLR-2 which in turn, induces a cascade of signaling events involving monocytes, other inflammatory cells and inflammatory cytokines.[32]

Inflammation

Inflammation is a key component of acne which largely accounts for its morbidity and sequelae (pigmentary disturbances and scarring). Inflammation, for long was believed to being a secondary process in the pathogenesis of acne. New data indicates that immunological events led by peri-follicular helper T-cells in genetically predisposed individuals may in fact be a primary process, initiating comedogenesis through elaboration of IL-1.[33] Further, inflammation may up-regulate sebum production through the production of inflammatory mediator leukotriene B4 that binds to the receptors of sebocytes.

Sebum production is also influenced by neuropeptides—substance P and its degrading enzyme neutral endopeptidase that may explain stress-induced aggravation of acne.[34]

EPIDEMIOLOGICAL AND CLINICAL FEATURES OF ACNE PATIENTS

Epidemiology

Acne vulgaris is a chronic condition that is almost universal during adolescence. Hospital-based studies carried out in Asian populations have shown that acne vulgaris constitutes 11.2% and 19.6% of the total new patients attending their hospitals.[35,36] The condition usually starts in adolescence, peaks at the ages of 14–19 years and frequently resolves by mid-twenties. In one study conducted in India, the frequency of acne vulgaris was found to being very low: 1.06% with a mean age of 19.78 years. Interestingly, the authors found a high incidence of scarring (39.5%) and post-acne hyperpigmentation (24.6%).[37] Acne vulgaris develops earlier in females than males, which may reflect the earlier onset of puberty in females. The most severe forms of acne vulgaris occur more frequently in males, but the disease tends to be more persistent in females. Severity of the disease varies markedly from one individual to the other, depending on the interplay of various factors involved in the development of acne vulgaris. Grading systems based upon the clinical appearance of lesions as well as "lesion counting" are useful in assessing the severity of acne vulgaris.

Clinical Manifestations

Acne affects areas containing the largest oil glands, including the face, back and trunk. Face is the major theater of action,[38] involved in 99% of acneic subjects. Back and chest are involved in 60% and 15% of cases, respectively. Typical adolescent acne involves the entire face but shows predilection for cheeks. In men with a grown beard, it relatively spares the lower face and neck. The onset of acne in adults is largely confined to the jaw area. In some cases, acne is largely confined to the torso with little or no involvement of the face (acne corporis). Acne corporis denotes severe acne and often involves the entire back and in some cases, extends to buttocks and thighs.

Acne shows a variable and fluctuating mix of comedones, folliculocentric inflammatory lesions, scars, and pigmentary disturbances (Fig. 1).[39] The precursor lesion is a microcomedo which is microscopic and cannot be clinically perceived. As comedones enlarge, they become apparent and evolve into open or closed comedones, and further into papules or nodules.[40]

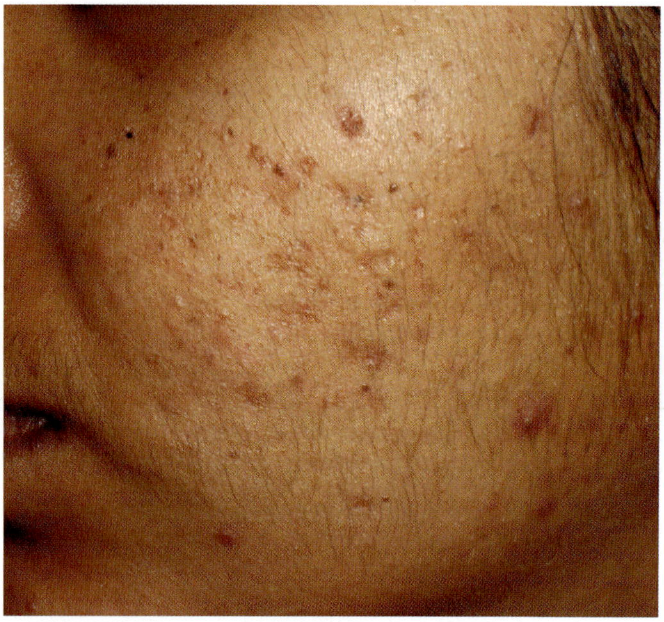

Figure 1: Facial acne with hirsutism
Courtesy: Dr Bajaj and Dr Saraswat

As a plug of sebaceous and keratinous material lodged within the outlet of a hair follicle, a comedo is an early non-inflammatory lesion of acne. Closed comedones are known as whiteheads since appearing as whitish to flesh-colored papules with an apparently closed overlying surface (although they do have minute follicular orifices). Open comedones (blackheads) appear as flat or slightly raised brown to black plugs that distend the follicular outlets; their dark color results from the presence of melanin.

Inflammatory lesions include papules, pustules, nodules and macules. Pustules and papules respectively result from superficial or deep inflammation associated with the rupture of the comedone "bag". Cysts or nodules are large, deep-seated abscesses that may be fluctuant when palpated. Macules are flat red spots left by acne lesions after healing. Although the diagnosis of acne is said to be untenable in the absence of comedones, 7% of acne patients do not present any comedo at first evaluation.[41] The severity of acne is not only gauged by the number and types of lesions but its immense palette of various clinical aspects among patients makes "The Acnes" a better generic.[42]

Acne Scars

Clearance of scars is the first request of acne patients. The two causes of acne scar formation can be broadly categorized as a result of increased tissue formation or loss or damage of dermal tissue.[43]

Two examples of excess tissue presence are hypertrophic scars and keloids. Hypertrophic scars are confined within the margins of the original injury. These scars are most prevalent within the first 2 months post-injury and, in contrast to keloids, tend to normally mature with occasional spontaneous regression. Keloids are a human-specific phenomenon characterized by disproportionate synthesis and deposition of collagen in excess outside the original margins of injury. These lesions are very persistent and are found almost equally among male and female patients. Both hypertrophic scars and keloids demonstrate thicker, more abundant collagen that is stretched and aligned in the same plane as epidermis. Suggested pathophysiology put forward the impact of various elements such as transforming growth factor-βI, platelet-derived growth factor, matrix metalloproteinases, interleukin-Iα, fibroblasts, altered microvascular regeneration, histamine, carboxypeptidase A, prostaglandin D2 and tryptase.[44]

The other cause of scars, loss or damage of tissue, is demonstrated by the three primary acne scar types described by Jacob et al.[45] icepick, rolling, and boxcar (Fig. 2). Icepick scars are usually small in diameter (<2 mm) and deep with tracts to the dermis or subcutaneous tissue possible. Depressed or boxcar scars are described as shallow (<0.5 mm) or deep (>0.5 mm) and are often 1.5–4 mm in diameter. They have sharply defined edges with steep, almost vertical walls. Soft rolling scars can be circular or linear, are often greater than 4 mm in diameter, and present gently sloped edges that merge with a clinically normal skin. Papular scars are somewhat less known subtypes of acne scars. Also variously called perifollicular elastolysis, postacne anetoderma-like scars, and papular elastorrhexis, these are seen mainly on the chin, chest and upper back. They are soft perifollicular hypopigmented to skin-colored papules that are easily distensible (Fig. 3).

Pigmented scars occur as a reaction to inflammation linked to the healing process. When acne develops, an inflammatory reaction confers either a red (in light skinned individuals) or a brown (in dark skinned individuals) color to the concerned region. The

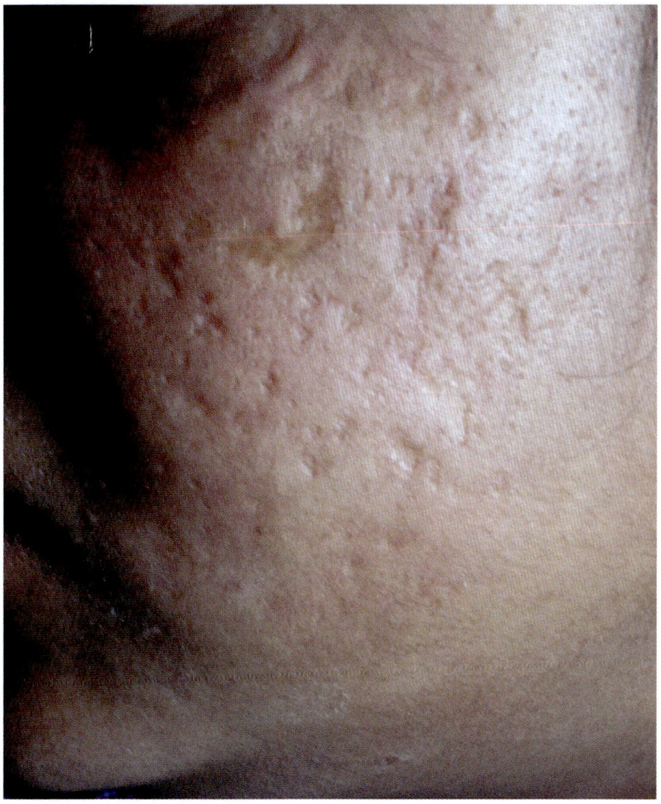

Figure 2: Boxcar and icepick scars after facial acne
Courtesy: Dr Bajaj and Dr Saraswat

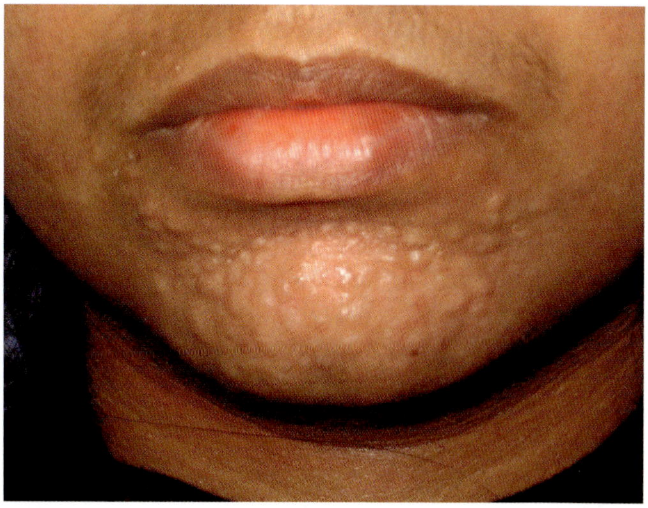

Figure 3: Papular acne scars
Courtesy: Dr Bajaj and Dr Saraswat

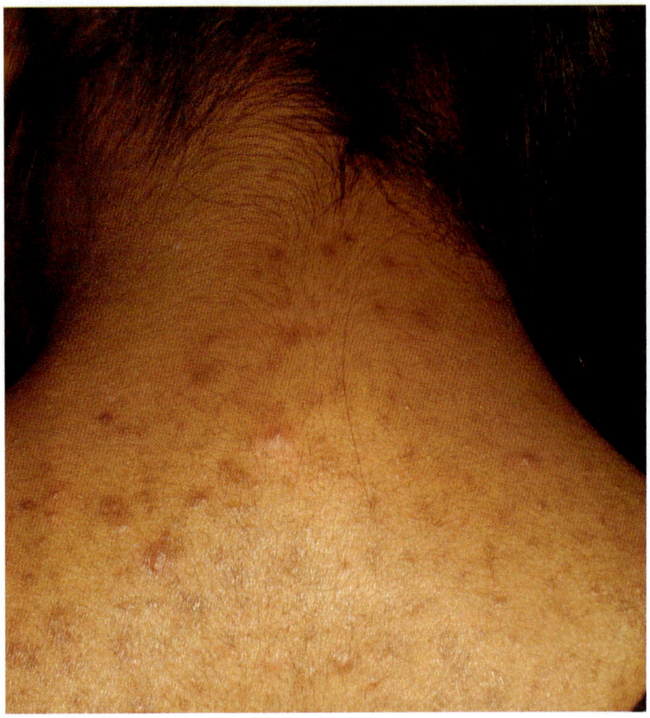

Figure 4: Truncal acne with post-inflammatory hyperpigmentation
Courtesy: Dr Bajaj and Dr Saraswat

development of color in reaction to the swelling is a very normal element among the healing process of acne, but unfortunately leads to colored acne scars (Fig. 4).

There is a correlation between the severity of scars and the delay between the onset of acne lesions and the start of acne treatment. Epidermal impairments, such as erythema and pigmentation are reversible, whereas dermal damage such as atrophic and hypertrophic scars is partially reversible.

Acne among Dark-skinned Patients

The active acne lesions in dark-skinned patients can clinically appear similar to those seen in light-skinned patients.[46] Dark-skinned patients can develop inflammatory papules, pustules, nodules, and cysts. These inflammatory lesions promote the development of post-inflammatory hyperpigmentation (PIH) and scarring. In dark-skinned patients, the most disturbing feature of acne is not the active lesion *per se* but the resulting PIH.[47,48] The latter appears as hyperpigmented macules and the higher the skin phototype, the more intense the pigmentation.[46]

Keloid formation and hypertrophic scarring are other sequelae of acne that are more commonly seen among the dark-skinned populations.

FACTORS PRECIPITATING OR AGGRAVATING ACNE

The course of acne is anything but monotonous. There are periodic flares, some of which being related to various triggering and aggravating factors as discussed below.

Oils

In India, the use of vegetable oils extracted from coconut, almond, olive and rye is popular. Such oils are traditionally used as moisturizers and revitalizers (as body rubs), and for hair grooming. Oils form an occlusive film over the applied area and when oxidized, may exacerbate acne.[5] In southern India, mineral-oil-based pomades are popular and frequently cause acne on the forehead.

Facials (Facial Massage)

Facials are popular and are regularly used by women in urban areas. A study in India[49] described facials as inducers of acneiform eruptions in 33.1% of subjects. These eruptions are characterized by deep nodules and closed comedones, showing predilection for the cheeks.

Repeated Irritation

Follicular irritation from shaving, waxing, threading, and laser hair removal is sometimes described as associated with the onset of papules and pustules.

Sweat

Sweating in a hot and humid environment exacerbates acne in 15% of patients.[50]

Menstruation

Premenstrual flare of acne has been reported in 70% of female acne patients.[51] It is noteworthy that progesterone and estrogens possess pro- and anti-inflammatory effects and that their alteration or modulation may be significant factors.[51]

Stress

Mental stress frequently aggravates acne,[52] complementary to the fact that acne itself induces such stress.

Sunlight

The effect of sun exposure upon acne comprises a double edge aspect. Sun exposures mitigate acne on short period (approximately 1 month post exposure) but, later, clearly worsens its severity. The first phase might relate to an anti microbial impact from UV's (partly killing *P. acnes*) but, on the other hand, later induces squalene oxidization that leads to comedogenesis.[53]

Season

In hot and humid summer, acne may worsen, due to acute blockage that results from an increased water content in the epithelial cells of the sebaceous follicle (ductal hydration).[54]

Diet

Some recent literature has suggested links between acne and diet. A retrospective analysis of a large database in the USA allowed a positive association to be established between the intake of diary products by high school female students and the severity of their acne, as diagnosed by physicians.[55] It was hypothesized that milk and dairy products carry hormones and bioactive molecules that have the potential to aggravate acne. In another epidemiologic study, data was presented to suggest that high glycemic load foods (sugary foods) rise up the prevalence of acne.[56] However, the precise role of diet in the pathogenesis of acne remains unclear and controversial.

Drugs

Some drugs are known to elicit acneic eruptions. These comprise halogenated compounds, progestogens, oral contraceptive pills, corticosteroids, isoniazid, and lithium. Recently, a new class of therapeutic agents, epidermal growth factors (EGF)-receptor antagonists (gefitinib, erlotinib, cetuximab), has been described as triggering acneiform eruptions.[57]

MEDICAL TREATMENT

The general principles of treatment are based upon four strategies that may be combined, according to the clinical aspect of acne of a patient (inflammatory, retentional): (i) decreasing the sebaceous gland secretion, (ii) correcting the ductal hypercornification, (iii) decreasing *P. acnes* population and associated flora and (iv) producing an anti-inflammatory effect. With regard to the vast mosaic feature of acne among all patients, it should be kept in mind that "One treatment does not fit all".[58]

Benzoyl Peroxide

It is a well-known and highly effective topical agent available in different formulations (washes, lotions, creams and gels) and concentrations (2.5–10%). Benzoyl peroxide (BP) is a broad-spectrum antimicrobial agent which exerts its effect via its oxidizing activity. BP has anti-inflammatory, keratolytic and comedolytic activities, and is indicated in mild-to-moderate acne vulgaris. The main limitations of BP relate to its dose-dependent cutaneous irritation, skin dryness and allergic contact dermatitis.[59] Besides, contacts between BP and garments, pillows, etc. often lead to their irreversible discoloration.

Topical Retinoids

These have been in use for more than 40 years. Topical retinoids target the microcomedo-precursor lesion of acne[59] with a high effectiveness upon the abnormal follicular epithelial hyperproliferation. Hence, they reduce follicular plugging, microcomedones and both noninflammatory and inflammatory acne lesions. Their biological effects are mediated through nuclear hormone receptors (retinoic acid receptor RAR and retinoids X receptor RXR with three subtypes α, β and γ) and cytosolic binding proteins. Tretinoin®, Adapalene®, Tazarotene®, Isotretinoin® (oral route only and restricted to male patients), Metretinide®, retinaldehyde and β-retinoyl glucuronide are currently available retinoids, most being topically applied, of which Tretinoin® and Adapalene® are the most studied and used worldwide. The main adverse effect with topical retinoid is a primary irritant dermatitis, at least at the start of applications, leading to erythema, scaling, burning sensation, all of variable intensities according to skin type, sensitivity and types of formulations.

Topical Antibiotics

Clindamycin and erythromycin are both effective against inflammatory acne in topical form in combination of 1–4% with or without the addition of Zinc.[59] Topical Clarithromycin®, Azithromycin® and Nadifloxacin® are available in India, but their efficacy and safety lack clinical reports. Side effects, though minor, include erythema, peeling, itching, dryness and burning. Pseudomembranous colitis is an extremely rare adverse effect of topical clindamycin. The most important side effect of topical antibiotic use is the development of bacterial resistance and cross resistance. They, therefore, should not be used as monotherapy.

Other Topical/New Agents

- *Salicylic acid* (SA) has been used since at least 60 years as a comedolytic agent, at variable doses (1–10%) but is less potent than topical retinoids
- *Azelaic acid* is available as 10–20% topical cream which has been shown to be slightly effective in inflammatory and comedonal acnes
- *Lactic acid/lactate lotion* is of some help in preventing and reducing acne lesion counts
- *Picolinic acid gel* 10% is an intermediate metabolite of the amino acid, tryptophan. When applied twice daily for 12 weeks, it was found to be effective in reducing both type of acne lesions
- *Dapsone gel* 5% is a sulfone compound with anti-inflammatory and antimicrobial properties that shows some efficacy in inflammatory acne.

Surgical Therapy: Chemical Peel

Chemical peeling, like retinoids, in patients with skin of color is another therapeutic option that can address both acne and PIH simultaneously.[46] Patients with skin photo-type IV–VI typically undergo superficial or (less commonly) medium-depth chemical peels. Their response to chemical peeling may vary and the selection of the peeling agent should then be done with caution. The two most commonly used superficial peeling agents in acne are glycolic acid (GA) and SA. GA is a naturally occurring alpha hydroxy acid (the fruit acids family) that acts by inducing epidermolysis, dispersing basal layer melanin and increasing collagen synthesis.[60,61] GA peels utilize concentrations ranging 20–70% and require neutralization to terminate the peel. GA peels are contraindicated in pregnancy and in glycolate-sensitive patients. SA causes keratolysis by disrupting intercellular lipid linkages between epithelioid cells. Superficial SA peels are usually performed with strengths ranging 20–30% without the need for neutralization and have very low potential to induce PIH. Medium depth peels with 15–30% trichloroacetic acid can also be used with, however, a significantly higher risk of inducing PIH.

Lasers and Light-based Therapies

Lasers and light sources can be an effective adjunct to topical or systemic management of acne.[46] There have been numerous case reports and a few clinical studies evaluating the use of devices including blue light, diode laser, intense pulsed light (IPL), and photodynamic therapy (PDT) for the treatment of acne in skins of color.[62-65] In blue light therapy, fluorescent porphyrins produced and excreted by *P. acnes* are targeted and destroyed by the blue light. The diode laser has been shown an effective acne treatment in two clinical studies conducted in Asian patients (skin photo-types III-V) with only a few patients experiencing transient PIH or erythema.[63,66]

COSMETICS AND SKIN CARE IN ACNE

Appropriate skin care contributes to successful management of acne.[5] The objective is to keep the skin and hair (scalp) clean, to control oiliness and prevent excessive dryness and to compensate for daily changes to maintain the skin in a near-ideal state. These objectives can be achieved by balancing cleansing, moisturizing and judicious use of supplemental skin care products.

Cleansers

The purpose of cleansing is to remove dirt, sebum and sweat present onto oily skin. Soaps are not recommended since drying up the skin when already dry and irritated with topical medications, such as retinoids and/ or BP. Too frequent washings to reduce oiliness is counterproductive as it leads to rebound oiliness through repeated irritation of the sebaceous gland. Steaming, scrubbing and the use of exfoliants make acne worse. Soap-free cleansers with pH 5–7 are the best. Cleansing milk is adequate for removing make-up, as compared to toners and astringents. Exfoliating agents speed-up the natural renewal of skin cells and help in the treatment of acne by alleviating comedones provided they are not used aggressively and if scrubbing is avoided.

Salicylic-acid-containing cleansers, exfoliators or creams are helpful in the early stages of treatment. Thanks to its keratolytic, comedolytic and anti-inflammatory effects, SA helps shedding corneocytes, opening clogged pores and neutralizing bacteria.

Some SA derivatives have been also developed for an increased effectiveness. For example, lipo hydroxy acid is a lipophilic derivative of SA with comedolytic properties. Several clinical studies have demonstrated its anti-comedogenic properties.[67,68]

Shaving

Daily shaving can irritate the skin. An electric shaver may be a better option than a mechanic razor. A shaving gel or cream affords better effect than shaving foam and moisturizing lotion is more adequate than a conventional after-shave lotion.

Moisturizers

Most topical anti-acne treatments lead to dryness or increased desquamation of the skin. Appropriate use of oil-free moisturizers should be permitted or even encouraged. The objective is to correct dryness so as to leave the skin feeling hydrated without causing oiliness.

Sunscreen Products

By globally affecting/decreasing the epidermal thickness, some acne treatments like retinoids, chemical peels and tetracycline antibiotics have the potential to increase photosensitivity, by lowering the minimal erythematous dose (MED). With regard to the deleterious effects of sun-exposures upon acne and, on longer objectives, upon a premature skin aging, broad-spectrum sun protection is strongly recommended. This requires identifying a suitable sunscreen product incorporated in the daily routine, according to daily habits (outdoor, indoor occupations). It is also imperative to emphasize the importance of photo-protection in the treatment and prevention of PIH.[46]

ACNE AND QUALITY OF LIFE

Acne-specific measures of QOL include acne disability index, cardiff acne disability index, assessment of the psychological and social effects of acne, and acne quality of life. These measurement tools can be used to monitor changes during therapy and to devise strategies for improving adherence to treatment.[5]

The impact of acne on QOL has been recognized for over 30 years. Acne is associated with greater psychological burden than a variety of disparate chronic disorders. The levels of social, psychological, and emotional impairments in acne compare with chronic diseases such as asthma, epilepsy, diabetes, and arthritis.[50] Acne impacts QOL irrespective of gender and age, but to a level showing some correlation with the severity of the disease. Besides anxiety and depression, acne patients are prone to a low self-esteem, low self-confidence, low self-assertiveness, embarrassment, social inhibition, affectation, shame, altered body image, psychosomatic symptoms (e.g. pain and discomfort), obsessive-compulsiveness and suicidal ideation. Younger patients are subject to scorn, teasing and stigmatization. The impact of acne upon the QOL of Indian patients remains unfortunately nondocumented. Indians appear to accept acne more readily and its impact on QOL in Indian population might be of lower magnitude according to a consensus established by IAA members.

REFERENCES

1. Leyden JJ. Therapy for Acne vulgaris. The New Eng J Med. 1997; 1156-62.
2. Leyden JJ. Current issues in antimicrobial therapy for the treatment of acne. J Eur Dermatol Venereol. 2001;15:51-5.
3. Cunliffe WJ, Gollnick HPM. Acne: Diagnosis and Management. London: Martin Dunitz; 2001.
4. Rademaker M, Garioch JJ, Simpson NB. Acne in school children: No longer a concern for dermatologists. BMJ. 1989;298:1217-9.
5. Kubba R, Bajaj AK, Thappa DM, et al. Acne in India: guidelines for management - IAA consensus document. Indian J Dermatol Venereol Leprol. 2009;75:1-62.
6. Koo J. The psychosocial impact of acne: patient's perceptions J Am Acad Dermatol. 1995;32:S26-30.
7. Thiboutot D, Gollnick H, Bettoli V, et al. Global alliance to improve outcomes in acne. New insights into the management of acne: an update from the Global Alliance to Improve Outcomes in Acne group. J Am Acad Dermatol. 2009;60:S1-50.
8. Zaenglein AL, Thiboutot DM. Acne vulgaris. In: Jorizzo JL, Rapini RP, Olognia JL, editors. Dermatology. 2nd ed. Edinburgh: Elsevier Mosby; 2009.
9. Cappel M, Mauger D, Thiboutot D. Correlation between serum levels of insulin-like growth factor-1, dehydroepiandrosterone sulfate, and dihydrotestosterone and acne lesion counts in adult women. Arch Dermatol. 2005;141:333-8.
10. Xu SX, Wang HL, Fan X, et al. The familial rish of acne vulgaris in Chinese Hans—a case-control study. J Eur Acad Dermatol Venereol. 2007;21:602-5.
11. Goulden V, McGeown CH, Cunliffe WJ. The familial risk of adult acne: a comparison between first-degree relatives of affected and unaffected individuals. Br J Dermatol. 1999;141:297-300.

12. He L, Yang Z, Yu H, et al. The relationship between CYP17-34T/C polymorphism and acne in Chinese subjects revealed by sequencing. Dermatology. 2006;212:338-42.
13. He L, Wu WJ, Yang JK, et al. Two new susceptibility loci 1q24.2 and 11p11.2 confer risk to severe acne. Nat Commun. 2014;5:2870.
14. Pochi PE, Strauss JS, Downing DT. Age related changes in sebaceous gland activity. J Invest Dermatol. 1979;73:108-11.
15. Pochi PE, Strauss JS. Endocrinologic control of the development and activity of the human sebaceous gland. J Invest Dermatol. 1974;62:191-201.
16. Gollnick HPM, Zouboulis CC, Akamatsu H, et al. Pathogenesis and pathogenesis-related treatment of acne. J Dermatol. 1991;18:489-99.
17. Pochi PE, Strauss JS. Sebum production, casual sebum levels, titrable acidity of sebum and urinary fractional 17-ketosteroid excretion in males with acne. J Invest Dermatol. 1964;43:383-8.
18. Burton JL, Shuster S. The relationship between seborrhea and acne vulgaris. Br J Dermatol. 1971;84:600-1.
19. Cunliffe WJ, Shuster S. Pathogenesis of acne. Lancet. 1969;1:685-7.
20. Deplewski D, Rosenfield RL. Role of hormones in pilosebaceous unit development. Endocrine Rev. 2000;21:363-92.
21. Akamatsu H, Zouboulis CC, Orfanos CE. Control of human sebocyte proliferation in vitro by testosterone and 5-alpha-dihydrotestosterone is dependent on the localization of the sebaceous glands. J Invest Dermatol. 1992;99:509-11.
22. Knutson DD. Ultrastuctural observations in acne vulgaris: The normal sebaceous follicles and acne lesions. J Invest Dermatol. 1974;62:288-307.
22. Cunliffe WJ, Holland DB, Clark SM, et al. Comedogenesis: Some new aetiological, clinical and therapeutic strategies. Br J Dermatol. 2000;142:1084-91.
24. Knaggs HE, Holland DB, Morris C, et al. Quantification of cellular proliferation in acne using the monoclonal antibody Ki-67. J Invest Dermatol. 1994;102:89-92.
25. Hughes BR, Morris C, Cunliffe WJ, et al. Keratin expression in pilosebaceous epithelia in truncal skin of acne patients. Br J Dermatol. 1996;134:247-56.
26. Downing DT, Stewart ME, Wertz PW, et al. Essential fatty acids and acne. J Am Acad Dermatol. 1986;14:221-5.
27. Thiboutot DM, Knaggs H, Gilliand K, et al. Activity of type 1 5-a reductase and 17-β-hydroxysteroid dehydrogenase in the infrainfundibulum of subjects with and without acne vulgaris. Dermatology. 1998;196:38-42.
28. Ingham E, Eady EA, Goodwin CE. Pro-inflammatory levels of interlukin 1-α like bioactivity are present in the majority of open comedones in acne vulgaris. J Invest Dermatol. 1992;98:895-901.
29. Guy R, Kealey T. Modelling the infundibulum in acne. Dermatology 1998;196:32-7.
30. Habif TP. Acne, rosacea, and related disorders, In: Habif TP, Editor. Clinical dermatology: A color guide to diagnosis and therapy, 4th ed. Edinburgh: Mosby; 2004. pp. 168-70.
31. Knor T. The pathogenesis of acne. Acta dermatovenerol Croat. 2005;13:44-9.
32. Kim J, Ochoa MT, Kruzik SR, et al. Activation of toll-like receptor 2 in acne triggers inflammatory cytokine responses. J Immunol. 2002;169:1535-541.
33. Jeremy AH, Holland DB, Roberts SG, et al. Inflammatory events are involved in acne lesion initiation. J Invest Dermatol. 2003;121:20-7.
34. Zouboulis CC, Bϕhm M. Neuroendocrine regulation of sebocytes: A pathogenetic link between stress and acne. Exp Dermatol. 2004;13:31-5.
35. Al-Ameer AM, Al-Akloby OM. Demographic features and seasonal variations in patients with acne vulgaris in Saudi Arabia: A hospital-based study. Int J Dermatol. 2002;41:870-1.
36. Tan HH, Tan AW, Barkham T, et al. Community-based study of acne vulgaris in adolescents in Singapore. Br J Dermatol. 2007;157:547-51
37. Adityan B, Thappa DM. Profile of acne vulgaris—a hospital-based study from South India. Indian J Dermatol Venereol Leprol. 2009;75:272-8.
38. Simpson NB, Cunliffe WJ. Disorders of the sebaceous glands. In: Burns T, Breathnach S, Cox N, Griffiths C, Editors). Rook's textbook of dermatology, 7th edition. Oxford: Blackwell Science; 2004. pp. 43.28-43.34.
39. Brown SK, Shalita AR. Acne vulgaris. Lancet. 1998;20;351:1871-6.
40. Kurokawa I, Danby FW, Ju Q, et al. New developments in our understanding of acne pathogenesis and treatment. Exp Dermatol. 2009;18:821-32.
41. Cunliffe WJ, Holland DB, Clark SM, et al. Comedogenesis: Some new aetiological, clinical and therapeutic strategies. Br J Dermatol. 2000;142:1084-91.
42. Plewig G, Kigman AM,. Acne and Rosacea. 3rd ed. Berlin: Springer Verlag; 2000.
43. Rivera AE. Acne scarring: a review and current treatment modalities. J Am Acad Dermatol. 2008;59:659-76.
44. Bouzari N1, Davis SC, Nouri K. Laser treatment of keloids and hypertrophic scars. Int J Dermatol. 2007;46:80-8.
45. Jacob CI, Dover JS, Kaminer MS. Acne scarring: a classification system and review of treatment options. J Am Acad Dermatol. 2001;45(1):109-17.
46. Davis EC, Callender VD. A review of acne in ethnic skin: pathogenesis, clinical manifestations, and management strategies. J Clin Aesthet Dermatol. 2010;3:24-38.
47. Taylor SC, Cook-Bolden F, Rahman Z, et al. Acne vulgaris in skin of color. J Am Acad Dermatol. 2002;46:S98-106.
48. Callender VD. Acne in ethnic skin: special considerations for therapy. Dermatol Ther. 2004;17:184-95.
49. Khanna N, Datta Gupta S. Rejuvenating facial massage: A bane or boon? Int J Dermatol. 2002;41:407-10.
50. Simpson NB, Cunliffe WJ. Disorders of the sebaceous glands. In: Burns T, Breathnach S, Cox N, Griffiths C, editors. Rook's textbook of dermatology. 7th ed. Oxford: Blackwell Science; 2004. pp. 43.31-32.
51. Cunliffe WJ, Gollnick HPM. Acne: Diagnosis and management. London: Martin Dunitz; 2001. pp. 49-67.
52. Ganceviciene R, Böhm M, Fimmel S, et al. The role of neuropeptides in the multifactorial pathogenesis of acne vulgaris. Dermatoendocrinol. 2009;1:170-6.
53. Saint-Léger D, Baque A, Cohen E, et al. A possible role for squalene in the pathogenesis of acne. Br J Dermatol. 1986;114:535-42.
54. Sardana K, Sharma RC, Sarkar R. Seasonal variation in acne vulgaris: myth or reality. J Dermatol. 2002;29:484-8.
55. Adebamowo CA, Spiegelman D, Danby EW, et al. High school dietary dairy intake and teenage acne. J Am Acad Dermatol. 2005;52:207-14.
56. Cordain L, Lindeberg S, Hurtado M, et al. Acne vulgaris: A disease of western civilization. Arch Dermatol. 2002;138:1584-90.
57. Degitz K, Placzek M, Borelli C, et al. Pathophysiology of acne. J Dtsch Dermatol Ges. 2007;5:316-23.
58. Longshore SJ, Hollandsworth K. Acne vulgaris: one treatment does not fit all. Cleve Clin J Med. 2003;70:670, 672-4, 677-8 passim.
59. Rathi SK. Acne vulgaris treatment: the current scenario. Indian J Dermatol. 2011;56:7-13.

60. Roberts WE. Chemical peeling in ethnic/dark skin. Dermatol Ther. 2004;17:196-205.
61. Song JY, Kang HA, Kim MY, et al. Damage and recovery of skin barrier function after glycolic acid chemical peeling and crystal microdermabrasion. Dermatol Surg. 2004;30:390-4.
62. Tzung TY, Wu KH, Huang ML. Blue light phototherapy in the treatment of acne. Photodermatol Photoimmunol PhotoMed. 2004;20:266-9.
63. Yeung CK, Shek SY, Yu CS, et al. Treatment of inflammatory facial acne with 1,450 nm diode laser in type IV to V Asian skin using an optimal combination of laser parameters. Dermatol Surg. 2009;35:593-600.
64. Kawana S, Tachihara R, Kato T, et al. Effect of smooth pulsed light at 400 to 700 and 870 to 1,200 nm for acne vulgaris in Asian skin. Dermatol Surg. 2010;36:52-7.
65. Oh SH, Ryu DJ, Han EC, et al. A comparative study of topical 5-aminolevulinic acid incubation times in photodynamic therapy with intense pulsed light for the treatment of inflammatory acne. Dermatol Surg. 2009;35:1918-26.
66. Noborio R, Nishida E, Morita A. Clinical effect of low-energy double-pass 1450 nm laser treatment for acne in Asians. Photodermatol Photoimmunol PhotoMed. 2009;25:3-7.
67. Bissonnette R1, Bolduc C, Seité S, et al. Randomized study comparing the efficacy and tolerance of a lipophilic hydroxy acid derivative of salicylic acid and 5% benzoyl peroxide in the treatment of facial acne vulgaris. J Cosmet Dermatol. 2009;8:19-23.
68. Léveque JL, Hamzavi I, Seite S, et al. Randomized trial comparing a chemical peel containing a lipophilic hydroxy acid derivative of salicylic acid with a salicylic acid peel in subjects with comedonal acne. J Cosmet Dermatol. 2011;10:174-8.

Chapter 11

Skin Aging and Antiaging Cosmetics

Michèle Verschoore, *L'Oréal Research and Innovation, Asnières, France*
Hema Jerajani, *MGM Medical College and Hospital, Mumbai, India*

INTRODUCTION

Like many other countries, India sees its population aging. As a result, geriatric dermatology is gaining a steady momentum. India has met the United Nation's definition of an aging country when the population aged over 60 years exceeds 7%, an already crossed threshold, thought to reach 25% by 2025.[1] The dermatologic issues of this aging population are strongly influenced by many social, economic, and cultural factors.[2]

Aging is a physiological phenomenon. It must be distinguished from some degenerative diseases whose prevalence increases with age. From a biological point of view, aging is defined as the irreversible changes in biological homeostasis which take place as a result of time-related events.

Skin and its aging show disparity, i.e. high inter-individual variations amongst humans. Skin aging underlines the concept of physiological or biological age which may not fit chronological age. The plurality of factors involved in skin aging could account for such differences.

In broad outline, two major types of factor are involved in skin aging process:

1. *Intrinsic or chronological factors:* They include different patterns: (i) a genetic determination at a cellular level as described by Hayflick;[3] (ii) a series of successive molecular errors during DNA transcription leading to alterations in protein synthesis, (iii) an increase in intercellular free radicals as postulated by Harman[4] cumulative damage caused by free radicals to mitochondria, eventually resulting in membrane damage and reduced energy production;[4,5] and (iv) exhaustion or dysfunction of stem cell reservoir.[6]
2. *Extrinsic factors:* Mostly linked to lifestyle, extrinsic factors relate to nutrition and smoking habits, exposure to toxics (including excessive consumption of alcoholic beverages) and environmental factors, especially sun exposure. Those factors could all speed-up physiological processes of aging although experimental data suggest that UV-induced alterations would be more specific.

Since skin is obviously accessible for examination, it is an organ of utmost interest for studying and understanding the aging process.

CLINICAL SIGNS OF SKIN AGING

Chronological Aging

It is wellknown that with age the dermal–epidermal junction (DEJ) flattens whereas epidermis and dermis become thinner. These alterations are associated with changes in microrelief of the skin surface, as described by Hashimoto.[7] However, the major changes related to chronological aging concern the superficial dermis where the amount of free water increases with age, while the content of its macrofibrillar proteins (elastin, collagens) and proteoglycans decreases.[8] Such changes in the balance between free water and macromolecules alter the viscoelastic properties of the skin.

It must also be taken into consideration that some of the age-related skin clinical changes could partly result from subcutaneous changes, mainly in hypodermis.

Signs of chronological skin aging must be observed on unexposed skin areas, such as inner forearms or lower back which are the areas usually investigated in most works related to this matter.

Three signs are linked to chronological aging:

1. *Epidermal and dermal atrophy*, which induces a change in skin appearance: To explore this skin condition, the clinician just needs inspection. With age, the skin loses its porcelain transparency and peachy appearance and becomes thinner which will later reflect in the visual appearance of cigarette paper or papyrus. Skin color also takes a duller tone (Fig. 1). In elderly subjects, usually over 80 years, atrophic skin can be associated with a scaly aspect, creating the whole clinical feature called "senile xerosis", sometimes accompanied by itching.

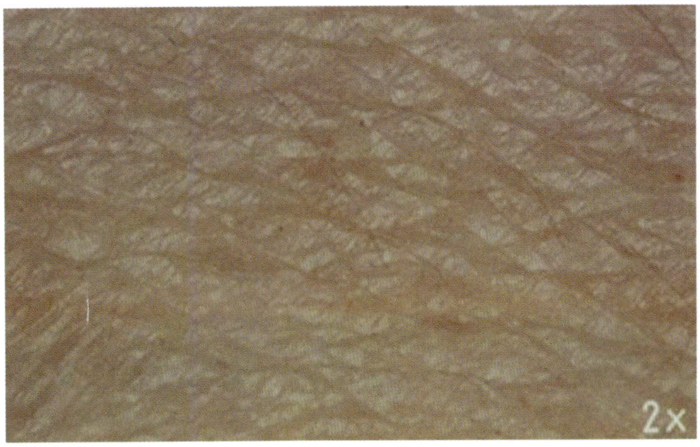

Figure 1: Epidermal atrophy aspect. With age, the skin loses its transparency and becomes thinner creating an appearance of cigarette paper or papyrus
©L'Oréal Research and Innovation

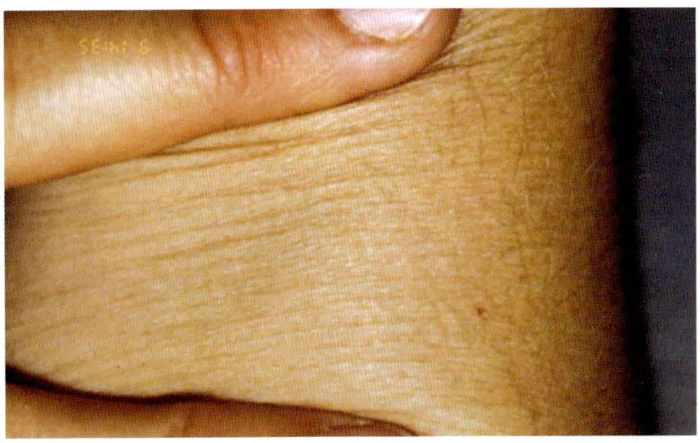

Figure 2: How to explore skin texture: To explore skin texture, the clinician must perform a gentle superficial pinching of skin with a scissor movement between index and middle finger
©L'Oréal Research and Innovation

2. *Crinkling skin*, a change in skin texture: To explore skin texture, the clinician must perform a gentle superficial pinching of skin with a scissor movement between index and middle finger (Fig. 2). In young people, skin texture is similar to satin. With age, the glazed texture is progressively lost, and the skin gets crinkled (Fig. 3). This can be quantitatively evaluated.

3. *Flaccidity*, a change in skin firmness: To explore skin firmness, the clinician must do a gentle pinching of skin

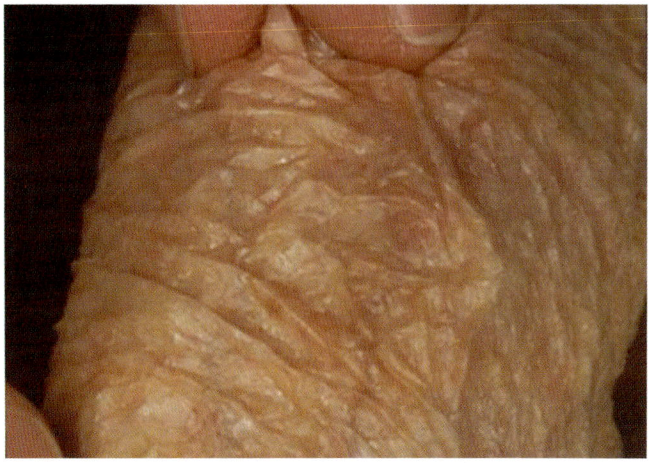

Figure 3: Crinkling skin: With age, the glazed texture is progressively lost, and the skin gets crinkled. Here, the skin of an 88-year-old woman
©L'Oréal Research and Innovation

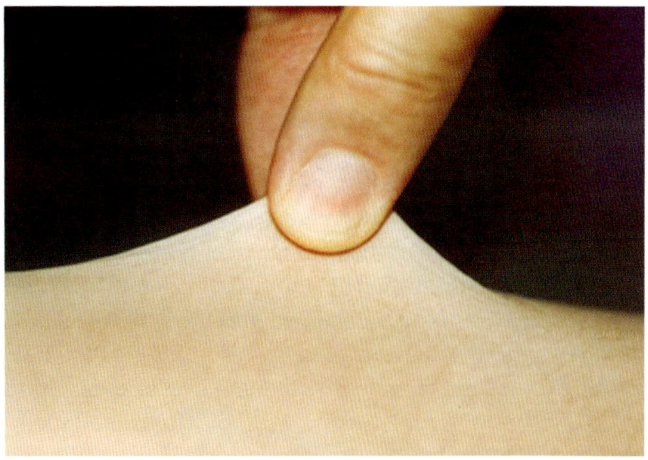

Figure 4: How to explore skin firmness: To explore skin firmness, the clinician must do a gentle pinching of skin between thumb and index, in a vertical movement
©L'Oréal Research and Innovation

between thumb and index, in a vertical movement (Fig. 4). Dermal changes induce loss of skin firmness. However, in old people, changes in subcutaneous compartments, such as hypodermis are also causative of skin flaccidity. As example, with age the loss of firmness is responsible for low-cheek sagging, increase in the facial nasolabial fold, and skin tissue sagging in the posterior part of arms.

Effect of aging in some parts of the body, like foot sole, may have functional consequences: the hardness of foot sole at later stage of life is mainly due to repeated mechanical trauma and could be prevented.[9]

Photoaging

Signs of photoaging are only seen on sun-exposed areas, such as face, neck, volar forearms, and dorsum of hands. They result from chronic sun exposures throughout life. Whilst some authors consider photoaging process as an acceleration of chronological aging, most admit that photoaging presents a specific biological pattern. Clinical and histological signs of photoaging are the results of acute skin damage induced by intensive exposure to sun UV rays along with lower daily exposures, repeated lifelong.[10] Durai et al. showed on phototype IV skin (the predominant type in India) that chronological aging symptoms are more prominent than photoaging clinical symptoms.[11]

Clinical Elastosis: A Change in Skin Appearance and Skin Texture

To understand the clinical appearance of elastosis, it is important to keep in mind what takes place at the histological level. Elastosis is the result of activation by chronic sun exposure (or smoking) of an unbalanced dermal-matrix remodeling, with a higher stimulation of collagenases and elastases. It ensues an overproduction of abnormal dermal matrix material resulting in dermal infiltration with "elastotic material". At a first step, the clinical consequence is the "orange peel skin appearance," which reflects skin stuffing by skin appendages. In a second step, there is a stuffing breakdown and the superficial part of skin dermis is totally invaded by this "elastotic material" causing important changes in cutaneous texture, resulting in a thick and swollen skin, with big folds and deep wrinkles. Whatever the stage, skin elastosis gives a yellowish appearance to facial skin. On the upper presternal area (V neck), skin elastosis could give a redness appearance to the skin.

Pigmented Disorders and Actinic Lentigos

The darker is the phototype, the more frequent are pigmented disorders and actinic lentigos.

Actinic lentigos are also called "solar lentigines", "sun spots" or "age spots". They are histologically characterized by an increase in the amount of melanin at the basal layer, epidermal extension into dermis and penetration of melanin granules within the dermis with melanophages. They appear at around 40 years of age. Their number is small (less than 10 on face), their diameter is up to 4 mm, and no seasonal changes in color are observed. They are localized on face, dorsal hand, and forearms.

In Asian population, specific freckles are also observed.[12] These spots, also called "Asian spots" appear at around 16–22 years. They are localized only on face, mainly on nose and cheek bones. They can be numerous (more than 30 on face) their diameter is less than 3 mm, and seasonal changes in color are observed.

Very often, pigmented disorders induced by photoaging are characterized by hyperpigmented areas, of variable color intensity. Such dyspigmentations give an uneven skin tone and play an important role in age perception.[13] A recent study performed in India on 1,204 women focused on the evolution of pigmentary disorders, with age[14] showing that hyperpigmented disorders, such as simplex lentigo, dark circles, and spread macules occur at early stages of life and increase with age, contributing to an overall facial unevenness.

Facial Aging

The face plays a major part in the age perception of an individual where clinical signs of chronologic aging and photoaging are mixed. Furthermore, anatomic specificities of the cephalic part of the body (bone cranial architecture, subcutis, muscles insertion) are responsible for specific facial aging signs such as wrinkles, sagging, and enlargement of skin pores.

Wrinkles

Wrinkles are one of the key sign of facial aging. They are the result of different processes.

(i) Subcutaneous muscle contraction.

Facial muscles are linked to the deep part of skin and their contractions are responsible for facial expression. Striae muscular fibers can be observed in the subcutaneous tissue, forming the "panniculus carnosus". The tension transmitted to the skin during facial muscle contractions, including contraction of "panniculus carnosus" leads to "expressional wrinkles", as illustrated by well-known counterbalance effect of botulinum toxin on wrinkles.

Since repeated all along the life, these contractions impact the structural organization of dermal collagen fibers. Finally, they determine the anatomic localization of wrinkles on face: crow's feet, glabella, forehead, perioral area.

(ii) Changes in texture and loss of firmness turn "expressional wrinkles" "into "permanent wrinkles".

(iii) Facial elastosis increases wrinkle depth and number, and makes "permanent wrinkles" worse.

Facial Sagging

From 35 years to 45 years, the changes in subcutaneous tissue (hypodermis and fascia) and the gravitation entailing lipid downward migration are responsible for facial sagging with fall of low cheek, fall of submental neck, increase of nasolabial folds and bags under eyes. From 60 years to 65 years, these signs become more and more visible.

Skin Pores

At around 40–50 years of age, skin pores become more visible on cheeks, forehead and chin, especially in women, found associated with menopause.

SKIN AGING IN INDIA

Clinical Evaluation

As previously mentioned, clinical signs of skin aging are not only linked to chronological age. Consequently, prior clinical assessment is very important for subject selection and signs' quantification when dealing with skin aging. Assessment can be done either directly on the subject (*in situ* evaluation) or on standardized photographs. With regard to inter-investigators variability, clinical assessment needs to consider the most reliable way to control and reduce this variability. Prime requirement is to involve experienced and trained clinicians.

For a clinician used to examine and deal with pathologic conditions to turn to and focus his expertise on the new field of semiology of normal skin is indeed a new and somewhat difficult task. Semiology of skin surface appearance, uneven pigmentation, etc. need to be learned and mastered. In addition, two other factors must be considered: (i) repeatability for the same investigator with time; and (ii) inter-investigator reproducibility.

Photographic reference rating scales are recommended to guide the clinicians and reduce investigators' variability. Among those, validated grading scales for assessment repeatability and reproducibility must be preferred. Again, to be used efficiently, they require trained clinicians. Two categories of scales could be used:

1. Global scales for facial aging, such as overall photoaging scales. These scales are particularly useful for including subjects in a controlled study.
2. Focused scales according to area and signs, such as wrinkle scales, actinic lentigo scales, etc. These scales are especially recommended when quantitative clinical assessment is required.

To assess the efficacy of products or ingredients, clinical scoring on standardized photographs (with same magnification, lighting and subject position) are of real interest. Blinded comparative clinical scoring can be done by one or a set of clinicians. Such comparative rating is easy to implement, and generated data is usually very consistent.

Noninvasive Methods

Numerous methods exist to quantitatively assess skin aging. In the 80s and 90s, the methods used were mainly based on biophysical measurements. Since the last decade, image analysis on standardized pictures has been increasingly used.

Most used and relevant methods are the following.

Skin Microrelief Assessment[15-17]

Skin microrelief changes with age (Fig. 5): the depth of skin furrows increases, resulting in decreased density. The reference method to study skin microrelief consists in taking skin replicas with elastomer gels, which are then assessed by image analysis software. Now, laser profilometry can be performed directly on skin.

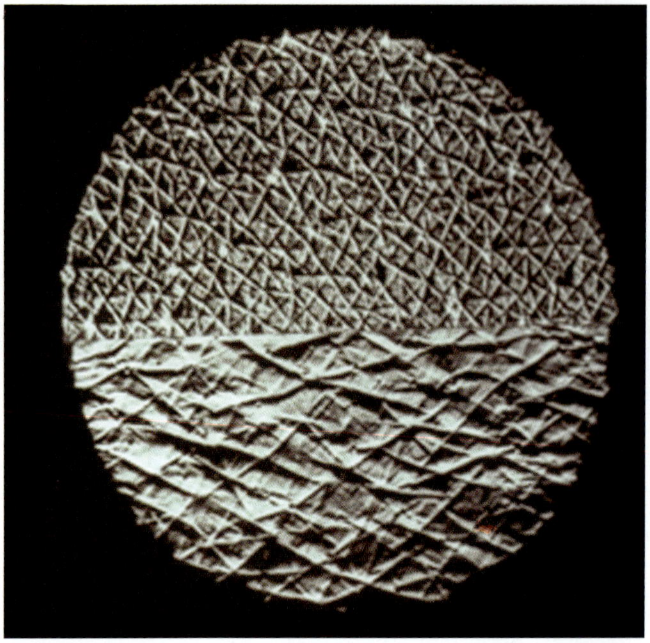

Figure 5: Skin microrelief on forearm. Upper half part represents skin microrelief of a young woman (23 years); lower half part shows skin microrelief of an old woman (82 years). Notice the enlargement of network with age and changes in the orientation of the lines

Skin Thickness[18,19]

Skin thickness can be measured with high resolution echography (up to 20 MHz). Ultrasound imaging allows the whole skin thickness (epidermis and dermis) to be quantified.

With confocal microscopy, it is possible to measure the thickness of the stratum corneum (SC) and of the malpighian epidermis and also to assess the amplitude of undulation of the DEJ.[20]

Optical coherent tomography (OCT) enables epidermal thickness and dermal thickness to be evaluated.

Skin Biomechanical Changes[19,21-25]

Several methods have been used including ballistometry and twistometry. The most often used method to measure changes in skin biomechanical properties is the Dermal-torquemeter® (Diastron, Broomal, PA, USA), which records parameters linked to skin elasticity and skin viscoelasticity.

Skin Color

The most widely used devices are Chromameter® (Konica-Minolta, Osaka, Japan) and Mexameter® MX18 (C-K Electronic, Köln, Germany). Chromameter® is a very useful device to measure color changes[26] using the L*a*b* reference system: L* represents lightness, from white (0) to black (100), a*b* reflect chromaticity. However, due to the great heterogeneity of pigmentation, it is the rule to perform multiple measurements on different adjacent areas, and to only consider their mean values. To improve color measurements, specifically on face, a Chromasphere® has been developed[27] allowing quantitative color measurements to be performed on the whole face with a completely controlled lighting of the face.

Image Analysis on Standardized Pictures

Repositioning method allows reproducible pictures of the same subject in the same position to be taken, with the same lighting conditions, at different times. The pictures can be obtained with normal light, cross-polarized light, parallel polarized light and UV light. Cross-polarized light is very useful to assess pigmented disorders whereas parallel polarized light enhances the oily aspects of the skin.

Automatic image analysis software programs are available for measuring various cutaneous parameters. However, although very significant improvements have been brought, the data obtained must be carefully checked by clinicians.

Biological and Histological Approaches

When biopsies are performed to assess skin aging, several parameters can be assessed:

- Histologic parameters. Thanks to histochemical staining or immunostaining against specific proteins, changes occurring within the tissue can be visualized and qualitatively or quantitatively evaluated. The most used parameters are epidermal thickness, renewal and differentiation markers but also changes in the dermal components, such as elastin, fibrillin-1 and collagens
- Transcriptomic analysis, completed with quantitative polymerase chain reaction (PCR) as well as proteomic analysis are new tools of interest to study specific biologic activation.

SKIN AGING IN INDIA

The sensitivity of the skin towards aging alterations, such as dermal damage, solar elastosis, and wrinkle formation, also depends upon constitutive pigmentation, the lighter skins being more prone to. Few studies have been specifically dedicated to understand Indian specific aging signs. Durai et al.[11] conducted a study in Puducherry, India, on 500 elderly individuals attending their dermatology outpatient department, to evaluate the severity of photoaging in this population (skin phototype IV–V). Photoaging changes were less common than chronological aging ones in studied population. They confirmed that in India the most important cutaneous change suggestive of photoaging is dyspigmentation. Interestingly, they also showed that chronological changes were more frequent in females than males, while photoaging was more frequent in males, linked to their outdoor occupational sun exposure. This discrepancy between men and women may be less prone in the future, as the outdoor lifestyles seem to reach more and more women in urban populations.

Facial skin color heterogeneity being a major issue in India, a recent study aimed at assessing facial Indian skin color and its changes with age.[28] 1,200 healthy Indian women aged 18–85 years from four cities (Mumbai, Chennai, Delhi and Kolkata) were recruited and their facial skin color was analyzed on several areas with Chromasphere® device. The study showed some facial specific heterogeneities in Indians that can change with age. Skin color of the cheek becomes darker with age irrespective of the city ($p > 0.005$) and is significantly less saturated and redder in Chennai. Dark circles appear as a major concern since becoming darker, less saturated and redder with age (Fig. 6). However, their color contrast with cheeks does not change with age, i.e. no conspicuous increase. Compared to other populations, a loss of saturation was observed with age, giving an overall impression of muted skin.

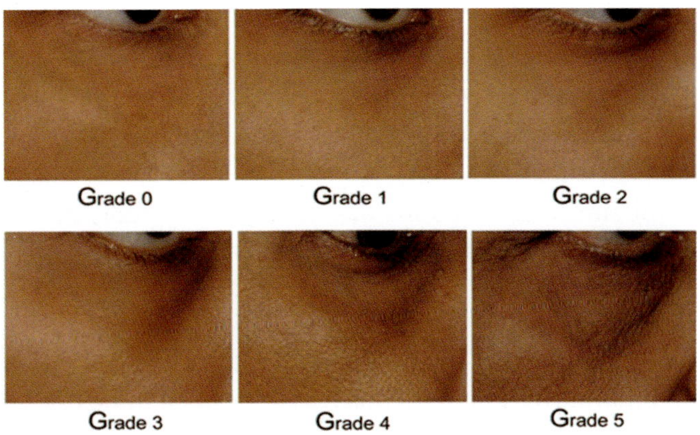

Figure 6: Dark circles in Indian population: 5 grades of severity ©L'Oréal Research and Innovation

ANTIAGING COSMETICS

α Hydroxy Acids

α Hydroxy acids (AHAs) correspond to acids of the general structure: R-CHOH-COOH. Widely used in skin creams and lotions, AHAs are well recognized as potent exfoliating agents with subsequent stimulation of cell renewal. Desquamation of dead cells, corneocytes, due to loosening of corneosome junctions is the core mechanism of action. They may also interact at both epidermal and dermal levels. Dermal effects include improvement in the quality of elastic fibers and collagen architecture, increase in collagen density and dermal thickness.

α Hydroxy acids are commonly used at concentrations ranging 4–15% in skincare creams and lotions for their clinical efficiency in smoothing out the effects of photoaging through improving wrinkles, skin hydration, elasticity and tone. But they can also be used by dermatologists at much higher concentration (such as 70% for glycolic acid) for peeling with outstanding results in resurfacing photoaged skin. However, some discomfort such as stinging, tingling and redness may appear in relation to AHA effectiveness depending on concentration level. Greasy skin seems to be more tolerant as compared to dry, sensitive skin.

α Hydroxy acids derivatives, such as polyhydroxy-acids, have been developed in order to increase tolerance or to optimize their properties.

β Hydroxy Acid Family

Salicylic acid (SA) belongs to the β hydroxy acid family and has been used for years to treat skin disorders like acne, hyperkeratosis... SA penetrates rather rapidly and the breakdown of corneodesmosomes, the intercellular "rivets" of SC, can occur throughout the SC as a result.

To refine the properties of SA, a new lipophilic derivative: *C8-lipohydroxyacid or C8-LHA*, has been developed and extensively studied in clinical trials[29] with skin relief evaluation (through skin replicas analyzed by a scanning microscope), confocal microscopy and biopsies. A 20% increase in epidermis thickness has been measured with a formulation containing 1.5% of C8-LHA. In fact biopsies show a thinning of the SC together with an increase in the thickness of Malpighian and germinative layers. Interestingly, the images of replica show a sequential loss of individual corneocytes instead of desquamation in clusters as generally seen with SA.[29] A review of the biologic properties and clinical benefits of this lipophilic derivative has been published.[30] Interestingly, it has been shown that 2% C8-LHA significantly reduce the number of clusters of melanosomes, increase basal epidermal thickness, and produce a variety of changes that resemble those induced by all-trans retinoic acid but smoothly controlled.[31]

Optimized formulations at the adequate concentration of C8-LHA with a slow penetration rate and good storage in the superficial layers of the SC are proven to be effective and safe.

Retinol

Retinol and carotenoids are the two most common forms of vitamin A found in Nature. Carotenoids are vitamin A precursors or provitamin A whereas vitamin A or retinol is further converted through metabolic pathways into various derivatives, such as retinoic acid, retinaldehyde, retinyl esters.[32] Retinol and its natural and synthetic derivatives form a class of substances known as retinoids, which bind to specific nuclear receptors of epidermal cells and are highly recognized by dermatologists for their well-known, statistically proven benefits in the care and prevention of skin ageing.[33,34] It is worth noting that their efficiency is restricted to topical applications and that 2–6 months are needed to see a clear and proven benefit.

Formulation/Penetration

Since highly unstable and sensitive to oxygen in the air which is amplified by light exposure and heat, retinol requires very specific formulation techniques, encapsulation for example, to prevent its degradation.

Indications and Mechanisms of Action of Retinoids

The reduced mottled hyperpigmentation by retinoids relates to an enhanced epidermal cell turnover, decreasing the time of contact between keratinocytes and melanocytes, promoting a decrease in melanosome transfer and a rapid loss of melanins via epidermopoiesis.[35] Fine lines and wrinkles are reduced through the reduction of collagen breakdown due to the decrease in matrix metalloproteinases (MMP) enzymes that degrade collagen whilst collagen synthesis and glycosaminoglycan (GAG) synthesis are stimulated. The decrease in skin roughness is explained by retinoids modulated expression of genes which are involved in differentiation and proliferation and which promote epidermal cell turnover.[36]

Clinical Trials Conducted with Retinol

A double blind study has shown a high level of evidence of retinol efficiency.[37] Retinol 0.4% was applied to the upper inner part of the arm in 36 elderly subjects 3 times a week for 24 weeks in a randomized vehicle-controlled study. At 24 weeks, the clinical grading scores of fine wrinkling were significantly improved and, in skin biopsy samples, GAG expression and pro-collagen I immunostaining significantly increased. We also found significant effects on crow's feet wrinkles with 0.1% retinol cream in a double blind study versus vehicle using fringe projection analysis (L'Oréal Research data, unpublished). On the other hand, Tesoriere et al.[38] suggested that retinol behaved as an effective antioxidant at low concentration (*in vitro* study).

Skin Tolerance

Whereas the acceptance of retinoic acid by patients is limited due to side effects including erythema, burning, scaling, pruritus,[34] irritation is not a major issue with topical retinol; only some sensitive skins may experiment slight irritation. Combining good moisturizer and effective sunscreen with retinol treatment is most appropriate.

In summary retinoids are important ingredients for treating chronologically and photo aged skin.

Hyaluronic Acid

Hyaluronic acid or hyaluronan (HA) is the most abundant GAG in cutaneous tissue[39] representing one of the major components of extracellular matrix of the skin into which cells and fibrous networks of collagen and elastin are embedded.[40] Keratinocytes and fibroblasts are the principal source of HA in the epidermis and dermis.[41]

Thanks to its very high capacity to bind to water, HA has a prominent role in the maintenance of the extra-cellular space and control of hydration. Cell responses to HA are primarily mediated by CD44, the major expressed HA receptor of the cell surface. The regulation of keratinocyte proliferation is linked to the presence of CD44 on keratinocytes. Cell surface receptors such as CD44 and TLR2[42] have been reported to inform cells about the size and content of hyaluronan at the cell surface and to mediate its effects.

The huge size of HA (up to 2,000 kDa), however, makes it hardly possible to penetrate the skin except in special conditions. To increase its penetration, fragmentation of HA has been proposed (down to 250/400 kDa) but the right choice of a low molecular fragment of HA is important since it has been shown that some HA fragments with a molecular size less than 20 kDa could have proinflammatory effect due to their binding to TLR2 and TLR4 receptors.[43,44] Skin Ethic® model was used to evaluate the effect of HA on gene expression.[45]

Appropriate HA fragments have been proven to reverse skin atrophy as early as one month after initiation of treatment and this effect is mediated through a CD44 dependent mechanism[46] but the increase in human thickness is observed only in case of skin atrophy which is a common sign of chronologically aged skin. Some low molecular weight (LMW) fragments of HA can influence the expression of many genes, including those contributing to keratinocyte differentiation and formation of intercellular tight junction complexes which are reported to be reduced in aged and photodamaged skin. Marked reduction of wrinkles has been demonstrated with LMW HA.[46]

Delayed wound healing is also a good indication for use of hyaluronan. HA is involved in tissue remodeling[46] and an activated synthesis of HA has been reported to occur in wounded adult epidermis.[47]

Moreover, HA may protect the skin against UV-induced oxidative stress through its free radical scavenging properties.[48]

Vitamin C

Vitamin C, also known as ascorbic acid, is a water soluble vitamin. Naturally unstable, ascorbic acid requires very specific types of formulation. Derivatives can also be used but the development of formulations with good skin penetration and bioavailability is mandatory.

The role of vitamin C is crucial in the synthesis of collagen and elastin.[33] It is a cofactor for both propyl and lysyl hydroxylases that catalyze the formation of hydroxyproline and hydroxylysine.[49] Proline and lysine are found throughout the collagen molecule and their hydroxylation facilitates the excretion of procollagen from the fibroblast.[50] It makes collagen structure more stable and less sensitive to heat.[51]

Ascorbic acid also acts as one of the most efficient antioxidants (free-radical scavenging properties) in aqueous medium. In the skin, vitamin C has been shown to modulate the effect of UV-induced ROS damage[52] and to potentially reverse the negative effect of UV rays.[53] DNA mutations are the first steps in carcinogenesis and a link between DNA repair and vitamin C has been suggested.

In *in vitro* reconstructed skin model, vitamin C has been shown to optimize the formation of the DEJ leading to a structure closer to that of normal human skin. DEJ has a major role in maintaining skin cohesion resistance to mechanical stress and exchanges between epidermis and dermis. It deteriorates in aged skin, where the rete ridges digitating with dermal papillae progressively disappear leading to an almost flat DEJ.[54]

Consequently, vitamin C has a number of utmost interesting properties for the treatment of aged and photoaged skin. Its level decreases with age, especially in the epidermis (Fig. 7).[55]

Well-controlled clinical trials have shown favorable results of vitamin C in aged human skin. A 3-month study in 19 subjects whose half face was treated either with L-ascorbic acid or vehicle[56] showed significant clinical improvement in fine wrinkling, tactile roughness, visual dryness, telangiectasia, laxity/tone, pigmentation with an objective improvement in optical profilometry analysis in L-ascorbic acid treated side versus vehicle-treated. Another double blind placebo-controlled study with 5% ascorbic acid formulation applied daily to facial skin showed clinical benefits after 3 months which further increased after 6 month treatment.[57] At the molecular

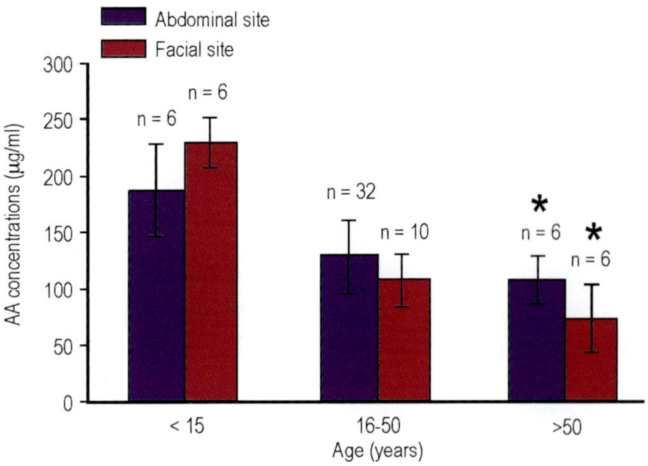

Figure 7: Ascorbic acid concentrations from two human skin sites according to age[55]
©L'Oréal Research and Innovation

level, a study on 10 postmenopausal women revealed a significant increase in mRNA levels of collagen I and III after 6 months in the biopsy samples of L-ascorbic acid treated skin compared to vehicle treated with increased levels of MMP-1 tissue inhibitor, which reduces collagen breakdown.[56] A study of the papillary index of aged skin measured by confocal microscopy in postmenopausal women showed that the number of nutritive capillary loops increased in the papillary dermis close to the basal level of epidermis in L-ascorbic acid treated samples vs. vehicle treated.[58]

Pro-Xylane®

It has been widely reported that superficial dermis is a major target in skin aging. Resonance magnetic imaging (RMI) has brought out a significant increase in free water content with age when comparing 2 age groups (<40 and >70 years of age).[8] On the other hand, the most frequent signs of aging include loss of texture, skin laxity, and alterations of viscoelastic properties.

Pro-Xylane® has been developed using a biomimetic approach in order to improve the proteoglycan and GAG content and restore age altered distribution to make skin firmer with toning up effects on skin texture.[59] *In vitro,* Pro-Xylane® increases GAGs expression in aged skin with an increase in procollagen I and fibrillin.[1] Moreover, Pro-Xylane® induces the synthesis of collagens VII and IV and laminin 5 which are glycoproteins of the DEJ involved in anchoring properties.[60,61] At the epidermal level, a significant increase in the expression of hyaluronan receptor CD44 at the surface of keratinocytes has been revealed in an atrophic skin model.[62]

A double blind randomized clinical study with a right/left comparison has been performed. One side was treated with Pro-Xylane® and the other one with its vehicle in 15 women (average 62-years-old) for a 3-month period of time. A significant reduction of the overall clinical score of aging was seen in the Pro-Xylane® treated side as early as 35 days after starting treatment. Overall score included mean score of pigmented spots, roughness, wrinkles, sagging. Viscoelasticity, as measured with the DTM device (Dermal Torque Meter®, Dia-Stron Ltd., Andover, United Kingdom) showed significantly improved at day 35 in the Pro-Xylane® treated side. On the biopsies performed from the Pro-Xylane® treated side, a comparison between before and after treatment revealed a statistically significant increase in GAGs. In another study on 50 healthy women (aged 45–65), twice daily application of a formulation containing Pro-Xylane® gave excellent results upon some biomechanical properties of the skin (tonicity, firmness) with a statistical reduction of skin relief (total number of wrinkles, total surface wrinkle area and length of wrinkles) (L'Oréal Research data, unpublished).

Antioxidants

As described in the first part of this chapter, free radicals play a crucial role in aging. They are highly reactive chemicals that can damage any structure in living cells. Every cell generates free radicals through its mitochondrial energetic metabolism but exogenous sources of free radicals can damage skin, such as those induced by sunlight, pollution, stress, smoking and excessive alcohol consumption, for example. Since skin must provide the first line of defense against environmental free-radical attack, it has developed a complex antioxidant network that includes enzymatic and nonenzymatic components.[63]

The efficacy of topical antioxidants depends upon their skin penetration. Some antioxidants, such as vitamin C, cysteine, methionine, selenium, glutathione are water soluble; others are lipid soluble, such as vitamin E, vitamin A, carotenoids, coenzyme Q10, and some others are both water and fat soluble such as lipoic acid, some polyphenols and flavonoids. The water soluble, category is effective mainly in extra- and intracellular fluid whereas the lipid soluble antioxidants mainly protect biological membranes.

Vitamin C is a paramount element for cells to develop efficient systems able to regenerate the active reduced form of vitamin C to get optimal intracellular concentration.[63] Free radicals can participate in signaling pathways, regulating cell proliferation, differentiation, and death. Antioxidants can antagonize the free radical–induced changes in gene expression.[64] The antioxidant vitamin C may interfere with UV-induced generation of reactive oxygen species (ROS). In humans, following UVB exposure, a significant reduction of the minimal erythemal dose (MED) with a less intense erythematous response was seen on vitamin C treated sites of the volar forearms in 10 volunteers[65] as compared to controls. Ascorbic acid acts by scavenging and quenching free radicals and by regenerating Vitamin E from its radical form.[66] By replenishing vitamin E, vitamin C indirectly inhibits lipid peroxidation.[67] Vitamins C and E are the major antioxidants in the human body.

Vitamin E is the principal lipid soluble antioxidant even though its concentration within epidermis is extremely low. It protects cellular membranes, lipoproteins. Free d,α- tocopherol is the most biologically active form. Vitamin E acts as an antioxidant when applied before sun exposure to protect skin from UV-induced photodamage in both *in vitro* and clinically controlled trials.[33] In a human clinical trial, vitamin E applied to the face (5–8%) for 4 weeks decreased skin roughness, length of facial lines and wrinkle depth compared to placebo.[68]

Flavonoids comprise a diverse group of plant pigments with antioxidant properties. As far as skin benefits are concerned, two classes of flavonoid appear to be especially beneficial: proanthocyanins and polyphenols. Soy isoflavones have a quadruple mechanism of action to fight oxidative process in the skin.[69] This class includes genistein and daidzein.[70] Silymarin is a strong antioxidant that prevents lipid peroxidation by scavenging free radical species.

Polyphenols compose the largest category of botanical antioxidants. Curcumin and its related compound resveratrol are used in topical preparation for their antioxidant properties. The most active antioxidant in any tea is EGCG (epigallocatechin-3-gallate) and green tea has the highest concentration of EGCG.

Resveratrol is a natural polyphenolic antioxidant found in more than 70 plant species such as berries, peanuts and grapes. In addition to being a powerful antioxidant, resveratrol has multiple biological activities, including antidiabetic, anti-inflammatory, antitumorigenic. It also acts as a vasodilator, platelet inhibitor and shows important cardioprotective effects. Working through multiple pathways this powerful antioxidant can improve the function of multiple organ systems including the skin. Resveratrol holds great promise as a topical ingredient for treating skin since it can both prevent and improve the clinical signs of aging.[71] It is now known that resveratrol and dietary restriction can improve health and longevity through activating sirtulins, an important group of enzymes. Many of its scientifically proven properties show great potential to ameliorate the esthetic problems of skin aging. *In vitro* studies have demonstrated that resveratrol effectively downregulates both activating protein (AP)-1 and NF-κB and thus serves a key role in preserving dermal collagen and reducing skin inflammation.[72] AP-1 is one of the prominent transcription factors responsible for the production of metalloproteinases, the enzymes that break down collagen, believed to be the primary cause of wrinkling. Likewise, NF-κB is paramount in the production of proinflammatory mediators that contribute to skin aging. Resveratrol is an effective agent for the prevention and treatment of skin aging, however to avoid photounstability skin has to be protected from UV rays when resveratrol is applied on the morning. Resveratrol can also be exclusively used at night for an optimized efficacy.

Jasmonic Acid Derivative

Jasmonic acid, a plant hormone derived from linolenic acid, is known to be involved in plant stress regulation, wound repair and defense.[73] A new derivative of jasmonic acid (THJ, TetraHydroJasmonic acid*), with amphiphilic properties, was synthesized by green chemistry processes. A recent study demonstrated its efficacy and performance *in vitro* and *in vivo*.[74] Using a skin equivalent model (REALSKIN®), the study showed that THJ was able to stimulate extra cellular matrix proteins that are altered during aging process causing a strong reduction

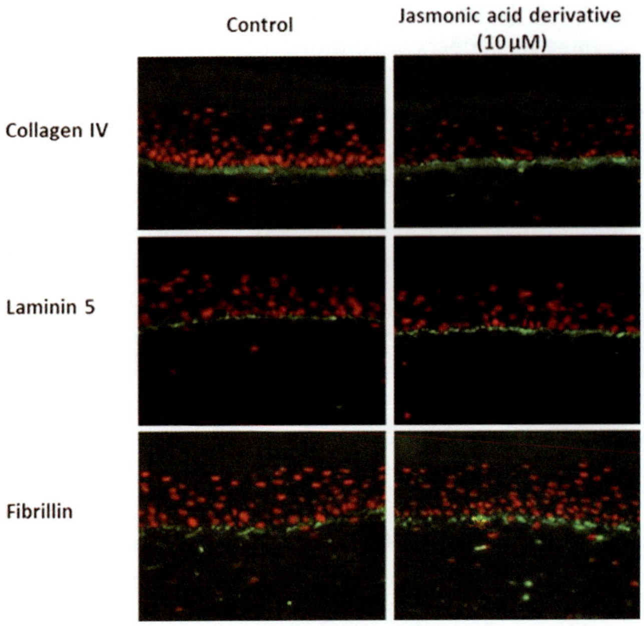

Figure 8: Immunohistochemistry of extracellular matrix proteins in REALSKIN®. Representative immunohistological sections of REALSKIN® (reconstructed human skin) after 5 days exposure to 10 µmol/L jasmonic acid derivative reveal compared with non-treated controls, an increased deposition of collagen IV and laminin-5 at the DEJ and fibrillin in the upper dermis ©L'Oréal Research and Innovation

of the DEJ surface area and the loss of dermal papillae.[75,76] Application of THJ to REALSKIN® (10 µmol/L) for 5 days increased the deposition of collagen IV, and laminin-5 at the DEJ level as well as the deposition of fibrillin in the upper dermis as revealed by immunohistochemistry (Fig. 8). These results were confirmed *in vivo*. In a validated double-blind patch test assay, THJ was applied to photoaged skin and compared with retinol and all-trans retinoic acid: THJ significantly increased the deposition of fibrillin-rich microfibrils in the papillary dermis proximal to the DEJ, the accumulation being at a similar level to that observed using retinol or tRA. The antiaging effect of THJ was proved in an in use clinical study performed on 42 women over 3 months: applying a product containing 2% THJ twice a day significantly reduced the area and length of crow's feet wrinkles on the face.

Sunscreens

Sun UV rays are the major etiological agent of most types of skin cancer and key factors in the photoaging process. There is an increasing evidence that UVA contributes to photoaging, which results in the accumulation of massive amounts of abnormal clusters of elastic material in the dermis of photoaged skin.[77] Even very small doses of UV have biological effects and the benefit of daily protection is well established.[78]

Sunscreens form a topical barrier to prevent sunlight from damaging the skin. Their value has been proven by an immense number of studies. Sun avoidance and sunscreen use are widely accepted strategies of primary prevention against photoaging. All skin types are concerned by UV-damage and can therefore be protected by rationale photoprotection strategies.[79-81]

Although initially developed to prevent sunburn, the use of sunscreens has since considerably broadened. Prevention of photoaging is a full claim of sunscreen and UVA protection became an utmost attribute for this prevention. But photostability of sunscreen products is a prime requisite for the efficiency of protection with regard to photoaging related endpoints.[82]

Mexoryl SX® is a photostable sunscreen that offers mid-range UVA protection. When combined with photostabilized avobenzone, UVA protection is significantly enhanced. Furthermore Mexoryl XL® increases the UVA protection level brought by Mexoryl SX® in a synergistic manner.[83]

The level of UVA protection in the prevention of photoaging is instrumental and the pivotal need for sunscreens with well-balanced UVA/UVB protection factors of a minimal 1/3 respective ratio above 1/3 providing a steadily efficient protection throughout the UV range have been fully demonstrated with a reconstructed 3D-skin model.[84]

Sunscreens are indispensable cosmetics in the prevention of skin aging, and for the first time clinically proven. In a recent study conducted in Australia for 4.5 years on 903 adults under the age of 55, the daily use of a sunscreen was shown to clearly prevent skin aging.[85] Regular sunscreen use by young and middle-aged adults younger than 55 years can retard skin aging. In more pigmented skin, such as Indian skin, despite its natural slight photoprotection with melanin, a full spectrum of photodermatoses can be observed,[86] including photoaging and UV-induced dyschromias. Specific instructions and counseling of parents with children suffering from photosensitivity is essential not only to decrease the morbidity but also to prevent accelerated skin aging and improve quality of life.[87]

CONCLUSION

Clinical and physiological changes observed during skin aging mainly concern superficial dermis and epidermis. Signs are clearly different for photoaging and chronological aging processes. According to population and climatic factors, facial skin aging show some specificities, which must be considered for prevention and care of skin aging.

With the increase in life expectancy, prevention of skin aging is essential for health reasons and for maintaining good appearance. Self-perception of healthy skin is essential for well-balanced mood. In addition, cosmetic ingredients and skincare products dealing with skin aging, such as sunscreens participate to the prevention of pigmentation disorders, which are a predominant sign of skin aging in India. Cosmetics have been significantly proven to decrease wrinkles and prevent dyspigmentation associated with aging. They are a mainstay in cutaneous health maintenance regimen.

REFERENCES

1. India: facing an ageing population. Developments Magazine. Available from www.developments.org.uk/articles/india-facing-an-ageing-population. [Accessed June, 2014].
2. Verma SB. Dermatology for the elderly: An Indian perspective. Clinics in Dermatology. 2011;29:91-6.
3. Hayflick L. The limited in vitro lifetime of human diploid cell strains. Exp Cell Res. 1965;37:614-36.
4. Harman D. Aging: a theory based on free radical and radiation chemistry. J Gerontol. 1956;11:298-300.
5. Yang JH, Lee HC, Lin KJ, et al. A specific 4977-bp deletion of mitochondrial DNA in human ageing skin. Arch Dermatol Res. 1994;286:386-90.
6. Gago N, Perez-Lopez V, Sanz-Jaka JP, et al. Age-dependent depletion of human skin-derived progenitor cells. Stem Cells. 2009;27:1164-72.
7. Hashimoto K. New method for surface ultrastructure: comparative studies of scanning electron microscopy and replica method. Int J Dermatol. 1974;13:367-81.
8. Richard S, Querleux B, Bittoun J, et al. Characterization of the skin in vivo by high resolution magnetic resonance imaging: water behaviour and age-related effects. J Invest Dermatol. 1993;100(5):705-9.
9. Periyasamy R, Anand S, Ammini AC. The effect of aging on the hardness of foot sole skin: a preliminary study. Foot (Edinb). 2012;22:95-9.
10. Battie C, Verschoore M. Cutaneous solar ultraviolet exposure and clinical aspects of photodamage. Indian J Dermatol Venereol Leprol. 2012;78:S9-14.
11. Durai PC, Thappa DM, Kumari R, et al. Aging in elderly: chronological versus photoaging. Indian J Dermatol. 2012;57: 343-52.
12. Li L, de Lacharrière O, Lian S, et al. Pigmented spots on face and hands: specific features in Chinese skin. A clinical study on 2000 Chinese women. Ann Dermatol Venereol. 2002;129:81-141.
13. Nkengne A, Bertin C, Stamats GN, et al. Influence of facial skin attributes on the perceived age of Caucasian women. J Eur Acad Dermatol Venereol. 2008;22:982-91.
14. Hourblin V, Nouveau S, Roy N, et al. Skin complexion and pigmentary disorders in facial skin of 1204 women in 4 Indian cities. Indian J Dermatol Venereol Leprol. 2014 [in press].
15. Lévêque JL, Corcuff P, de Rigal J, et al. In vivo studies of the evolution of physical properties of the human skin with age. J Invest Dermatol. 1984;23:322-9.
16. Corcuff P, de Lacharrière O, Lévêque JL. Extension-induced changes in the microrelief of the human volar forearm: variations with age. J Gerontol. 1991;46:223-7.
17. Zou Y, Song E, Jin R. Age-dependent changes in skin surface assessed by a novel two-dimensional analysis. Skin Res Technol. 2009;15:399-406.
18. de Rigal J, Escoffier C, Querleux B, et al. Assessement of aging of the human skin by in vivo ultrasonic imaging. J Invest Dermatol. 1989;93:621-5.
19. Richard S, de Rigal J, de Lacharriere O, et al. Non invasive measurement of the effect of lifetime exposure to the sun on the aged skin. Photodermatol Photoimmunol Photomed. 1994;10: 164-9.
20. Nouveau-Richard S, Monot M, Bastien P, et al. In vivo epidermal thickness measurement : ultrasound vs. confocal imaging. Skin Res Technol. 2004;10:136-40.
21. Agache P, Monneur C, Leveque JL, et al. Mechanical properties and Young's modulus of the skin in vivo. Arch Dermatol Res. 1980;269:221-32.
22. Escoffier C, de Rigal J, Rochefort A, et al. Age related mechanical properties of human skin. An in vivo study. J Invest Dermatol. 1989;93:353-7.
23. Smalls LK, Randall Wickett R, Visschner MO. Effect of dermal thickness, tissue composition and body site on skin biomechanical properties. Skin Res Technol. 2006;12:43-9.
24. Ryu HS, Joo YH, Kim SO, et al. Influence of age and regional differences on skin elasticity as measured by the Cutometer. Skin Res Technol. 2008;14:354-8.
25. Zhang Y, Brodell RT, Mostow EN, et al. In vivo skin elastography with high-definition optical videos. Skin Res Technol. 2009;15: 271-82.
26. Malacara D. Color Vision and Colorimetry: Theory and Applications. Society of Photo-Optical Instrumentation Engineers; Bellingham, USA: 2002
27. De Rigal J, Abella ML, Giron F, et al. Development and validation of a new Skin Color Chart. Skin Res Technol. 2007;13:101-9.
28. Cointereau-Chardon S, Flament F, Hourblin V, et al. " Indian Facial Skin color: age and latitude effect". Poster: International Congress of Dermatology 2013, New Delhi, India.
29. Leveque JL, Corcuff P, Rougier A, et al. Mechanism of action of a lipophilic salicylic acid derivative on normal skin. Eur J Dermatol. 2002;12:XXXV- XXXVIII.
30. Saint-Leger D, Leveque JL, Verschoore M. The use of hydroxy acids on the skin : characteristics of C8-lipohydroxy acid. J Cosmet Dermatol. 2007;6:59-65.

31. Pierard GE, Kligman AM, Stoudmayer T, et al. Comparative effects of retinoic acid, glycolic acid and a lipophilic derivative of salicylic acid on photodamaged skin. Dermatology. 1999;199:50-3.
32. Duell EA, Derguini F, Kang S, et al. Extraction of human epidermis treated with retinol yields retro-retinoids in addition to free retinol and retinyl esters. J Invest Dermatol. 1996;107:178-82.
33. Zussman J, Ahdout J, Kim J. Vitamins and photoaging: Do scientific data support their use. J Am Acad Dermatol. 2010;63:507-25.
34. Mukherjee S, Date A, Patravale V, et al. Retinoids in the treatment of skin aging: an overview of clinical efficacy and safety. Clinical Interventions in Aging. 2006;1:327-48.
35. Ortonne JP. Retinoid therapy of pigmentory disorders. Dermatol Ther. 2006;19:280-8.
36. Serri R, Iorizzo M. Cosmeceuticals: focus on topical in photoaging. Clin Dermatol. 2008;26:633-5.
37. Kafi R, Kwak HS, Schumacher WE, et al. Improvement of naturally aged skin with vitamin A (Retinol). Arch Dermatol. 2007;143:606-12.
38. Tesoriere L, D'arpa D, Re R, et al. Antioxidant reactions of all-trans retinol in phospholipids bilayers: Effect of oxygen partial pressure, radical fluxes, and retinol concentration. Arch Biochem Biophys. 1997;343:13-8.
39. Laurent TC, Fraser JR. Hyaluronan. FASEB J. 1992;6:2397-404.
40. Wegmann M, Santonnat B, Lersch P, et al. Low molecular weight hyaluronic acid: Its effect on epidermal gene expression and skin aging. SOFW-journal. 2008;134:17-22.
41. Wang C, Tammi M, Tammi R. Distribution of hyaluronan and its CD44 receptor in the epithelia of human skin appendages. Histochemistry. 1992;98:105-12.
42. Jiang D, Liang J, Noble PW. Hyaluronan in tissue injury and repair. Annu Rev Cell Dev Biol. 2007;23:435-61.
43. Jiang D, Liang J, Fan J, et al. Regulation of lung injury and repair by Toll-like receptors and hyaluronan. Nat Med. 2005;11:1173-9.
44. Pivarcsi A, Bodai L, Rethi B, et al. Expression and function of Toll-like receptors 2 and 4 in human keratinocytes. Int Immunol. 2003;15:721-30.
45. Mehul B, Asselineau D, Bernard D, et al. Gene expression profiles of three different models of reconstructed human epidermis and classical cultures of keratinocytes using cDNA arrays. Arch Dermatol Res. 2004;296:145-56.
46. Kaya G, Tran C, Sorg O, et al. Hyaluronate Fragments reverse skin atrophy by a CD44-dependent mechanism. PLoS Med. 2006;e493.
47. Tammi R, Pasonen-Seppänen S, Kolehmainen E, et al. Hyaluronan synthase induction and hyaluronan accumulation in mouse epidermis following skin injury. J Invest Dermatol. 2005;124: 898-905.
48. Trommer H, Wartewig S, Bottcher R, et al. The effects of hyaluronan and its fragment on lipid models exposed to UV irradiation. Int J Pharm. 2003;254:223-34.
49. Ronchetti IP, Quaglino DJr, Bergamini G. Ascorbic acid and connective tissue. In: Harris JR, ed. Biochemistry and biochemical cell biology. New York: Plenum Press; 1996. p. 41.
50. Dehm P, Prockop DJ. Synthesis and extrusion of collagen by freshly isolated cells from chick embryo tendon. Biochim Biophys Acta. 1971;238:536-46.
51. Berg RA, Prockop DJ. The thermal transition of the non hydroxylated form of collagen : evidence for the role of hydroxyproline in stabilizing the triple helix of collagen. Biochem Biophys Res Commun. 1973;52:115-20.
52. Wenstrup RJ, Murad S, Pinnell SR. Ehlers-Danlos syndrome type V: clinical manifestations of collagen lysyl hydroxylase deficiency. J Pediatr. 1989;115:405-9.
53. Roshchupkin DI, Pistsov MY, Potapenko AY. Inhibition of ultraviolet light-induced erythema by antioxidants. Arch Dermatol Res. 1979;266:91-4.
54. Marionnet C, Vioux-Chagnoleau C, Pierrard C, et al. Morphogenesis of dermal-epidermal junction in a model of reconstructed skin: beneficial effects of vitamin C. Exp Dermatol. 2006;15:625-33.
55. Leveque N, Muret P, Mary S, et al. Decrease in skin ascorbic concentration with age. Eur J Dermatol. 2001;12:XXI-XXII.
56. Traikovich S. Use of topical ascorbic acid and its effects on photodamaged skin topography. Arch Otolaryngol Head Neck Surg. 1999;125:1091-8.
57. Humbert P, Haftek M, Creidi P, et al. Topical ascorbic acid on photoaged skin: clinical topographical and ultrastructural evaluation; double-blind study vs placebo. Exp Dermatol. 2003;12:237-44.
58. Sauermann K, Sören J, Koop U, et al. Topically applied vitamin C increases the density of dermal papillae in aged human skin. BMC Dermatology. 2004;4:13.
59. Pineau N, Carrino DA, Caplan AI, et al. Biological evaluation of a new C-xylopyranoside derivative (C-Xyloside) and its role in glycosaminoglycan biosynthesis. Eur J Dermatol. 2011;21:359-70.
60. Sok J, Pineau N, Dalko-csiba M, et al. Improvement of the dermal epidermal junction in human reconstructed skin by a new c-xylopyranoside derivative. Eur J Dermatol. 2008;18:297-302.
61. Vassal-Stermann E, Duranton A, Black AF, et al. A New C-Xyloside induces modifications of GAG expression, structure and functional properties. PLoS One. 2012;7:e47933.
62. Pineau N, Bernerd F, Cavezza A, et al. A new C-xylopyranoside derivative induces skin expression of glycosaminoglycans and heparan sulphate proteoglycans. Eur J Dermatol. 2008;18:36-40.
63. Catani MV, Savini I, Rossi A, et al. Biological role of vitamin C in keratinocytes. Nutrition Reviews. 2005;63:81-90.
64. Ushakova T, Melkonyan H, Nikonova L, et al. Modification of gene expression by dietary antioxidants in radiation-induced apoptosis of mice splenocytes. Free Radic Biol Med. 1999;26:887-91.
65. Murray J, Darr D, Reich J, et al. Topical vitamin C treatment reduces UV radiation-induced erythema in human skin. J Invest Dermatol. 1991;96:587.
66. Chan AC. Partners in defense, vitamin E, and vitamin C. Can J Physio Pharmacol. 1993;71:725-31.
67. Wefers H, Sies H. The protection by ascorbate and gluthatione against microsomal lipid peroxidation is dependent on vitamin E. Eur J Biochem. 1988;174:353-7.
68. Mayer P. The effects of Vitamin E on the skin. Cosmet Toiletries. 1993;108:99-109.
69. Sharma S, Sultana S. Modulatory effect of soy isoflavones on biochemical alterations mediated by TPA in mouse skin model. Food Chem Toxicol. 2004;42:1669-75.
70. Draelos ZD. The power of antioxidants. Healthy-aging.advanceweb.com. [Accessed June 2014].
71. Oresajo C, Pillai S, Manco M, et al. Antioxidants and the skin: understanding formulation and efficacy. Dermatol Ther. 2012;25:252-9.
72. Kundu JK, Shin YK, Surh YJ, et al. Reveratrol modulates phorbol ester-induced pro-inflammatory signal transduction pathways in mouse skin in vivo: NR-kappaβ and AP-1 as prime targets. Biochem Pharmacol. 2006;72:1506-15.
73. Browse J. Jasmonate: an oxylipin signal with many roles in plants. Viam Horm. 2005;72:431-56.
74. Tran C, Michelet JF, Simonetti L, et al. In vitro and in vivo studies with tetra-hydro-jasmonic acid (LR2412) reveal its potential to correct signs of skin ageing. J Eur Acad Dermatol Venereol. 2014;28:415-23.

75. Lavker RM, Zheng PS, Dong G. Aged skin: a study by light, transmission electron, and scanning electron microscopy. J Invest Dermatol. 1987;3:44s-51s.
76. Langton AK, Sherratt MJ, Griffiths CEM, et al. A new wrinkle on old skin: the role of elastic fibres in skin aging. Int J Cosm Sci. 2010;32:330-9.
77. Takeuchi T, Uitto J, Bernstein EF. A novel in vivo model for evaluating agents that protect against ultraviolet A-induced photoaging. J Invest Dermatol. 1998;110:343-7.
78. Seité S, Fourtanier A. The benefit of daily photoprotection. J Am Acad Dermatol. 2008;58:160-6.
79. Antoniou C, Kosmadaki MG, Stratigos AJ, et al. Photoaging: prevention and topical treatments. Am J Clin Dermatol. 2010;11:95-102.
80. Konda D, Thappa DM. Age reversing modalities: an overview. Indian J Dermatol Venerol Leprol. 2013;79:3-8.
81. Kaimal S, Abraham A. Sunscreens. Indian J Dermatol Venerol Leprol. 2011;77:238-43.
82. Marrot L, Belaïdi JP, Lejeune F, et al. Photostability of sunscreen products influences the efficiency of protection with regard to UV-induced genotoxic or photoageing-related endpoints. Br J Dermatol. 2004;151:1234-44.
83. Bissonnette R. Update on sunscreens. Skin Therapy Letter. 2008;13:2.
84. Fourtanier A, Bernerd F, Bouillon C, et al. Protection of skin biological targets by different types of sunscreens. Photodermatol Photoimmunol Photomed. 2006;22:22-32.
85. Hughes MC, Williams GM, Baker P, et al. Sunscreen and prevention of skin aging: A randomized trial. Ann Intern Med. 2013;158:781-90.
86. Sharma VK, Sahni K, Wadhwani AR. Photodermatoses in pigmented skin. Photochem Photobiol Sci. 2013;12:65-77.
87. Inamadar AC, Palit A. Photosensitivity in children: an approach to diagnosis and management. Indian J Dermatol Venerol Leprol. 2005;71:73-9.

Chapter 12

New Insights in Hair Research

Bruno A Bernard, *L'Oréal Research and Innovation, Asnières, France*

INTRODUCTION

The hair follicle is a unique structure, characteristic of mammals. Microscopically, the follicle can be divided into four compartments, namely, from the scalp surface deeper inwards- the infundibulum, the sebaceous gland, the isthmus and the bulbar region, which itself should be divided into upper, central and lower parts. If one considers terminal scalp hair, it penetrates 4 mm deep into the dermis, down to the hypodermis. Histologically, the hair follicle is composed of different cell types of either mesenchymal or epithelial origin, organized into well defined compartments. The dermal compartment includes the connective tissue sheath (CTS) and dermal papilla (DP). The epithelial compartment includes hair matrix and three concentrical structures, namely, the outer root sheath (ORS), the inner root sheath (IRS) and the hair shaft (HS).

The hair follicle is also a fascinating organ, since it encompasses most of the rules that control body homeostasis, as well as cell and tissue integration into an organized, autonomous and self-renewing biological entity. In the adult scalp, each of the 150,000 (estimated) follicles undergoes, on its own, a cyclical process of growth, degradation and renewal which partly recapitulates the sequence of events which takes place during its formation during fetal life.

Indeed, from the time it is formed, human hair follicle produces a HS at an average rate of 367 + 56 µm/day, 280 + 50 µm/day and 418 + 51 µm/day in Caucasian, African and Asian groups, respectively.[1] A 3-year average period of growth (anagen phase) is followed by a 3-week involution period (catagen phase) followed by a 3-month resting period (telogen phase). After a 2–5 months latency period[2], in the course of which the HS is shed without regrowth[3], a new cycle is turned on. Interestingly, hair cycles are asynchronous from one follicle to another and the phase durations of the "nth" cycle has no influence on the "nth +1" cycle.[4] A mathematical model—the follicular automaton has been developed, which takes into account the stochastic transition of each follicle between successive phases.[4] While a decrease in the mean duration of anagen phase as well as a lengthening of latency period was demonstrated in the course of natural aging,[5] a parallel decline in average hair diameter was also observed.[6]

Another fascinating feature of the hair follicle is its high degree of autonomy with respect to its dermal environment since it is apparently able to drive its own androgen metabolism,[7] its own inflammatory response,[8] and maintain both structure and function, namely, hair fiber production when dissected out and kept under *in vitro* culture conditions.[9] The hair follicle must be looked at as a unique dynamic biological structure as well as a paradigm of tissue homeostasis and integration, harboring most of the clues of normal organogenesis and development. Its self-controlled organization reflects a perfectly tuned internal communication network, the understanding of which could certainly lead to new approaches to biologically control hair growth, hair shape and hair color.

NEW INSIGHTS IN HAIR BIOLOGY

Thanks to new technologies and new tools, decisive advances have been made in the knowledge of hair cycle, hair growth control, and androgenic alopecia.

Hair Cycle

It is clear today that human hair cycle is far from having "clock" regularity and that duration of anagen, catagen and telogen phases: 3 years, 3 weeks, 3 months, respectively, are only average values. In fact these are values around which phase effective durations fluctuate. It is now accepted that hair follicles follow a stochastic behavior, at the origin of hair permanence on the scalp.[4]

Recently, telogen phase received a renewed attention from hair biologists. As a result, telogen phase appeared less quiescent than previously suspected.[10] Indeed, during telogen phase, a competition between inducers and inhibitors controls the hair regrowth onset.[11] A strong expression of "bone morphogenic protein" (BMP)[12] and "fibroblast growth factor-18" (FGF-18)[13] characterizes a telogen refractory period, preventing any neo-morphogenetic process to take place. The progressive increase of noggin, a BMP antagonist, of Wnt ligands, activators of the canonical Fzz/β-catenin pathway, and TGF-β2[14] then permits the inducers' signal to reach a critical threshold,[11] which triggers the transition of telogen follicle from refractory to permissive state and, in synergy with increased FGF-7 production from the DP,[15] the onset of a new cycle. Through interaction with vitamin D3 VDR receptor, the transcription-coactivator called "mediator" (MED) will then modulate, among others, the expression of Dlx3 homeotic gene as well as sonic hedgehog, BMP and hairless pathways' genes,[16] all involved in hair fiber and IRS[17] differentiation programs.

On top of refractory and permissive periods, telogen phase can be subdivided into three sub-phases: one during which the hair fiber is still present, a second called exogen[18] during which proteases actively release the fiber[19] and a third called kenogen,[20] during which the empty follicle has not yet triggered a new morphogenetic process. This kenogen phase can last for 2–12 months.[21] As a consequence of this follicular dynamics, the density of visible hairs is always less than total hair follicle density.

From the above results, a new vision of hair follicle behavior emerged. In fact, we recently proposed that the hair follicle can be considered as a bistable organ which, under a stochastic manner, transits from a stable active steady-state (anagen) to a stable dormant steady state (telogen), through quick remodeling phases, one involving active involution process (catagen) and one named neogen, involving active neomorphogenesis (Fig. 1).[22] Of note, this bistability hypothesis was recently mathematically confirmed.[23]

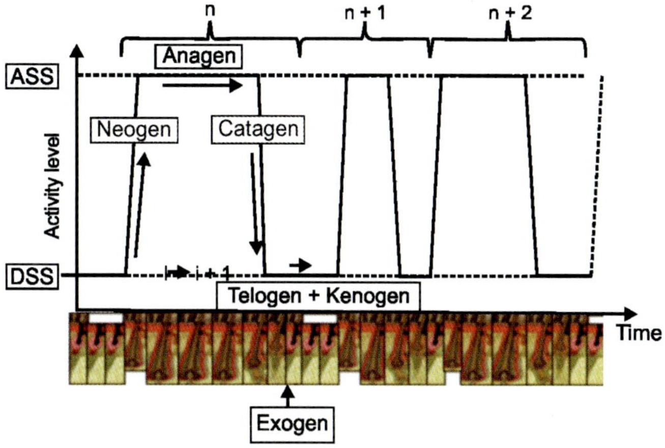

Figure 1: New representation of the hair follicle behavior, with an active steady state of fiber production (anagen) and a dormant steady State (telogen/kenogen), interspaced by short lasting phases of neomorphogenesis (neogen) and regression (catagen). Three successive periods (n, n + 1, n + 2) are represented ©L'Oréal Research and Innovation

Hair Growth Control

The list of factors positively or negatively influencing hair growth is long already,[24,25] and among them, insulin like growth factor-1 (IGF-1) was described as a key factor for anagen maintenance.[26] The importance of IGF-1 in hair growth control was further supported by the fact it was secreted by the dermal papilla (DP).[27] From a mechanistic point of view, IGF-1 was shown to induce PDGF-A and –B ("platelet derived growth factor"-A and-B) synthesis and to increase the Bcl2/Bax ratio thus preventing apoptosis.[28] Of note, 1,763 MHz radiofrequency was able to induce increased IGF-1 synthesis in DP cells and consequently to stimulate *in vitro* human hair growth.[29] A possible new field of androgenic alopecia treatment is open.

But if the quest for new hair growth promoters is still strongly active, the understanding of intimate hair fiber structure remains an open field, with promising issues in terms of hair quality. For example, mass spectrometry analysis of hair fiber has revealed the catalog of keratins and keratin-associated proteins (KAPs) actually present in human hair cortex and cuticle,[30] paving the way to a better understanding of their macromolecular organization and possible role in hair fiber physical properties. Another study, focused on KAP-2 family confirmed that KAPs indeed interacted with subsets of hair keratins and other KAPs.[31,32] Finally, known to be the only transglutaminase expressed in the hair fiber,[33] transglutaminase 3 was shown to play a major functional role in hair fiber structure, confirming that hair fiber was not only stabilized by disulfide bonds but also by isopeptide linkages.[31]

Androgenic Alopecia

If the role of hormonal context in androgenetic alopecia is rather well established, it remains that the list of dihydrotestosterone (DHT) targets keeps increasing. In response to DHT, DP fibroblasts secrete diffusible factors which affect follicular keratinocyte proliferation and differentiation. Among these effectors, TGFβ1 was identified,[34] but also Interleukin-6 (IL-6), the production of which is increased in alopecic dermal papilla.[35] IL-6 would inhibit hair matrix keratinocyte proliferation and induce follicle regression.

Besides androgens, prostaglandin D2 (PGD2) has been identified as a new diffusible factor, which could play a role in androgenic alopecia. It was already known that hair follicle was endowed with a full prostaglandin (PG) metabolism[36] and that hair follicle expressed the whole spectrum of PG receptors, including GPR44 PGD2 receptor.[37] A recent study[38] described the inhibitory effect of PGD2 on hair growth and an increased PGD2 synthesis in alopecic zones. Altogether these results suggest that hair growth is under the control of a subtle balance between positive and negative influence of PGE2 and PGF2α on the one hand[39] and PGD2 on the other hand.

If androgenic alopecia development clearly appears today as a multifactorial process, it was recently found that stem cells, in charge of follicle renewal, might also play a role. Though it has been known for quite a long time that human hair follicle harbored two stem cell reservoirs,[40] it's only recently that these two reservoirs were characterized as not identical.[41-43] Indeed, the upper reservoir harbors CD200+, CD27+, K15+, K19+ stem cells, while the lower reservoir harbors CD34+, CD27+, K19+, AC IX+, GLUT1+ stem cells (Fig. 2).[42] The expression of AC IX, GLUT1 further suggested that the lower reservoir bathed in an hypoxic environment.[44,45] These two reservoirs fuse during telogen phase and ultimately respond to DP activating signals to trigger neogen phase. Of note, a recent study showed that human hair follicle CD34+ progenitor cell population dramatically decreased in alopecic follicles,[46] suggesting that the CD34+, CD27+, K19+, AC IX+, GLUT1+ stem cell population was key for an optimal hair follicle cycle to take place. Indeed, in androgenic alopecia, the anagen duration is shortened while the kenogen phase is increased.[11] Moreover, with aging, a decline in clonogenic potential of human hair follicle keratinocytes and earliest precursors, holoclones, was observed.[47] This could be linked to a decrease in stem cell functionality with aging and more precisely to the decrease in CD34+ progenitor cell population,[46] possibly due to a change in hair follicle hypoxic environment. From this point of view, an active like diethyl pyridine-2,4-dicarboxylate, able to mimic the beneficial effect of hypoxia,[42] might help maintaining a full activity of human hair follicle epithelial stem cell population and favor the shortening of kenogen phase.[48]

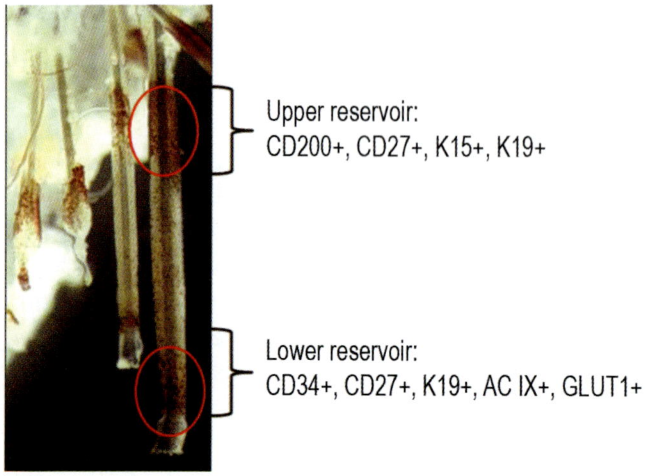

Figure 2: The two epithelial stem cell reservoirs of human hair follicle, as revealed by keratin 19 expression. Dispase extracted whole hair follicles were reacted with Ks19.1 monoclonal antibody and revealed by streptavidin-peroxidase complex. Note that the upper reservoir harbors CD200+, CD27+, K15+, K19+ stem cells, while the lower reservoir harbors CD34+, CD27+, K19+, AC IX+, GLUT1+ stem cells
©L'Oréal Research and Innovation

Finally, it is obvious that androgenic alopecia development is influenced by the genetic background. Indeed, two androgenic alopecia-linked loci were unequivocally identified: one on X chromosome, harboring both AR (androgen receptor) and EDA2R ectodysplasin A2 receptor genes,[49] and another one on chr20p11, harboring PAX1 ("paired box 1") gene.[50] A third locus was localized on chr3q26[51] and another one on chr7p21.1, harboring HDAC9 (histone deacetylase-9) gene,[52] known to be in functional interaction with AR. Recently, four additional androgenic alopecia risk loci were identified, among which Wnt10A locus on chr2q35.[53] Altogether, these results further confirm that androgenic alopecia is a multigenic trait.

REFERENCES

1. Loussouarn G, El Rawadi C, Genain G. Diversity of hair growth profiles. Int J Dermatol. 2005;44 (Suppl.1):6-9.
2. Courtois M, Loussouarn G, Hourseau C, et al. Hair cycle and alopecia. Skin Pharmacol. 1994;61:84-9.
3. Stenn K, Parimoo S, Prouty S. Growth of the hair follicle: a cycling and regenerating biological system. In: Chuong CM (Ed). Molecular basis of epithelial appendage morphogenesis. Austin, TX, USA: RG Landes Co; 1998. pp.111-30.
4. Halloy J, Bernard BA, Loussouarn G, et al. Modeling the dynamics of human hair cycles by a follicular automaton. Proc Natl Acad Sci USA. 2000;97:8328-33
5. De Lacharrière O, Deloche C, Misciali C, et al. Hair diameter diversity, a clinical sign reflecting the follicle miniaturization. Arch Dermatol. 2001;137:641-6.
6. Courtois M, Loussouarn G, Hourseau C, et al. Ageing and hair cycles. Br J Dermatol. 1995;132:86-93.
7. Gerst C, Dalko M, Pichaud P, et al. Type-1 steroid 5α-reductase is functionally active in the hair follicle as evidenced by new selective inhibitors of either type-1 or type-2 human steroid 5α-reductase. Exp Dermatol. 2002;11:52-8.
8. Mahé Y, Buan B, Billoni N, et al. Pro-inflammatory cytokine cascade in human plucked hair. Skin Pharmacol. 1996;9:366-75.
9. Thibaut S, Collin C, Langbein L, et al. Hair keratin pattern I human hair follicles grown *in vitro*. Exp Dermatol. 2003;12:160-4.
10. Geyfman M, Gordon W, Paus R, et al. Identification of telogen markers underscores that telogen is far from a quiescent hair cycle phase. J Invest Dermatol. 2012;132:721-4.
11. Plikus MV. New activators and inhibitors in the hair cycle clock: targeting stem cells' state of competence. J Invest Dermatol. 2012;132:1321-4.
12. Botchkarev VA, Botchkareva NV, Nakamura M, et al. Noggin is required for induction of the hair follicle growth phase in postnatal skin. FASEB J. 2001;15:2205-14.
13. Kimura-Ueki M, Oda Y, Oki J, et al. Hair cycle resting phase is regulated by cyclic epithelial FGF18 signaling. J Invest Dermatol. 2012;132:1338-45.
14. Oshimori N, Fuchs E. Paracrine TGF-β signaling counterbalances BMP-mediated repression in hair follicle stem cell activation. Cell Stem Cell. 2012;10:63-75.
15. Greco V, Chen T, Rendl M, et al. A two-step mechanism for stem cell activation during hair regeneration. Cell Stem Cell. 2009;4:155-69.
16. Oda Y, Hu L, Bul V, et al. Coactivator MED1 ablation in keratinocytes results in hair-cycling defects and epidermal alterations. J Invest Dermatol. 2012;132:1075-83.
17. Kim BK, Lee HY, Choi JH, et al. Hairless plays a role in formation of inner root sheath via regulation of Dlx3 gene. J Biol Chem. 2012;287:16681-8.
18. Stenn K. Exogen is an active, separately controlled phase of the hair growth cycle. J Am Acad Dermatol. 2005;52:374-5.
19. Higgins C, Westgate GE, Jahoda CAB. Modulation in proteolytic activity is identified as a hallmark of exogen by transcriptional profiling of hair follicles. J Invest Dermatol. 2011;131:2349-57.
20. Rebora A, Guarrera M, Kenogen. A new phase of the hair cycle? Dermatology. 2002;205:108-10.
21. Courtois M, Loussouarn G, Hourseau C, et al. Hair cycle and alopecia. Skin Pharmacol. 1994;7:84-9.
22. Bernard BA. The human hair follicle: a bistable organ? Exp Dermatol. 2012;21:401-3.
23. Al-Nuaimi Y, Goodfellow M, Paus R, et al. A prototypic mathematical model of the human hair cycle. J Theor Biol. 2012;310:143-59.
24. Stenn K, Paus R. Controls of hair follicle cycling. Physiol Rev. 2001;81:449-94.
25. Peters EM, Ericson ME, Hosoi J, et al. Neuropeptide control mechanisms in cutaneous biology: physiological and clinical significance. J Invest Dermatol. 2006;126:1937-47.
26. Philpott M, Sanders DA, Kealey T. Cultured human hair follicles and growth factors. J Invest Dermatol. 1994;102:857-61.
27. Itami S, Inui S. Role of androgen in mesenchymal epithelial interactions in human hair follicle. J Invest Dermatol Symp Proc. 2005;10:209-11.
28. Ahn S-Y, Pi L-Q, Hwang ST, et al. Effect of IGF-I on Hair Growth Is Related to the Anti-Apoptotic Effect of IGF-I and Up-Regulation of PDGF-A and PDGF-B. Ann Dermatol. 2012;24:26-31.
29. Yoon SY, Kim KT, Jo SJ, et al. Induction of hair growth by insulin-like growth factor-1 in 1,763 MHz radiofrequency-irradiated hair follicle cells. PLoS One. 2011;6(12):e28474.
30. Barthelemy N, Bednarczyk A, Schaeffer-Reiss C, et al. Proteomic tools for the investigation of human hair structural proteins and evidence of weakness sites on hair keratin coil segments. Anal Biochem 2012;421:43-55.
31. Thibaut S, Cavusoglu N, de Becker E, et al. Transglutaminase-3 enzyme: a putative actor in human hair shaft scaffolding? J Invest Dermatol. 2009;129:449-59.
32. Fujikawa H, Fujimoto A, Farooq M, et al. Characterization of the human hair keratin-associated protein 2 (KRTAP2) gene family. J Invest Dermatol. 2012;132:1806-13.
33. Thibaut S, Candi E, Pietroni V, et al. Transglutaminase 5 expression in human hair follicle. J Invest Dermatol. 2005;125:581-5.
34. Inui S, Itami S. Molecular basis of androgenetic alopecia: From androgen to paracrine mediators through dermal papilla. J Dermatol Sci. 2011;61:1-6.
35. Kwack MH, Ahn JS, Kim MK, et al. Dihydrotestosterone-inducible IL-6 inhibits elongation of human hair shafts by suppressing matrix cell proliferation and promotes regression of hair follicles in mice. J Invest Dermatol. 2012;132:43-9.
36. Colombe L, Vindrios A, Michelet JF, Bernard BA. Prostaglandin metabolism in human hair follicle. Exp Dermatol. 2007;16:762-9.
37. Colombe L, Michelet JF, Bernard BA. Prostanoid receptors in anagen human hair follicles. Exp Dermatol. 2008;17:63-72.
38. Garza LA, Liu Y, Yang Z, et al. Prostaglandin D2 inhibits hair growth and is elevated in bald scalp of men with androgenetic alopecia. Sci Transl Med. 2012;4:126ra34.
39. Sasaki S, Hozumi Y, Kondo S. Influence of prostaglandin F2alpha and its analogues on hair regrowth and follicular melanogenesis in a murine model. Exp Dermatol. 2005;14:323-8.

40. Commo S, Gaillard O, Bernard BA. The human hair follicle contains two distinct K19 positive compartments in the outer root sheath: a unifying hypothesis for stem cell reservoir? Differentiation 2000;66:157-64.
41. Inoue K, Aoi N, Sato T, et al. Differential expression of stem-cell-associated markers in human hair follicle epithelial cells. Lab Invest. 2009;89:844-56.
42. Rathman-Josserand M, Genty G, Lecardonnel J, et al. Hypoxia and human hair follicle stem/progenitor cells. J Invest Dermatol. 2013;133:2094-7.
43. Purba TS, Hasalm IS, Poblet E, et al. Human epithelial hair follicle stem cells and their progeny: current state of knowledge, the widening gap in translational research and future challenges. Bioessays. 2014;63:513-25.
44 Dayan F, Roux D, Brahimi-Horn C, et al. The oxygen sensor factor-inhibiting hypoxia-inducible factor-1 controls expression of distinct genes through the bifunctional transcriptional character of Hypoxia-Inducible Factor 1 alpha. Cancer Res. 2006;66:3688-98.
45. Kaluz S, Kaluzova M, Liao SY, et al. Transcriptional control of the tumor- and hypoxia-marker carbonic anhydrase 9: a one transcription factor (HIF-1) show? Biochim Biophys Acta. 2009;1795:162-72.
46. Garza LA, Yang CC, Zhao T, et al. Bald scalp in men with androgenetic alopecia retains hair follicle stem cells but lacks CD200-rich and CD-34 positive hair follicle progenitor cells. J Clin Invest. 2011;121:613-22.
47. Lecardonnel J, Deshayes N, Genty G, et al. Ageing and colony-forming efficiency of human hair follicle keratinocytes. Exp Dermatol. 2013;22:604-6.
48. Reygagne P. Evaluation Clinique de la stemoxydine à 5% en lotion sur la densité capillaire. Ann Dermatol Venereol. 2013;140:9-12.
49. Brockschmidt FF, Hillmer AM, Eigelshiven S, et al. Fine mapping of the human AR/EDA2R locus in androgenetic alopecia. Br J Dermatol. 2010;162:899-903.
50. Hillmer AM, Brockschmidt FF, Hanneken S, et al. Susceptibility variants for male-pattern baldness on chromosome 20p11. Nat Genet. 2008a;40:1279-81.
51. Hillmer AM, Flaquer A, Hanneken S, et al. Genome-wide scan and fine-mapping linkage study of androgenetic alopecia reveals a locus on chromosome 3q26. Am J Hum Genet. 2008b;82:737-42.
52. Brockschmidt FF, Heilmann S, Ellis JA, et al. Susceptibility variants on chromosome 7p21.1 suggest HDAC9 as a new candidate gene for male-pattern baldness. Br J Dermatol. 2011;165:1293-302.
53. Heilmann S, Kiefer AK, Fricker N, et al. Androgenetic Alopecia: Identification of Four Genetic Risk Loci and Evidence for the Contribution of WNT Signaling to Its Etiology. J Invest Dermatol. 2013;133:1489-96.

Chapter 13

Human Scalp and Related Cosmetic Care Products

Didier Saint-Léger, *TING SA, Paris, France*
Cécile Clavaud, *L'Oréal Research and Innovation, Aulnay-sous-Bois, France*
Lionel Breton, *L'Oréal Research and Innovation, Aulnay-sous-Bois, France*
Suresh Talwar, *Lucknow, India*

INTRODUCTION

The human scalp, of a surface ranging 600–700 cm^2 in adults, is a specific skin area usually hidden, which is one of its major typical features. The slow unveiling of the scalp during the course of alopecia, being male or female pattern, is a frequent source of stress at the individual level.[1,2] In today's society, the active shaving of hair has social consequences, viewed either as a form of provocation, a stigma of social rejection or a religious obedience.

Although normally unseen, our sensory system is almost constantly perceived by an itching or tingling scalp. About a quarter of people—both genders—claim having a sensitive or reactive scalp, without any evident correlation with the regular use of cosmetic products of any type, most of them being destined to hair care. Nevertheless, it is noteworthy that about half of the human population has dandruff, irrespective of ethnicities and gender. This largely explains the high demand and regular use of antidandruff shampoos that efficiently clean hair and make this scalp condition to vanish in the same simple procedure.

In overall, the human scalp appears a particular site among the skin "planet", offering a medium of a unique microecology. This chapter attempts to depict its specificities.

STRUCTURE AND CHARACTERISTICS OF THE SCALP

The structure of the scalp is broadly similar to that of other skin areas, with a comparable cell population (keratinocytes, melanocytes, Langerhans cells, Merkel cells, etc.). However, the scalp differs from other skin sites by the following criteria:

- The surface microrelief is much less pronounced than in other sites
- Epidermis is about twice thicker than in other skin sites, together with a highly undulated dermal-epidermal junction, resulting from a faster turnover
- All other associated functions (sebaceous and sweat glands, hair follicles, etc.) can be found on scalp, showing a high and permanent activity
- The presence of about 200 follicles/cm^2 (ostia of about 100–120 μm), by including the intrafollicular surface, roughly doubles the total developed scalp surface
- Scalp is the skin territory of the richest hydrolipidic "film", supplying a high amount of various constituents (keratin debris, sebum, sweat and their byproducts). Logically, such medium provides a favorable ecological niche to an intense microbial colonization (bacteria, yeasts, etc.)
- Scalp is a source of frequent and unpleasant sensorial feelings such as itching, pruritus.

Most of these features are altered in some scalp disorders such as dandruff.

SEBORRHEA OF THE SCALP

Sebaceous Gland

This gland almost systematically annexes the hair follicle (Fig. 1). Its size, which reflects its lipid-producing activity, is generally inversely correlated with the diameter of its associated hair.[3] Sebaceous gland is considered as a secondary sexual organ with regard to its strong dependence on androgens. From a dormant phase during the first ten years of life, sebaceous gland enlarges and becomes progressively active, under the initial

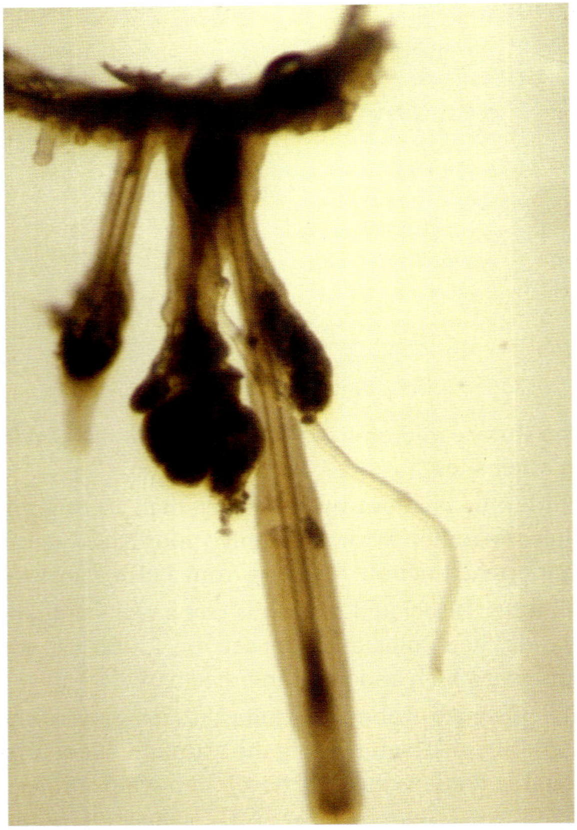

Figure 1: Pilosebaceous unit, the postbiopsy preparation ©L'Oréal Research and Innovation

influence of dehydroepiandrosterone (DHEA) and, later, the sudden flux of gonadal androgens delivered at sexual puberty. Logically, such period opens a new era of greasy hair, acne, dandruff, all disorders being closely linked to the sebaceous function.

Sebaceous glands associated with hair follicles are distributed throughout the skin. They are found in greatest abundance on the face and scalp while absent on palms and soles.[4] Sebaceous glands can also form independently from the hair follicle such as Meibomian glands of the eyelid, ectopic sebaceous gland of the glans penis[5] and Fordyce spots of the oral epithelium. However, the immense majority of sebaceous glands is associated to the hair follicle to such extent that both are most described under the generic "pilosebaceous unit". These sebaceous glands secrete an oily substance (sebum) in the hair follicles to lubricate the skin and hair of animals.[6] Their function within the epidermis is to prevent the skin from dehydration and protect the body against infections and physical, chemical and thermal assaults of the environment. Sebum production is regulated throughout life, and decreases dramatically with age,[7] a decline associated with an increased dryness of the skin. Moreover, several human diseases, such as acne vulgaris, atopic dermatitis, seborrheic dermatitis and primary scarring alopecia are thought to be associated with a dysfunction of sebaceous glands.[8-10]

There is a crucial interdependency of sebaceous glands with hair follicles and epidermis as sebocyte dysfunction results in degeneration of hair follicle structures and a defective skin barrier.[10,11] This is illustrated in the asebia mutant mouse, which lacks the SCD1 enzyme that desaturates fatty acids. This mutant displays rudimentary sebaceous glands and an altered profile of skin surface lipids leading to chronic inflammatory reactions, alopecia and dermal scarring.[11] With age, the latter remains rather stable, of a higher intensity in males than females, albeit declines rather regularly in both genders from the 40's.[7] The role of sebaceous gland (and sebum, its major production) remains, to date, a topic of much speculation. For some authors, this gland represents a vestigial remnant of human skin which, glabrous for most of its surface, remains the greasier, as compared to animal species.

With regard to cosmetics, the approach to modify sebaceous gland function differs from 20 years ago, especially since the research of topical "antiseborrheic" yielded disappointing results. Even a drug highly effective by the oral route (13-cis-retinoic acid), appears inefficient when topically applied. Despite the ordinary and daily visible consequence of seborrhea of the scalp, i.e. a greasy hair progressively seen as "dirty", is gradually improved by the increasing frequency of shampooing. This is mostly linked to the tremendous advances in the chemistry of surfactants, especially in terms of tolerance and efficacy. At present time, hairwashing tends to be considered as important—and mundane—as teeth brushing or handwashing. However, although the skin surface sebum can be regularly removed, the continued presence of a few mg/cm^2 of sebum in the depths of the follicular canal[12-14] and its derivatives are sources of ongoing problems that will be addressed below.

Sebum Composition

Native and sterile (within the gland), sebum is an unusual lipidic mixture of wax esters (esters of long chain fatty alcohols and fatty acids, 25–26%), squalene (12–15%), triglycerides (of highly complex and rare fatty acids, 57–60%)[8] that behaves as an oil under normal conditions of temperature. With regard to lipid synthesis, the sebaceous gland (SG) does not follow the traditional laws of other organs (e.g. liver) that produce lipids of conventional structures, since able to use other lipidic chain starters than the classic Acetyl-CoA.

Sebum is mostly unsaturated, i.e. the fatty chains produced are fluid (saturated lipids are at solid state) in normal conditions, explaining its particular behavior and rheology.[4,15] However, this property also implies that such lipids are particularly vulnerable to oxidation like butter and other vegetable oils prone to become rancid. Oxidization process also generates highly reactive compounds (e.g. squalene peroxides) which may be aggressive toward living tissues.

In addition to these changes, sebum "fuels" an intense lipophilic bacterial and fungal colonization, through their lipolytic activity that hydrolyze triglycerides. They, thereby, supply glycerol, a rich source of carbon that can be used in both aerobic or anerobic conditions.

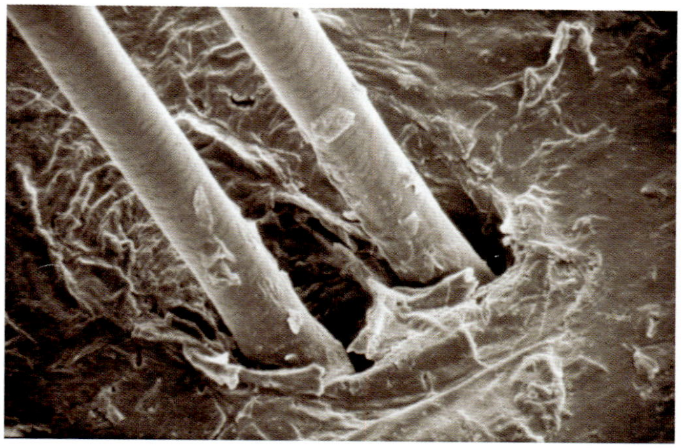

Figure 2: Human scalp and follicular ostia, right after a shampoo Scanning Electron Microscopy (SEM)
©L'Oréal Research and Innovation

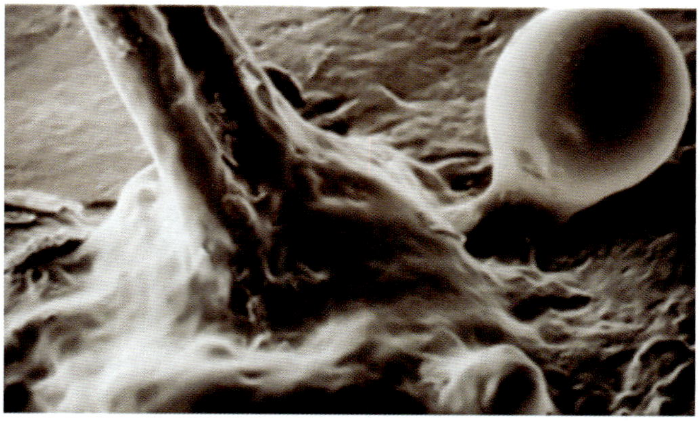

Figure 3: Same site (as shown in Figure 2), 24 hours after shampooing. The sebum excretion diffuses on the surface of the hair and scalp. The sphere elevation is water/sweat (SEM)
©L'Oréal Research and Innovation

Sebum Excretion

The production of sebum by the SG is continuous. As holocrine process, sebum is released by the lysis of the sebaceous cells that discharge their content into the follicular duct from which it is excreted.

Sebum flows and covers the surface of the scalp and the hair root, contributing to make adjacent hairs stuck together (Figs 2 and 3). Globally, 2 days after shampooing, the total amount of re-excreted sebum (scalp + hair) ranges from 500 mg to 2 g, according to individuals.[12,14]

Being continuously excreted, sebum can spread onto "unlimited" surfaces since hair represent a total surface area that can reach several square meters according to length. This explains in a large part the hyperbolic-like kinetics of scalp regreasing, where sebum level generally reaches a plateau (the so-called casual level) 2–3 days post shampoo.[14] Such kinetics was recently confirmed on a large number of subjects from seven different ethnic groups (Indians, Chinese, African-Americans, European-Caucasians, European-Americans, Japanese and Thais) by L'Oreal Research (to be published). Interestingly, compared to the six other ethnic groups, subjects from India show a much lower sebum casual level. Such observation clearly deserves further additional works.

Removal of surface hair and skin lipids by shampooing (discussed further in this chapter) does not impact the physiology of the sebaceous function. Some thirty-five years ago, the "reactive seborrhea" theory claimed that an exaggerated frequency of shampooing would induce an increased sebum production, but was soon ruled out by experimental facts.[12,14] In fact, the propensity of sebaceous lipids to spread onto scalp surface and hair, involves a third element, the stratum corneum, that acts like a "sponge" toward sebum. When the scalp stratum corneum becomes unable to fulfill such function, the surface of the scalp becomes oilier and hair regreasing appears faster. This phenomenon is particularly evident following an anti-dandruff action, since dandruff scales can absorb lipids up to about one-third of their weight. The removal and further absence of scales resulting from the use of the antidandruff shampoo, prevents the reabsorption of a substantial fraction of sebum which then becomes partially transferred to the hair surface. However, these phenomena are now strongly masked by the greater frequency of shampooing.

A potential new candidate for human sebocyte regulation is transforming growth factor β (TGFβ).[16,17] The TGFβ pathway is ubiquitous and involved in the control of growth and differentiation of many cellular and tissue types. The two major receptors of the TGFβ signaling pathway, TGFβ receptor I (TGFβ RI) and TGFβ receptor II (TGFβ RII), are expressed in mouse sebaceous glands.[18,19] In human and mouse epithelial cell lines, TGFβ acts as a potent inhibitor of proliferation.[20,21] In a new culture system associated with skin samples from pediatric donors, McNairn et al. demonstrated that reduced expression of TGFβ RII increased lipid production.[22]

FLORA AND FAUNA OF THE SCALP

Scalp Microflora

Scalp is permanently colonized by a microbial flora the level of which ranges from 10^4 to 10^8 organisms per cm^2 depending on individuals.[23-25] This colonization, established at birth, is mainly localized in the depths of the follicular duct, where sebum accumulates.

This permanent and commensal flora, varying in nature and abundance with skin sites, is now depicted as a "microbiome", increasingly identified through genetic tools (discussed further in this chapter). Comparable to the case of icebergs, the respective proportion of settlement between surface and depth is estimated at 10/90, but no quantitative data has been published yet. Scalp flora can be divided into two groups: (i) resident flora; and (ii) transient flora, where resident flora clearly predominates (>90%). The latter is indeed the only one able to thrive on and expand in the scalp as it is equipped with enzymes capable of using the available nutrients (lipids, amino acids, organic acids, etc.). Old publications based on cultivation methods to identify and quantify the resident flora have shown that it consists of two main types, with a relative ratio of approximately 50/50 on a normal scalp:

1. Lipophilic bacteria (*Propionibacterium* spp., *Staphylococcus* spp.).
2. Yeasts (*Malassezia* spp.), the major agents of dandruff (Fig 4).

Recent reports using Sanger sequencing and next-generation sequencing methods that are culture-independent methods, confirmed the predominance of *Propionibacterium* spp., *Staphylococcus* spp. and *Malassezia* spp. on the scalp (Fig. 5).[26-28] Thanks to the better accuracy of those new methods as compared to culture-based methods, the microorganisms were identified at the species level. *Propionibacterium* spp. consisted in *P. acnes* (99.7%) and *P. granulosum* (0.3 %). *Staphylococcus* spp. mainly included *S. epidermidis* (99.1%) and *Malassezia restricta* was the major fungal species (97%). Quantitative polymerase chain reaction (qPCR), showed that the relative ratio of bacteria to yeast was approximately 100 bacteria per one yeast on a normal scalp.[28]

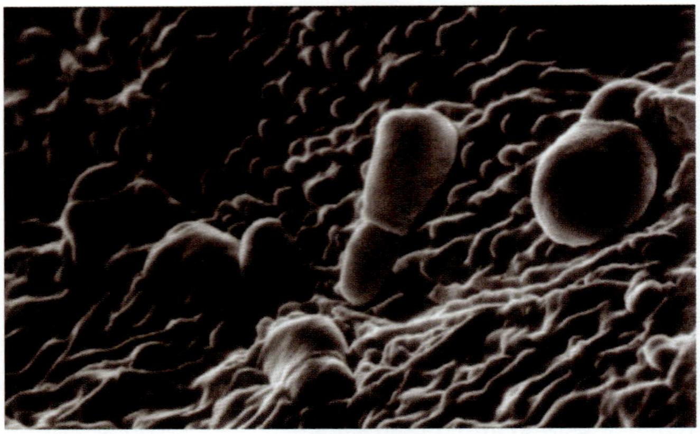

Figure 4: Units of *Malassezia* yeasts on the surface of a corneocyte (SEM)
©L'Oréal Research and Innovation

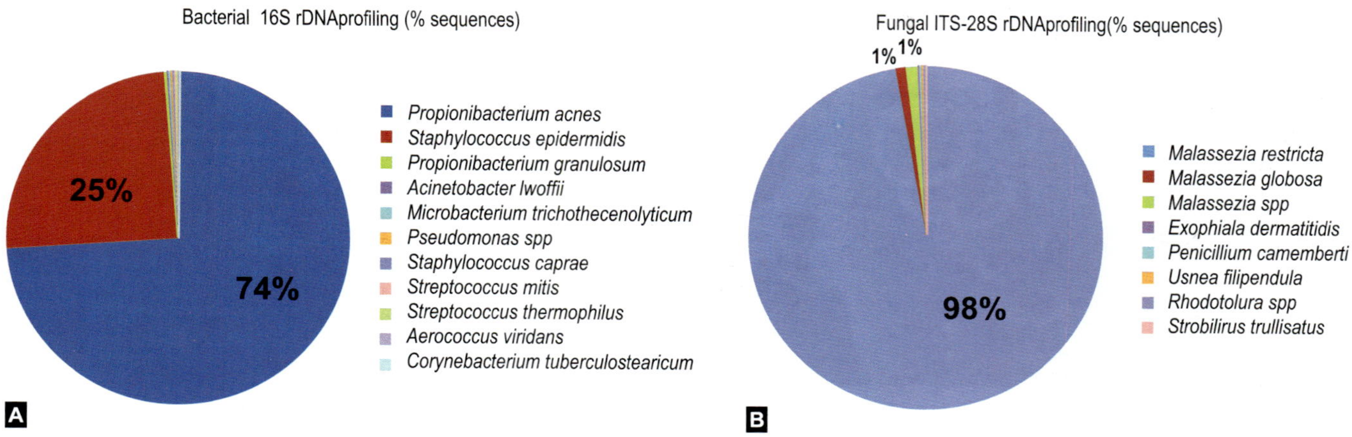

Figure 5: Distribution of bacterial and fungal species in normal scalp. **A,** Distribution of 1,241 sequences (~1500 bp) of 16S rDNA and **B,** 1,173 sequences (~1500 bp) of ITS-28S rDNA. Results are presented as the percent (%) of total sequences recovered per species ©L'Oréal Research and Innovation

This resident flora is generally considered to be saprophytic, i.e. not harming host. However, the multiplication of bacteria, fungi or of their metabolites may affect the skin of some predisposed people.

In contrast, transient flora may lead to potential infectious problems, brought by a temporary flora that is spread by contact or air-borne. *Staphylococcus aureus* spp. *(S. aureus)*, among others, is its most common representative. However, it cannot thrive long on the surface of the scalp and does not survive more than a few hours in normal conditions. If a more favorable environment (e.g. wounds as entrance gates) is found during such latency period, serious infections may then arise.[29,30] From this perspective, the human scalp can be seen as a potential reservoir of infectious agents, hence contributing to the spread of nosocomial infections responsible for about 80,000 deaths each year in Europe. Such fact largely supports the rationale of Louis Pasteur's requirements regarding wearing of a hat where hygiene should be as rigorous as possible (hospitals, canteens, etc.). In this regard, shampooing appears more than a simple cleaning process, but possibly be viewed as a preventive (and simple) measure against nosocomial infections, as well as frequent handwashing.[31]

Scalp Fauna

Colonization of the scalp by parasites is more discrete than flora and usually very temporary. Lice (pediculosis) are the most obvious examples (Fig. 6) of infestations commonly seen on children; schools being "efficient" transmission fields. Eradicating such disorder is most of the time successful, albeit long and tedious. It requires topical applications of specific drugs (e.g. Lanthane) that are obviously excluded from the cosmetic regulatory status.

It is worth noting the almost constant presence of certain mites, *Demodex folliculorum*, which colonize the follicle, sebum being their preferred nutrient (Fig. 7). This colonization seems affecting almost all individuals, but occurs in a very small proportion of hair follicles.[32,33] Nevertheless, *Demodex* induce inflammatory local skin reactions (Demodecia) and, since often present on eyelids, is the causative agent of blepharitis.

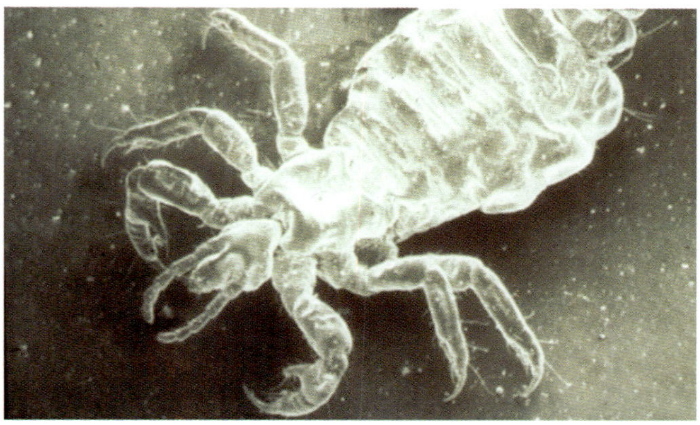

Figure 6: The head louse (*Pediculus humanus capitis*) (SEM) ©L'Oréal Research and Innovation

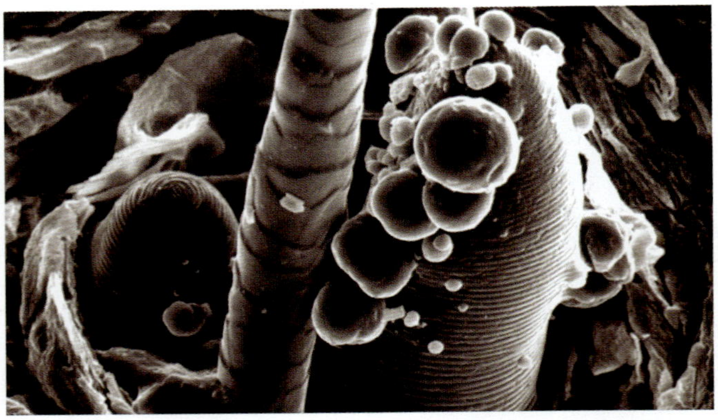

Figure 7: Two Demodex immersing their bodies in the follicular canal (SEM)
©L'Oréal Research and Innovation

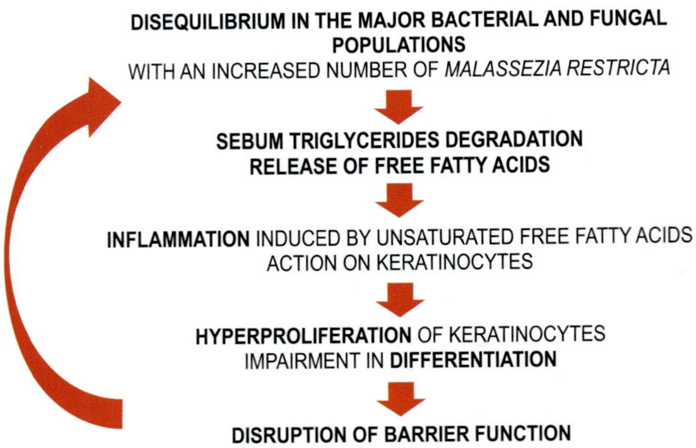

Figure 8: Summarized dandruff etiology factors
©L'Oréal Research and Innovation

DANDRUFF

This unesthetic disorder of the scalp affects about half of the world population, regardless of gender and ethnic groups, and is exacerbated during winter and stress periods. Dandruff is accompanied by sensory manifestations, such as itching and irritation, although prone scalps rarely show clinical signs that are usually associated with inflammation *(rubor, calor, tumor, dolor)*. Dandruff scalps are rarely red, hot, or painful. Seen by some authors as a disease,[34,35] the etiology of dandruff has been reviewed in a chapter of the book *The Science of Hair Care*[36] and more recently in 2013 two review articles were published, indicating the importance of dandruff in the field of cosmetic hair care market.[37,38]

In short, dandruff results from an abnormal desquamation of the scalp. Dandruff condition produces flakes composed of 1,000–10,000 horny cells still stuck together whereas normal scaling implies that horny cells are eliminated imperceptibly, as single entities. Such scaling is the classical result of the subclinical underlying inflammatory process where some blood cells (polymorphonucleocytes) infiltrate the dermis.

Although previous reports have suggested that dandruff was only due to the presence of *M. restricta* and *M. globosa*, the etiology of dandruff is not completely understood, especially because of its multifactorial nature. Though the colonization of the scalp by lipophilic *Malassezia* spp. has a major role in dandruff development, bacterial colonization, sebum and individual susceptibility are additional contributing factors (Fig. 8).

Malassezia was found representing about half of the resident flora of a normal scalp, increasing to 75% in dandruff.[23,39] Following reclassification of the *Malassezia* genus in the 1990s,[40] and the development of molecular methods it has become clear that the most abundant species on dandruff scalps were *M. restricta* and, to a lesser extent, *M. globosa*.[28,41,42] Species profiling of the dandruff scalp microflora using Sanger sequencing showed variable relative ratios between major bacterial species *P. acnes* and *S. epidermidis* (Fig. 9). This qualitative observation was further confirmed, using qPCR quantification of *M. restricta* and *P. acnes* indicated that *M. restricta* was ten times more prominent in dandruff subjects and that the amount of *P. acnes* was significantly lower in dandruff subjects, suggesting that these altered relative ratios between both species are linked to dandruff. In brief, dandruff scalps qualitatively and quantitatively favor the settlement of yeasts from the *Malassezia* spp., to the detriment of bacterial populations.

The production of sebum is also widely accepted as a contributing factor, since all prepubertal children (i.e. almost sebum-free) are dandruff-free. Being highly lipophilic, *Malassezia* spp. degrade sebum components through its lipase and lipoxygenase activities and release inflammatory unsaturated free fatty acids and lipoperoxides that disturb skin homeostasis.[43] However, scalp seborrhea and metabolization of related products by *Malassezia* appears a necessary but insufficient criterion of dandruff condition, for

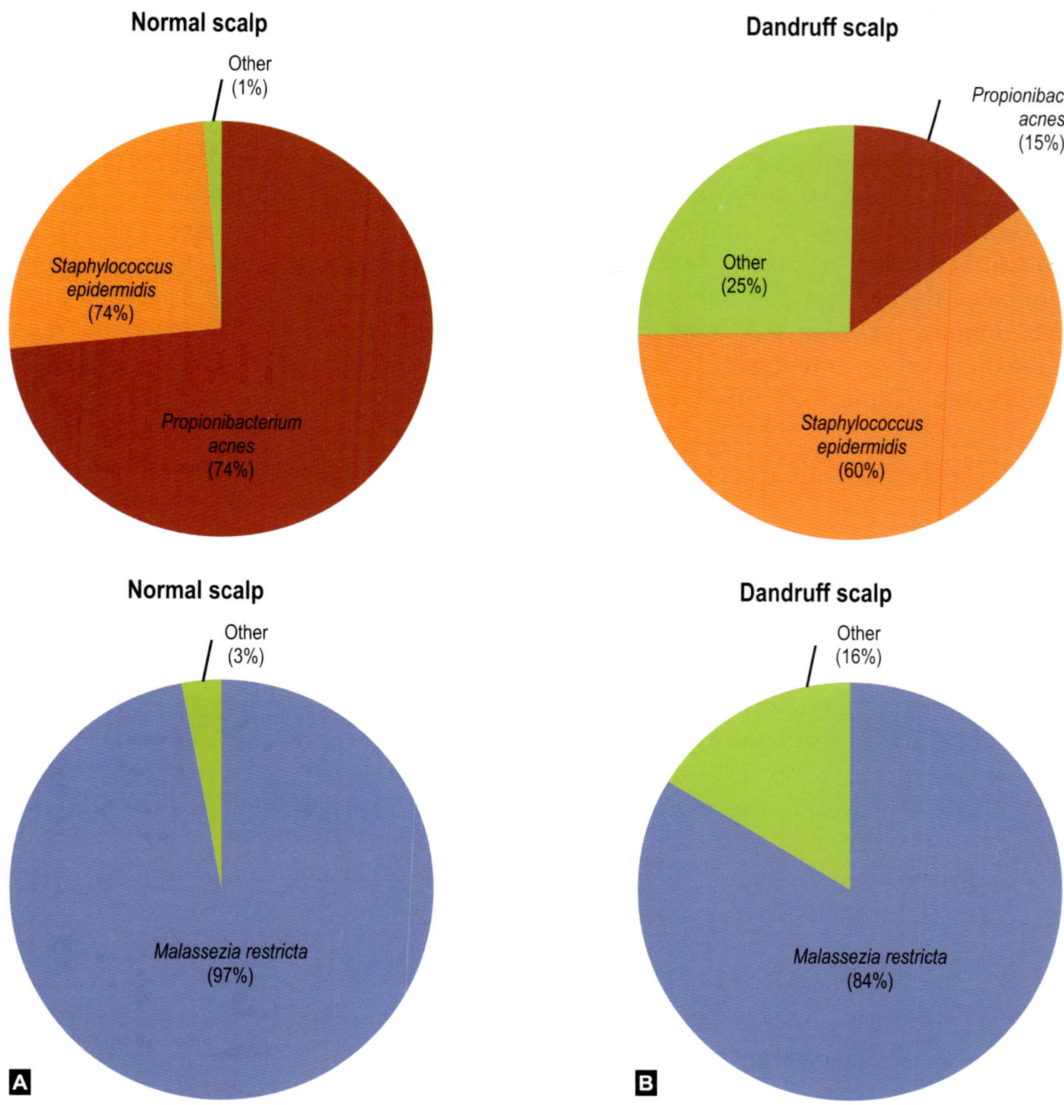

Figure 9: Distribution of bacterial and fungal species in 10-normal and 9-dandruff scalps. **A,** Distribution of 2,122 sequences (~1500 bp) of 16S rDNA. **B,** 2,225 sequences (~1500 bp) of ITS-28S rDNA between the normal scalps and dandruff-affected scalps. Results are presented as the percent (%) of total sequences recovered per species
©L'Oréal Research and Innovation

three main reasons: (i) A large proportion of humans with greasy scalp are dandruff-free;[44] (ii) Applying oleic acid on the scalp of nondandruff subjects did not induce flaking;[43] and (iii) Even though inhibitors of the *Malassezia globosa* lipase have been patented as new antidandruff compounds since 2001, no clinical study has been reported yet suggesting a limited efficacy of these compounds.[45,46]

Together with scalp microflora and sebum, individual susceptibility is the third important factor, particularly with respect to stratum corneum barrier integrity. Individual susceptibility could be involved in various steps of the disorder: (i) initiation and propagation of inflammation; (ii) disruption of proliferation and differentiation processes of the epidermis; and (iii) physical and functional skin barrier disruption. *Malassezia* spp. cells contain antigenic molecules, i.e. able to induce a host immune reaction.[47-50] Dandruff is not a cutaneous infection, therefore not transmissible. It may reflect a slight immune incompetency toward this yeast in about half of the human population. Immunization (competent or not) against *Malassezia* spp. seems initiated at an early stage: *Malassezia* antibodies can be detected in the blood of young healthy children.[51] It is noteworthy that a significant number of infants present similar disorders to dandruff, such as Cradle cap, at a period when scalp is still rich in sebum.[52]

SCALP AND COSMETIC PRODUCTS

Washing with Shampoos

The very word "shampoo" derives from the Hindi word *Champo* (massage). This act is the most common method to clean both hair and scalp and is performed billions of times every year, at home or during a hairdresser session. Hairwashing being the primary purpose, the emulsification of lipids and dirt during washing also ensures a cleaning of the scalp. Depending on countries, habits, climate and seasons, the frequency of shampooing may vary widely, from 2 times per week to 14 times per week (mornings and evenings), as observed in some Korean women. This traditional cleaning meets the following criteria:

- Shampoos are safe. Surfactant chemistry has made tremendous progress and now offers many effective and safe cleaning agents to the cosmetics industry, exhaustively reviewed in *The Science of Hair Care* book.[53] As simple illustration, it allowed the development of children's shampoos totally devoid of eye irritation potential, with regard to a possible contact of the product with the eye region.
- Contrary to some popular folklore, the use of shampoo and its frequency do not cause any negative effect upon the excretion of sebum, hair loss or epidermal physiology
- The act of washing is heavily dependent upon access to water (especially hot water). A wash in salon requires 30–50 liters of water, a lesser volume when performed at home, since most of the time included within the shower ritual.
- Usually of a short duration (few minutes), shampooing is remarkably effective. As the surface area of the hair and scalp can represent a few square meters (depending on hair length), the process of shampooing is a quick cleaning process of a surface comparable to a small kitchen.
- The routine of shampooing varies from country to country. In China, as an example, a now traditional "dry wash" is performed in salons: massaging and washing are combined, using the shampoo base deprived of water, a procedure which lasts 30 minutes, at the end of which 10–15 mL of water are added to allow foam to develop.[54]
- At home, shampooing is most often carried out under shower, often followed by dry heat, much determined by the volume of the hair, i.e. a possibly lengthy process. The latter is often perceived as a serious penalty in view of personal or professional activity. It largely explains lower shampooing frequency among women with long hair.
- The primary goal of a shampoo is obviously a cleaning effect. However, since the 1980s, additional attributes were brought to shampoos.[55] These include detangling, conditioning, smooth feeling, styling, fiber protection, shape or color protection, repairing damaged hair fibers, etc. usually covered by marketing claims such as "2- or 3-in-1".
- In addition to their cleansing function, antidandruff shampoos obviously target scalp. Among many commercial shampoo brands, antidandruff's are in the top-selling series.

Anti-dandruff Agents

Effective treatments for dandruff/seborrheic dermatitis require: (i) a potent active material; (ii) efficient topical delivery while maintaining bioavailability; and (iii) long-term product compliance to prevent the natural recurrence. The most widely used active strategy is to control yeasts of the genus *Malassezia* using antifungal agents. The sequence: *Malassezia→ inflammatory response→abnormal desquamation* is obviously broken by controlling yeast colonization, cutting water at source. Cause and symptoms disappear simultaneously. The most common agents, zinc pyrithione (ZPT), piroctone olamine, selenium sulfide (SeS_2) and ketoconazole, are usually used at 1% in a shampoo base (e.g. in the

Table 1: Main antifungal agents used against dandruff and/or seborrheic dermatitis

Active Ingredient	*Activity*	*Legal Status (Europe/USA)*	*Dandruff (D) or Seborrheic Dermatitis (SD)*
Zinc pyrithione	Antifungal Antibacterial Keratolytic	Europe: Cosmetic use 0.5–2% USA: OTC at 0.3–2%	SD/D
Tar	Regulator of keratinization	Europe: Not accepted USA: OTC at 0.5–5%	SD/D
Selenium sulfide	Antifungal Keratolytic	Europe: Cosmetic use up to 1% USA: OTC use up to 1%	SD/D
Ketoconazole	Antifungal Antibacterial Anti-inflammatory	Europe: prescription drug USA: OTC use up to 1% and prescription at 2%	SD/D
Piroctone olamine	Antifungal	Europe: cosmetic use up to 1% USA: Not accepted	SD/D

products providing the famous "2-in-1 action", in which care and antidandruff actions are provided in a single shampoo), although two of them (SeS_2, ketoconazole) are classified as OTC (Over the Counter, prescription-free) according to their concentration in the shampoo in the USA[34] (Table 1).

The active compounds are deposited onto the scalp surface and will later inhibit the growth of *Malassezia spp*. ZPT and selenium disulfide have additional keratolytic effect that participate in their antidandruff efficiency. Some keratolytic agents like salicylic acid can also be added. Studies showed good results with shampoos containing the exfoliating ingredient lipohydroxy acid.[56] Interestingly, the topical use of a traditional Indian medicine (Unani medicine) has been shown possessing an antidandruff activity, the efficacy of which being found similar to that of a standard drug (2% ketoconazole).[57]

In most cases, significant improvement in dandruff condition appears after 2–3 shampoos, sensory manifestations (itching) being the earliest to decline. Stopping treatment leads to restore scaling within 2–3 weeks, along with the scalp recolonization by the yeast. It should be noted that in some countries (United States, Japan), antidandruff strategy has been classified as drug action. Therefore, its active ingredients should be developed as drugs and registered accordingly. And yet used (often daily) by billions of people for over 40 years, antidandruff ingredients clearly appear "safe and efficient".

Cosmetics Destined to Scalp

Cosmetics exclusively "scalp-oriented" are in fact scarce, as compared to hair products. They, however, include:

- Products aiming at fighting seasonal hair loss or increasing hair density—(Aminexil®, and later Stemoxydin®) and medicinal or OTC products to promote hair regeneration—(Minoxidil®). Their topical application requires great care: they are often applied onto scalp line by line to deliver the product onto the scalp surface, avoiding its absorption by the hair fibers, i.e. giving privilege to scalp surface.
- Scalp comfort and moisturizing products are often offered as "hair masks" which also provide hair conditioning properties. All in all, the development of these products faces a major challenge: after application, with or without rinsing (leave on product), hair must look perfectly clean, shiny and by no way greasy. Similarly, hair coloring products (direct or oxidation) and perm products, even in contact with the scalp should not, in any way, stain or alter scalp and be a source of discomfort. Their development phases include such imperatives.

METHODS OF STUDYING THE HUMAN SCALP

Clinical and Sensorial Testings

Clinical

A clinical examination of the scalp is necessary in most studies. Given the possible "mosaic" appearance of the scalp, the examination should cover almost all scalp regions (temples, vertex, nape, etc.), releasing the hair area by area, using a comb and an inert spatula (Teflon or wood). Direct observation of different signs (erythema, pigmented spots, scars, warts, abrasions, etc.) can be performed with the naked eye or coupled with a magnifying glass or a video microscope.[58] In dermatology, such examination is paramount in the early detection of highly serious skin diseases such as melanoma[59] possibly present on scalp.

Apart from needs of a standardized visible light, illuminating the scalp by long range UVA's (Wood lamp type) allows locating melanin pigmentation or fluorescence to detect compounds related to flora such as porphyrins, synthetized by *Propionibacterium*.

Sensory

Given the numerous and frequent sensory events experienced on the scalp, an analog scale (e.g. a 0–10 range with 0 being "no itch" and 10 being "severe itch") questionnaire filled by the subjects, can be developed and further analyzed by nonparametric statistical tests of pair-wise comparison.

Instrumental Analysis

A fully hair covered scalp is of a difficult access for obvious reasons. Most research studies, therefore, require shaving the hair on a small area (1–2 cm^2) creating a free access to scalp. For a normal hair (density > 150 hairs/cm^2), this procedure does not impact at all the overall appearance of the hair and will not be noticed by the subject himself or his entourage. The small shaved area will allow a large number of observations or biophysical measurements to being carried out, such as:

- The Phototrichogram and Phototrichoscan.[60,61] These methods involve taking two successive pictures at a 2-day interval, which allows the hair formula to be established and parameters related to hair growth (% of hair in telogen phase, % in anagen phase, hair density, hair diameter, rate of growth, etc.) to be evaluated, all criteria being automatically processed by an adequate software.
- The measurement of scalp color that may reflect inflammation (erythema). This can be performed with conventional colorimetric devices using the L*, a*, b* space color, whose probes are consistent with the size of shaved area.
- Measurement of scalp temperature (32–34°C under normal conditions). Measurement methods with or without contact (infrared) can be performed.
- Measurement of scalp blood microcirculation (photoplethysmography, laser Doppler, etc.). This can be carried out by direct contact with the shaved area. Nevertheless, based upon our experience, such measurements are of a questionable reproducibility. The same holds true with the measurement of surface hydration with Corneometer® or equivalent devices. This is likely due to the presence of large size hairs which interfere with the electric waves, inversely to accessible sites free from terminal hairs, such as forearm.
- In contrast with the above measurements, the measurement of transepidermal water loss (TEWL), expressed in g/m^2/h, is well reproducible and remarkably informative regarding the status of the scalp barrier. This measure clearly separates dandruff from nondandruff subjects and is a helpful endpoint in the monitoring of various cosmetics effects.[54]
- Exploring the sebaceous function can easily be performed via the small area approach. Applying frosted glass or plastic film onto this surface, using the Lipometer® or the Sebumeter®, is simple to implement and allows the kinetics of scalp regreasing to be assessed.[14]
  - From a microbiological or biochemical point of view, two methods are to be preferred:
  - The Scrub method,[25] also known as Williamson-Kligman method can provide a lot of information. It consists of applying a small open ring (steel or Teflon) into which a small volume of sterile phosphate buffer detergent (Triton X100) is delivered. For 1–2 minutes, a Teflon policeman rubs the surface of the scalp, stirs the environment and extracts a complex mixture of bacteria, yeasts, corneocytes, proteins, enzymes, salts, etc. Originally designed for microbiological purposes, this technique can be extended to many other applications (proteomics, cytology, etc.). It is clearly the semiquantitative reference method of acceptable reproducibility.
  - The stripping method is also a reference method.[62-64] Applying an adhesive film on the small area leads to harvest the outermost layers

of the scalp, allowing various parameters to be subsequently quantified. The semiquantification of yeasts, scales, epidermal lipids, markers or biological messengers becomes possible. Widely used, this clever method has contributed significantly to our understanding of the physiology of the human scalp.

CONCLUSION

The human scalp, although normally hidden to our eyes, illustrates an important and symbolic pathway between skin and hair domains. As host of a precious head of hair, its supplying "soil", scalp faces permanent assaults that need permanent care or preventing actions. As such, the act of regular shampooing is the simplest example of an external help combining needs of cleaning a skin surface and adorning hairs, whose shiny aspect is often viewed as healthy symbol. With regard to dandruff prone scalps, controlling a slight subclinical inflammatory reaction through efficient and easy to use products, offers an adequate answer to physiological needs, esthetical and sensorial comfort.

Researches from these last two decades have witnessed many advances in the physiology of the human scalp, a too long time ignored skin site. New methods of investigation afforded an enlarged vision of its structure, properties and authorized great improvements in its related cosmetic products.

REFERENCES

1. Bouillon C, Wilkinson J. Hair: a psychoanalytical perspective. In: Lai W (Ed). The Science of Hair Care, Chinese Edition; 2009.
2. Colon EA, Popkin MK, Callies AL, et al. Lifetime prevalence of psychiatric disorders in patients with alopecia areata. Compr Psychiatry. 1991;32:245-51.
3. Pierard GE, Pierard-Franchimont C, Nikkels-Tassoudji N, et al. Improvement in the inflammatory aspect of androgenic alopecia. J Dermatol Treat. 1996;7:53-7.
4. Thody AJ, Shuster S. Control and function of sebaceous glands. Physiol Rev. 1989;69(2):383-416.
5. Hyman AB, Brownstein MH. Tyson's "glands." Ectopic sebaceous glands and papillomatosis penis. Arch Dermatol. 1969;99(1):31-6.
6. Smith KR, Thiboutot DM. Thematic review series: skin lipids. Sebaceous gland lipids: friend or foe? J Lipid Res. 2008;49(2):271-81.
7. Pochi PE, Strauss JS, Downing DT. Age-related changes in sebaceous gland activity. J Invest Dermatol. 1979;73(1):108-11.
8. Picardo M, Ottaviani M, Camera E, et al. Sebaceous gland lipids. Dermatoendocrinol. 2009;1(2):68-71.
9. Huang JT, Abrams M, Tlougan B, et al. Treatment of Staphylococcus aureus colonization in atopic dermatitis decreases disease severity. Pediatrics. 2009;123(5):e808-14.
10. Stenn KS. Insights from the asebia mouse: a molecular sebaceous gland defect leading to cicatricial alopecia. J Cutan Pathol. 2001;28(9):445-7.
11. Zheng Y, Eilertsen KJ, Ge L, et al. Scd1 is expressed in sebaceous glands and is disrupted in the asebia mouse. Nat Genet. 1999;23(3):268-70.
12. Kligman AM, McGynley KJ, Leyden JJ. Studies on the effects of shampoos on scalp lipids and bacteria. In: Orfanos C, Montagna W, Stutten G (Eds). Hair Research. Berlin: Springer-Verlag; 1981. pp. 592-601.
13. Piérard-Franchimont C, Piérard GE. Physiopathological approach to seborrhea of the scalp. Ann Dermatol Venereol. 1988;115(4):451-3.
14. Saint-Leger D, Leveque JL. A comparative study of refatting kinetics on the scalp and forehead. Br J Dermatol. 1982;106(6):669-75.
15. Saint-Leger D. Physiology of the pilosebaceous follicle. Rev Prat. 1993;43(18):2315-9.
16. Furue M, Kato M, Nakamura K, et al. Dysregulated expression of transforming growth factor beta and its type-I and type-II receptors in basal-cell carcinoma. Int J Cancer. 1997;71(4):505-9.
17. Downie MM, Sanders DA, Kealey T. Modelling the remission of individual acne lesions in vitro. Br J Dermatol. 2002;147(5):869-78.
18. Wollina U, Lange D, Funa K, et al. Expression of transforming growth factor beta isoforms and their receptors during hair growth phases in mice. Histol Histopathol. 1996;11(2):431-6.
19. Paus R, Foitzik K, Welker P, et al. Transforming growth factor-beta receptor type I and type II expression during murine hair follicle development and cycling. J Invest Dermatol. 1997;109(4):518-26.
20. Pietenpol JA, Stein RW, Moran E, et al. TGF-beta 1 inhibition of c-myc transcription and growth in keratinocytes is abrogated by viral transforming proteins with pRB binding domains. Cell. 1990;61(5):777-85.
21. Guasch G, Schober M, Pasolli HA, et al. Loss of TGFbeta signaling destabilizes homeostasis and promotes squamous cell carcinomas in stratified epithelia. Cancer Cell. 2007;12(4):313-27.
22. McNairn AJ, Doucet Y, Demaude J, et al. TGFbeta signaling regulates lipogenesis in human sebaceous gland cells. BMC Dermatol. 2013;13:2.
23. McGinley KJ, Leyden JJ, Marples RR, et al. Quantitative microbiology of the scalp in non-dandruff, dandruff, and seborrheic dermatitis. J Invest Dermatol. 1975;64(6):401-5.
24. Saint-Leger D, Kligman AM, Stoudemeyer TJ. The role of the resident microflora in the pathogenesis of dandruff. J Soc Cosmet Chem. 1989;40:109-17.
25. Williamson P, Kligman AM. A new method for the quantitative investigation of cutaneous bacteria. J Invest Dermatol. 1965;45(6):498-503.
26. Findley K, Oh J, Yang J, et al. Topographic diversity of fungal and bacterial communities in human skin. Nature. 2013;498(7454):367-70.
27. Conlan S, Kong HH, Segre JA. Species-level analysis of DNA sequence data from the NIH Human Microbiome Project. PLoS One. 2012;7(10):e47075.
28. Clavaud C, Jourdain R, Bar-Hen A, et al. Dandruff is associated with disequilibrium in the proportion of the major bacterial and fungal populations colonizing the scalp. PLoS One. 2013;8(3):e58203.
29. Noble WC. Microflora and Microbial Skin Diseases. Cambridge, UK: Cambridge University Press;1993.
30. Blanc D. Scalp Dermatosis. The Science of Hair Care (Lai Wei, Chinese Edition; 2009).

31. Chen YC, Chiang LC. Effectiveness of handwashing teaching programs for families of children in paediatric intensive care units. J Clin Nurs. 2007;16(6):1173-9.
32. Forton F. Demodex and perifollicular inflammation in man: review and report of 69 biopsies. Ann Dermatol Venereol. 1986;113(11):1047-58.
33. Elston DM. Demodex mites as a cause of human disease. Cutis. 2005;76(5):294-6.
34. Manuel F. Is dandruff a disease? Int J Trichology. 2010;2(1):68.
35. Ranganathan S, Mukhopadhyay T. Dandruff: the most commercially exploited skin disease. Indian J Dermatol. 2010;55(2):130-4.
36. Saint-Leger D. Dandruff (Pityriasis Capitis Simplex): of yeasts and men. In: Lai W (Ed).The Science of Hair Care, Chinese Edition; 2009.
37. Schwartz JR, Messenger AG, Tosti A, et al. A comprehensive pathophysiology of dandruff and seborrheic dermatitis - towards a more precise definition of scalp health. Acta Derm Venereol. 2013;93(2):131-7.
38. James AG, Abraham KH, Cox DS, et al. Metabolic analysis of the cutaneous fungi Malassezia globosa and M. restricta for insights on scalp condition and dandruff. Int J Cosmet Sci. 2013;35(2):169-75.
39. Saint-Leger D, Kligman AM, Stoudemeyer TJ. A new method to quantify scaling in dandruff. J Soc Cosm Chem. 1988;39:179-90.
40. Batra R, Boekhout T, Gueho E, et al. Malassezia Baillon, emerging clinical yeasts. FEMS Yeast Res. 2005;5(12):1101-13.
41. Gemmer CM, DeAngelis YM, Theelen B, et al. Fast, noninvasive method for molecular detection and differentiation of Malassezia yeast species on human skin and application of the method to dandruff microbiology. J Clin Microbiol. 2002;40(9):3350-7.
42. Paulino LC, Tseng CH, Strober BE, et al. Molecular analysis of fungal microbiota in samples from healthy human skin and psoriatic lesions. J Clin Microbiol. 2006;44(8):2933-41.
43. DeAngelis YM, Gemmer CM, Kaczvinsky JR, et al. Three etiologic facets of dandruff and seborrheic dermatitis: Malassezia fungi, sebaceous lipids, and individual sensitivity. J Investig Dermatol Symp Proc. 2005;10(3):295-7.
44. Burton JL, Pye RJ. Seborrhoea is not a feature of seborrhoeic dermatitis. Br Med J (Clin Res Ed) 1983;286(6372):1169-70.
45. US Patent 7,101,889 (Sept 2003).
46. DeAngelis YM, Saunders CW, Johnstone KR, et al. Isolation and expression of a Malassezia globosa lipase gene, LIP1. J Invest Dermatol. 2007;127(9):2138-46.
47. Baroni A, Orlando M, Donnarumma G, et al. Toll-like receptor 2 (TLR2) mediates intracellular signalling in human keratinocytes in response to Malassezia furfur. Arch Dermatol Res. 2006; 297(7):280-8.
48. Akaza N, Akamatsu H, Takeoka S, et al. Increased hydrophobicity in Malassezia species correlates with increased proinflammatory cytokine expression in human keratinocytes. Med Mycol. 2012;50(8):802-10.
49. Shibata N, Saitoh T, Tadokoro Y, et al. The cell wall galactomannan antigen from Malassezia furfur and Malassezia pachydermatis contains beta-1,6-linked linear galactofuranosyl residues and its detection has diagnostic potential. Microbiology. 2009;155:3420-9.
50. Saunders CW, Scheynius A, Heitman J. Malassezia fungi are specialized to live on skin and associated with dandruff, eczema, and other skin diseases. PLoS Pathog. 2012;8(6):e1002701.
51. Ashbee HR, Fruin A, Holland KT, et al. Humoral immunity to Malassezia furfur serovars A, B and C in patients with pityriasis versicolor, seborrheic dermatitis and controls. Exp Dermatol. 1994;3(5):227-33.
52. Sulcova J, Starka L, Jirasek JE. Age and sex differences in the metabolism of C19-delta5-steroids in human amniotic epithelium. J Dev Physiol. 1980;2(6):389-99.
53. Dubief C, Mellul M, Loussouarn G. Hair Care Products. In: Lai W (Ed). The Science of Hair Care, Chinese Edition; 2009.
54. Liu Y, Liu C, Collaudin C, et al. Challenging the scalp with 'dry' wash shampooing (DW) on Chinese men: an in vivo study. Int J Cosmet Sci. 2010;32(2):127-33.
55. Madnani N, Khan K. Hair Cosmetics. Indian J Dermatol Venereol Leprol. 2013;79(5):654-67.
56. Seite S, Rougier A, Talarico S. Randomized study comparing the efficacy and tolerance of a lipohydroxy acid shampoo to a ciclopiroxolamine shampoo in the treatment of scalp seborrheic dermatitis. J Cosmet Dermatol. 2009;8(4):249-53.
57. Shah AH, Haji A, Rather SA, et al. Clinical study on the management of Huzaz/Abria (Dandruff) with a pharmacopoeal preparation of a Unani medicine and its cosmetic evaluation. Anc Sci Life. 2009;29(2):24-7.
58. Rogers NE. Scoping scalp disorders: practical use of a novel dermatoscope to diagnose hair and scalp conditions. J Drugs Dermatol. 2013;12(3):283-90.
59. Larson DL, Larson JD. Head and neck melanoma. Clin Plast Surg. 2010;37(1):73-7.
60. Saitoh M, Uzuka M, Sakamoto M. Human hair cycle. J Invest Dermatol. 1970;54(1):65-81.
61. Guarrera M, Fiorucci MC, Rebora A. Methods of hair loss evaluation: a comparison of TrichoScan(®) with the modified wash test. Exp Dermatol. 2013;22(7):482-4
62. Pierard GE, Arrese JE, Pierard-Franchimont C, et al. Prolonged effects of antidandruff shampoos - time to recurrence of Malassezia ovalis colonization of skin. Int J Cosmet Sci. 1997;19(3):111-7.
63. Perkins MA, Cardin CW, Osterhues MA, et al. A non-invasive tape absorption method for recovery of inflammatory mediators to differentiate normal from compromised scalp conditions. Skin Res Technol. 2002;8(3):187-93.
64. Pierard-Franchimont C, Arrese JE, Pierard GE, et al. Correlation between Malassezia ovalis load and dandruff severity. J Mycol Med. 1998;8:83-6.

Chapter 14

Peelings and Fillers

Christian Oresajo, *L'Oréal Research and Innovation, Clark, USA*
Niti Khunger, *VM Medical College and Safdarjung Hospital, New Delhi, India*
Vinay Saraf, *Dr. B. Nanavati Hospitals and Research Center, Mumbai, India*
Claire Battie, *L'Oréal Research and Innovation, Asnières, France*

INTRODUCTION

For centuries, physical and chemical procedures have been used to improve and smooth the texture of the facial skin.

Chemical peelings are used worldwide and have proven their efficacy and safety. It is perhaps the most commonly performed cosmetological office procedure. Although newer rejuvenating procedures and devices arrive frequently, chemical peels have withstood the test of time for various dermatological indications. More recently, aging signs have been corrected through filling with different types of agents. Dermal fillers are now the third most common cosmetological procedure performed in the West to correct dermatological conditions like lip augmentation, fine lines to deeper nasolabial folds and volume correction of the cheeks. When treating dark-skinned patients, it is important to keep the goal according to the patient's expectations and to understand what is culturally acceptable to them and what they really desire, while trying to avoid every complication.[1]

This chapter gives an overview of peelings and fillers with a special focus for dark-skinned patients.

CHEMICAL PEELING

As an ancient method, chemical peeling has been diversified and improved, and become a part of the correction strategy against skin aging, which remains its main indication. Chemical peeling is a common office procedure that has evolved over the years, using the scientific knowledge of wound healing after controlled chemical skin injury. It can also be proposed for its "brightening up" effect, which revives and unifies a dull complexion, in evolutionary acne or acne scars, in the correction of other scars, or in dyschromias such as melasma or ageing spots. A sound knowledge of the skin type, indication, type of chemical peels used, good pre-peel and post-peel care in the hands of a competent dermatologist are important in accomplishing cosmetically good results.

Mode of Action

Chemical peeling agents are mostly acids that are applied to the skin to remove the outer damaged layers, thus accelerating the normal process of exfoliation. The regenerated skin is smoother and less wrinkled providing the skin with an improved appearance.[2] The objective of peeling is not only to smooth the skin surface, but also, and especially, to induce a better regeneration of destroyed layers and an anabolic stimulation of underlying layers.

Chemical peels generally cause a skin inflammatory response within a day of treatment.[3] The severity of inflammation correlates with the nature and concentration of the peeling agent and is directly proportional to the amount of collagen deposition at 21 days, suggesting that the inflammatory response is the driving force for subsequent skin improvement.[4] It is likely that pro-inflammatory mediators have a positive effect on skin matrix metabolism and are responsible for this improvement. The role of injury-induced cytokines in epidermal pathophysiology is established, although the importance of individual cytokines in chemical peel-induced skin rejuvenation has not been clearly defined yet.[5]

Four types of peeling can be distinguished depending on the depth of peeling effect: very superficial peeling (limited to stratum corneum only), superficial peeling (epidermis), medium peeling (papillary dermis) and deep peeling (reticular dermis).[6]

Depending on their concentration, certain substances can be used for both superficial and medium peelings. In the combined peeling, the combination of several products raises the penetration level. The efficiency rises with the depth and is inversely proportional to the tolerance. Superficial peeling presents very little risk, but the medium and especially the deep peeling require an experienced operator. Using the correct depth chemical peel is a critical component for success.[7]

Superficial Peeling

Superficial peels affect the epidermis and dermal-epidermal interface. It is an ambulatory technique, which can be easily performed in dermatologist's office and does not require any social eviction. Superficial peels are useful in the treatment of mild dyschromia, acne, post-inflammatory pigmentation, and actinic keratoses and help in achieving skin radiance and luminosity. Because of their superficial action, superficial peels can be used in nearly all skin types. After a superficial peel, epidermal regeneration can be expected within 3–5 days, and desquamation is usually well accepted.[7]

The peeling can be:

- *Very mild*: Penetration to the level of Malpighian layer [α-hydroxy acids (AHAs) with moderate concentration level, β hydroxyacids (BHA) such as salicylic acid (SA) and lipohydroxy acid C8-LHA, all-trans retinoic acid, 10–20 % trichloroacetic acid (TCA)].
- *Mild*: Penetration into the whole epidermis [70% glycolic acid (GA), Jessner's solution (JS), 20–30% TCA].

Although these peelings do not penetrate deeper than the epidermis, the induction of a discrete neocollagenesis has been histologically demonstrated within superficial dermis.[8] Their efficiency, particularly with AHAs, depends on repeat performance (4 or 5 consecutive peelings at about 1 month interval).

Peeling with α Hydroxy Acids

α Hydroxy acids are the most commonly used agents for superficial peeling. They are organic acids of natural origin, such as GA, lactic acid, malic acid, and pyruvic acid, generally used at 40–70% concentrations.[9]

They are indicated for very moderate facial photoaging (Glogau type I or II), very superficial acne scars skin seborrhea and decrease in enlarged pores. They are also useful for "brightening up", particularly the dull skin of smokers, post-lesion dyschromia, pilaris keratosis of face or extremities, and melasma. This series of peelings is effective on shallow and small wrinkles and dyschromia. It can replace the greyish and yellowish complexion induced by UV exposure or smoking, by a pinker complexion. Actinic keratosis can also be clearly attenuated by these peels alone or combined with 5-fluorouracil.

The complications are rare: epidermolysis, due to an excessive penetration of exfoliating factors, often linked to patients' untimely prior treatment; acneiform perioral dermatitis; painful erosion that evokes herpes; hyperpigmentation on dark phototype and/or on areas traumatized by friction.

Peeling with β Hydroxy Acids

Studies show that BHA peelings control oil and acne, as well as remove dead skin cells to a certain extent, better than AHAs.

Salicylic acid is applied particularly to dark phototypes, as 20–30% solutions or more rarely, ointment containing 50% SA. It can reach deeper layers than AHA, penetrate well the sebaceous follicles and can be very interesting for acne prone oily skins.

Lipohydroxy acid C8-LHA, where a C8 fatty chain has been grafted on SA, is thereby endowed with great affinity for inter-corneocytes lipids, making the detachment of cells more efficient and smooth. This chemical agent has been demonstrated to be an excellent exfoliant and useful for the treatment of photoaged skin and acne.[10] C8-LHA shows a better efficacy for skin peeling at a lower concentration than SA and GA.[11,12]

Jessner solution is a combination of resorcinol 14%, lactic acid 14%, SA 14%. The advantages of this formulation are that there is a synergetic effect caused by three keratolytic agents, as well as the additional benefit of a phenolic skin-lightening agent (resorcinol) as one of the components.[13] This peel is more powerful than AHA peels and is thought to break intracellular bridges between corneocytes, leading to an increased exfoliation.

A variety of other combinations with peeling agents has been used for skin benefits. For example, combinations of vitamin C or kojic acid with AHA are used for the treatment of melasma and other pigmentation problems; combinations of kojic acid/hydroquinone with AHA are used for solar lentigos, melasma and hyperpigmented spots. Combinations of AHA with azelaic acid have been used for the treatment of acne. The benefit of a combination peel product is based upon synergetic effect brought about by the unique blend of the agents.

Medium Peeling

Medium-depth peels may be used in the treatment of dyschromias, such as solar lentigines, multiple keratoses, superficial scars, pigmentary disorders, and textural changes. The healing process is longer, with full epithelialization occurring in about 1 week.[7] The penetration level includes the epidermis and the upper limit of superficial dermis, where the peeling produces a neo-collagen which is able to mitigate wrinkles, shallow scars and improve skin texture. On the skin surface, the complexion will be pinker and of a more uniform color, with the disappearance of solar lentigos and the erasure or mitigation of keratosis.

Thirty to fifty percent TCA is used as an intermediate to deep peeling agents. Depth of penetration is increased as concentration increased. Concentration over 35% is now less used because of poor tolerance and risk of scarring.

Another agent used for intermediate peeling is resorcinol, which penetrates as deep as the stratum granulosum. The turn-over of basal cells is increased, leading to a thickened epidermis. The fibroblasts of the papillary dermis are stimulated and they produce new collagen and glycosaminoglycans (GAGs).

Before peeling, all authors insist on the advantage of preparing the skin with topical retinoic acid or AHA for several weeks and of applying a cream with high sun protection level (SPF > 15).

For this type of rather painful peeling, a pre-medication with an oral sedative drug is proposed, and cooling the skin with electric fan during the whole procedure is recommended. In case of keratosis, these are beforehand surgically removed in order to facilitate the penetration of TCA.

With this combined peelings, just like with 35–50% TCA alone, desquamation is intense, brownish and in large clusters, necessitating a social eviction for over 1 day.

Sun protection after a medium-depth peel is recommended for several weeks. Because of the risk of prolonged hyperpigmentation, medium-depth peels should be conducted with caution in patients with dark skin.[14]

Deep Peeling

Deep peel may be used for severe photoaging, deep or coarse wrinkles, scars, and sometimes precancerous skin lesions.[15] It penetrates the skin as deep as the superficial part and sometimes even the medium part of reticular dermis. Penetrating the reticular dermis, the deep peel maximizes the regeneration of new collagen. Epithelialization occurs in 5–10 days, but deep peel requires significant healing time, usually 2 months or more, and sun protection must imperatively be used.

High concentration of TCA (over 50%) should be avoided. Phenol alone or combined with croton oil is one of the strongest chemical peeling solutions and produces a deep skin peel. Several formulas are available the most classic being that of Baker-Gordon [88% phenol: 3 mL, Septisol (liquid soap): 8 drops, croton oil: 3 drops]. More than phenol concentration, it is the presence of croton oil that assures deep penetration of the exfoliating solution. Peelings with phenol are forbidden in patients having a cardiopathy, a nephropathy or some severe diabetes.[16]

Other complications include hypopigmentation, hyperpigmentation, scarring, and keloid formation. Due to the increased risk of prolonged or permanent pigmentary changes, deep peels are not recommended for most dark-skinned individuals. The complications depend upon the depth of peeling and sometimes on the lack of experience of the operator.

Indications of Chemical Peels for Darker Skins

Chemical peels in darker skin population are mostly used for mottled dyschromia, acne, post-inflammatory hyperpigmentation (PIH) and melasma.[17] Even if a wide variety of agents are available for chemical peels, the choice becomes relatively limited when treating a patient with a Fitzpatrick skin type IV or above, since the risk of prolonged hyperpigmentation increases in dark-skinned patients.[1,14,17] Although various depths of peeling have been described, superficial and medium depth peels are safer for dark skinned patients. Deep chemical peelings should be avoided because of the risk of permanent pigmentary changes.[18] Even medium-depth peelings need to be used with extreme caution.[19]

Pigmentary Disorders (Figs 1 and 2)

Chemical peeling is a well-known modality of treatment for melasma. The basic mechanism of the action of chemical peeling in melasma is the removal of unwanted melanin by causing a controlled chemical burn to the skin.[20] Peeling has proved being a useful treatment for melasma on dark skin, as a sole treatment or an adjunct to other topical therapies. In a pilot study by Grimes et al.[21] on dark-skinned individuals, 20–30% SA peel was used to treat acne, PIH and melasma. It was observed that almost two-thirds of the patients with melasma showed a moderate improvement and all patients with PIH had a moderate to significant improvement. Only mild side effects were noted in 16% patients, which were transient and resolved within 1–2 weeks. Tretinoin peels also showed some good results on darker skin. Khunger et al. compared 1% tretinoin peel with a standard 70% GA peel.[22] Ten female patients with melasma were taken up for an open left-right comparison study of 12 weeks. One percent tretinoin peel was applied to one-half of the face, whereas 70% GA was applied to the other side at weekly intervals. The fall in melasma area severity index (MASI) at 6 weeks and 12 weeks with tretinoin peel was similar to that achieved with the standard glycolic solution, with only minimal side effects. Another study conducted by Safoury et al.[23] compared the therapeutic effect of combined 15% TCA and modified JS with 15% TCA on 20 Indian female patients (phototypes III and IV) with melasma. The result

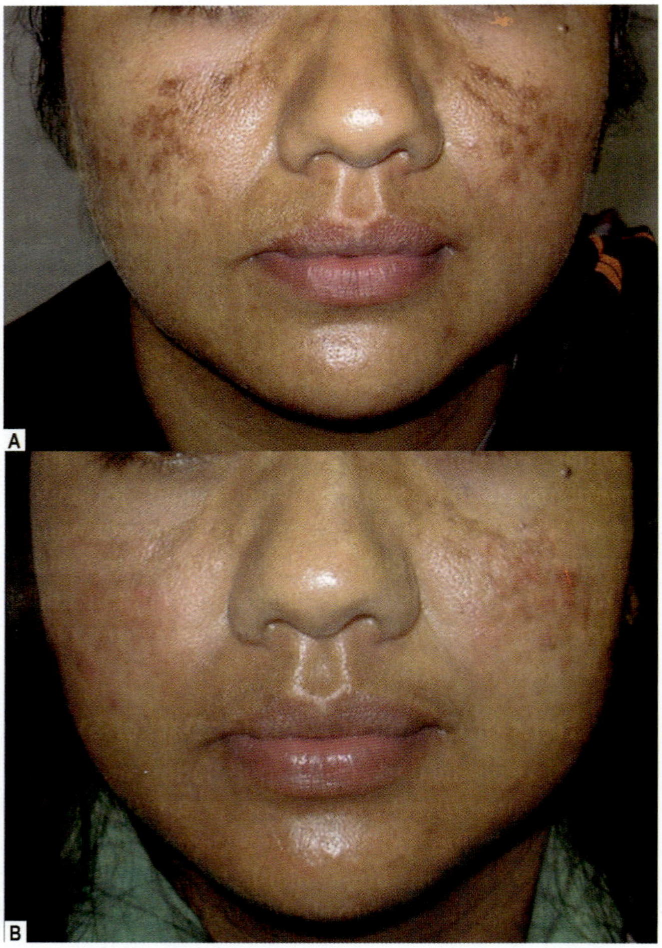

Figure 1: A, Melasma not responding to topical therapy with skin-lightening agents. **B,** After 10 sessions of sequential peels, salicylic acid 20% followed by 15% trichloroacetic acid
Courtesy: Dr Niti Khunger

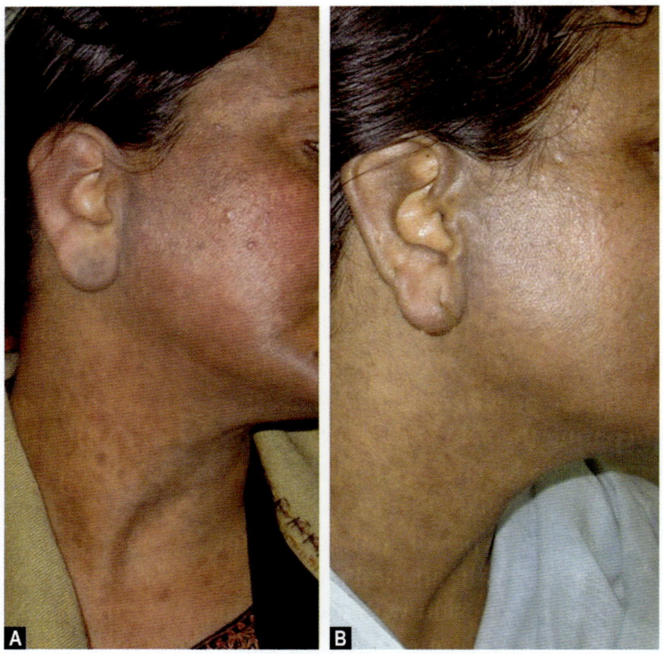

Figure 2: A, Dermal pigmentation following Riehl's melanosis. **B,** Improvement following 20 sessions of sequential peel, 20% salicylic acid followed by combination peel containing glycolic acid, kojic acid and hydroquinone
Courtesy: Dr Niti Khunger

was better on the side of the combination peel. Superficial GA peels showed to be a good adjunct to topical therapy in melasma in Indian patients; they provide an additional effect to a topical regimen.[24]

Acne (Fig. 3)

Clinicians and patients often use chemical peels as an adjunct to medical therapy in acne because they produce complementary rapid therapeutic effects and improvements in skin appearance and texture.[25,26] The most commonly used chemical peels in treating acne and acne scars include SA, GA, JS, resorcinol, and TCA. With good technique, peels may also be beneficial for dark-skinned patients who have pigmentary changes due to acne.[26] SA can be used to treat comedones and inflammatory lesions.[27] SA has shown good effects in dark-skinned Asian, African-American, and Hispanic patients with acne.[21,28] In addition, this treatment regimen facilitated resolution of PIH as well as a decrease in the overall pigmentation of the face.[21]

Mandelic acid (German mandel–almond) is an AHA, which can be derived from amygdalin, a glycoside found in bitter almonds, peaches and apricots. It is an excellent peel for acne and post acne pigmentation as it has dual properties of being comedolytic as well as antibacterial. It also has skin-lightening effects. Since mandelic acid has a larger molecular size as compared to GA, penetration is slower and hence less irritant and thus it is safer in darker skins. For chemical peeling, 30%, 40% and 50% mandelic acid is used. It can be combined with SA to give additional benefit. The lack of irritation, burning and erythema are advantages over GA, making it an excellent lunchtime peel and also safer for darker skins and sensitive skins.

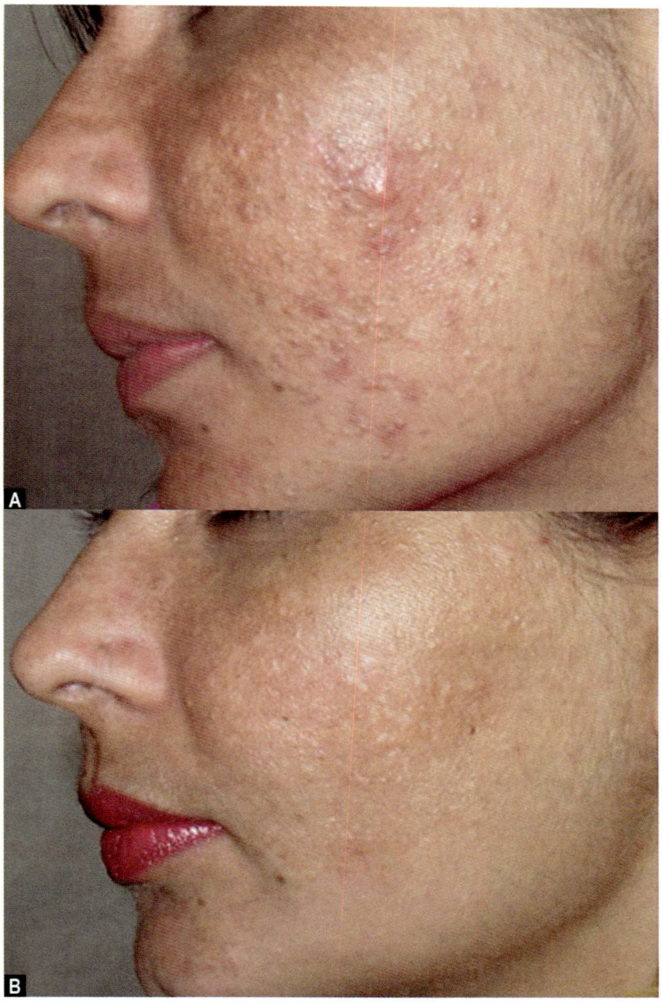

Figure 3: **A,** Acne with melasma. **B,** Improvement after 6 sessions of combined salicylic-mandelic acid peel
Courtesy: Dr Niti Khunger

Pre- and Post-peel Regimens

The biggest drawback with the use of chemical peels in dark skin is PIH which can either occur between the treatment sessions or after stopping treatment. Priming or preparing the skin prior to the peel is a useful adjunctive measure which also enhances the effect of the peeling agent apart from decreasing PIH. It involves the application of a topical depigmenting agent like hydroquinone, tretinoin or GA 2 weeks prior to the planned day of peel. Priming ensures uniform penetration of the peeling agent, enhances healing and maintains the effects achieved with the chemical peel.[29] In a study by Garg et al.[30] Indian patients with melasma were randomly allocated into three groups, receiving GA peel without priming, or following priming with 0.025% tretinoin or 2% hydroquinone, respectively. The fall in MASI was highest in the group receiving 2% hydroquinone as a priming agent with minimum relapse and PIH. In another study by Nanda et al.[31] better improvement was seen with 2% hydroquinone as a priming agent as compared to 0.025% tretinoin when used as an adjunct with 10–30% TCA peels.

Patients should be aware of the risk of skin dryness, irritation and erythema. Photoprotection may reduce the risk of PIH. Patient education is essential to reduce the risk of complications. Post-peel instructions include an efficient photoprotection and bland emollients.[32]

Evaluation of the Efficacy and Tolerance of Chemical Peels

In Vitro Methods to Study Efficacy of Peels

Monolayer cultures of keratinocytes and fibroblasts, as well as 3D reconstructed skin models can be used to evaluate "targets" for peel treatment using genomic as well as proteomic analysis of cell/tissue extracts. At the genomic level, valuable information can be obtained via cDNA microarray analysis. This method allows novel genes and proteins to be identified in keratinocytes or fibroblasts after exposure to potential peeling agents. This type of model can provide insight into the mode of action of a peeling agent. In addition to the *in vitro* monolayer culture models, 3D tissue models are available to test peel compounds. As an example of reconstructed epidermis model, EpiSkin™ has been used to evaluate the tolerance and efficacy of cosmetic products.[33] This *in vitro* model was developed and validated as a reproducible and predictive alternative method to animal testing for the safety of cosmetic ingredients. Using this model, it was possible to develop a cytotoxicity profile for cosmetic ingredients by evaluating the cell viability and the release of inflammatory mediators into the culture medium.[34,35] The tolerance of peeling agents can be assessed by topical application onto the EpiSkin model. In addition, efficacy of the peeling agents can be evaluated using an ex vivo desquamation test (release of squames from the Episkin model after topical application of peel agents), and by quantifying the corneodesmosine (a component of the corneodesmosomes) in the released squames. The efficacy of peel agents, especially LHA and GA, has been tested *in vitro* using this model. It then became possible to classify different peel agents based upon their efficacy and tolerance. In addition, this 3D model can be used to evaluate the interaction of peeling agent with the lipids and proteins of the stratum corneum and its depth of penetration into the different skin layers.

Clinical Testing Methods in Defining Peel Tolerance and Efficacy

Numerous clinical studies have been reported in the literature for the use of chemical peels in the treatment of various skin conditions (as discussed in the applications section above). In addition, histological and biochemical studies have been carried out both in humans and animal models to understand the mechanistic details of chemical peel action. In spite of all these studies, large gaps still exist in our knowledge on the mode of action of peels on human skin. Controlled studies, comparing the tolerance and efficacy of different peel regimens, are sparse. Relationship between the controlled aggression of the skin by different peeling agents and skin re-epithelialization and subsequent clinical improvement are not well documented.

A general outline for designing a peel clinical study is shown in Table 1. This general outline can be used for comparison of efficacy and tolerance of different peels. It is important to evaluate the tolerance of the treatment using a patch test at different times of the treatment period. The patch area has to be examined for dryness, erythema, edema and peeling level. In addition, subjective evaluation for skin reactions such as stinging, tingling, itching, and burning also has to be noted. The peel application can be continued for up to 14 weeks on a biweekly basis, depending on the strength of peeling agent and the pH of the final composition. Facial grading and instrumental evaluations can be done before the peeling agent is applied and at each time point following application. A self-assessment questionnaire is also important to document the subject's reactions at each treatment time.

FILLERS

Recent Developments and Basis for Dermal Fillers

Over the last 20 years, dermal fillers technology has expanded from autologous tissues and animal-derived collagens to bacterially-fermented biopolymers and synthetic implants. Beyond their physical composition, their recommended depth of injection, suitability for different facial areas, and duration of aesthetic improvement can further differentiate currently available products. While older dermal fillers rely upon the integrity of the injected material to achieve their clinical effects, some newer products are postulated to act by stimulating the patient's own biological and cellular processes.[36]

Table 1: General outline for a peel clinical study

Procedures	*Pre-treatment*	*Patch Test*	*Peel Application Week 4*		*Peel Applications * Weeks 6, 8, 10, 12, and 14*		*Follow-up 1–2 Weeks*
	2 Weeks	30–60 min after, 24 hours after, 1 week after	Before peel	30–60 min after peel	Before peel	30–60 min after peel	
Paperwork (informed consent, medical form, etc.)	X						
Product distribution/ collection	D		D				C
Peel application			X		X		
Facial grading • Fine lines and wrinkles • Radiance • Skin roughness • Skin tone • Hyperpigmentation			X		X		X
Tolerance evaluations: (objective irritation) dryness, erythema, edema and peeling		X	X	X	X	X	X
Tolerance evaluations: (subjective irritation) stinging, tingling, itching , burning		X		X		X	
Instrumental measurements • Firming • Hydration • Replicas • VISIA • Chromameter			X				X
Self-assessment questionnaire			X	X		X	X

The difference in facial appearance between the young and the elderly primarily lies in the following indices; smoothness in facial profile curvature, symmetry of tissue structures, adequacy in skin tension, fineness of skin texture, and pigmentation. Changes in facial profile curvature and symmetry are closely related to change in facial volume, and changes in facial volume are related to osteolysis, abnormal distribution of fat, and abnormalities in dermal collagen and elastic fibers due to aging.[37]

Today, dermal fillers constitute one of the most commonly performed cosmetic procedures for the rejuvenation of the aging face, with botulinum toxicum type A injections topping the list. Some of the injectable fillers most commonly used are hyaluronic acid (HA) derivatives, human-derived collagen, other biopolymers such as polylactic acid, or silicones. Also, autologous fat is used as an injectable filler for facial volume augmentation. Fillers can be used individually or in combination. The aging face can be divided into upper, middle, and lower third and correction treatments are usually designed considering the three different facial sections. For example, in the upper facial section, fronto transverse wrinkles, glabellar frownlines, and wrinkles around eyes are the focus for correction. In the middle section, lipid distribution around the cheeks and orbits is the key point. For the lower section of the face, nasolabial folds, labial lines and the plumpness of the lips are important for adjustment.[38]

Using this framework, treatment strategies for addressing each facial region are different. Generally, specific approaches and techniques for each anatomic region have to be separately evaluated, with particular emphasis and focus on the end benefit.[39]

Esthetic Augmentation

Tissue augmentation can be classified according to the material used; fat, collagen, HA, or silicone (Table 2).[40] Based on the biodegradability of the material, whether easy or difficult, fast or slow, it can be classified into: non-permanent (collagen, HA) or permanent [silicone, silica gel, poly(methyl methacrylate) (PMMA), and hydroxyapatite]. In addition, heterogeneous transplants (bovine collagen and HA from cockscomb), allogenic transplants, and autologous transplants (autologous fat or collagen) are used.

Collagen

Collagen is the major structural component of the dermis and is responsible for providing strength and support to human skin.

- *Animal-derived collagen:*[41] Bovine collagen was the first collagen product approved for human use. In 1981, Zyderm I was the first to be approved by FDA for marketing. Later, Zyderm II and Zyplast were also approved by FDA. Zyderm I is more suitable for finer wrinkles and the level of injection is at the layer of dermal papilla. Zyderm II is for medium wrinkles where the level of injection is at the layer of dermal mesoderm. Zyplast is specifically designed for deep wrinkles and the level of injection is at the dermal sub-corium. Regardless of collagen type, patient must undergo the skin test twice with a 2-week interval. According to statistics, 1–2% of patients, after multiple treatments with collagen, can still develop allergic reaction. For patient who had injection of collagen over 1 year, skin test would be required and injection can only be performed after 2 weeks of observation. Augmentation with bovine collagen requires over-injection of approximately 150% of the original amount.[42] The effect of bovine augmentation usually does not exceed 6 months. At sites with frequent motion, such as the lips, the effect can hardly last more than 3 months.
- *Bioengineered human-derived collagen:* This category of product comes from single fibroblasts in culture and is the fruit of tissue engineering. In 2003, FDA approved two products of this type: CosmoDerm I and CosmoPlast. These two products do not require skin test. The former is applied to finer wrinkles at the layer of dermal papilla and the latter is designed like Zyplast for deeper wrinkles at dermal sub-corium.
- *Autologous collagen:* Isolagen company provides a unique service, where a 3 mm^2 piece of skin is obtained from patient for tissue culturing. The fibroblasts in the sample, after stimulation, proliferate to millions in quantity and can be woven into collagen. The process takes several weeks. Products from single experiment can fill in a space of 1–1.5 cm^3. The technology is already patented in the USA and should be marketed soon. The advantage is absence of allergic reaction and no risk of infection from donor. Also, fibroblasts are unlimited to produce collagens. The effect of collagen injection usually can last 6 months.
- *Other collagen dermal fillers:* Dermicol-P35 is a novel cross-linked, fibrillar type I collagen isolated from porcine tendons that has not been associated with the same degree of immunogenicity as bovine collagen. Dermicol-P35 was shown in one study on 12 subjects to be associated with high tolerance, as well as a high degree of satisfaction.[43]

Dermicol-P35 27G and 30G are purified advanced collagen dermal fillers that are effective and well tolerated for cosmetic procedures. The majority of patients (63.4%) felt very comfortable or comfortable returning to their daily routine immediately post-procedure: 86.7% of patients participated in normal work or social events within 2 days post treatment. Adverse events were mild to moderate and were resolved or tolerable by day 7. The clinician assessed that most patients had between 50% and 100% improvement over baseline for all procedures at all-time points.[44]

Hyaluronic Acid

Hyaluronic acid is a naturally occurring linear polysaccharide of very high molecular weight (up to

Table 2: Facial fillers[40]

Filler	*Function*	*Uses*	*Pros*	*Cons*	*Comments*
Collagen-based products (Cosmoderm and Cosmoplast)	Human derived, bioengineered collagen injected to fill facial wrinkles	Anywhere; effective contouring agent (lips, line etched lines)	Immediate results with no downtime; formulated with lidocaine for patient comfort	Limited Longevity (lasts 3 months)	An FDA-approved collagen dermal filler that does require a skin test
Hyaluronic acid (Restylane, Perlane, Juvederm, Captique)	Non-animal-derived hyaluronic acid engineered to resist degradation for wrinkle filler and volume replacement	Volume and contouring (periorbital, nasolabial, lips, cheeks, etc.)	Results are immediate and last 6–18 months, reversible	May be visible or palpated if injected superficially; less effective for treating lipoatrophy or very large volume correction	Stimulates de novo collagen formation; FDA-approved for filling moderate to severe wrinkles around the nose and mouth; all other uses considered off-label; no risk of animal-based disease transmission
Calcium hydroxylapatite (Radiesse)	Microspheres of calcium hydroxylapatite inducing production of collagen	Volume enhancer (nasolabial and cheeks)	Biocompatible and ultimately biodegradable; long lasting (12 months and may be beyond); moldable	Clumping lumping and nodules can appear when injected into the lips	Do not use Radiesse in the lips; FDA approved for facial lipoatrophy and moderate to severe wrinkles around the mouth
Poly-L-Lactic acid (Sculptra and New-Fill)	Synthetic material is injected into the face; causing body to produce its own collagen	Volume enhancer (nasolabial and cheeks, and temples)	Long-lasting (18–24 Months)	Results not immediate, may require multiple treatments; skin nodules and granulomatous reactions possible	In a clinical study of Sculptra, the treatment results lasted for up to 2 years after the first treatment session; FDA approved for facial lipoatrophy
Fat Transfer	Fat cells are harvested from one part of the body and injected into the face to replenish volume	Volume augmentation (Cheeks, periorbital, and temple); not used for finer contouring	Most natural filler, fat can be stored for touch-ups	For volume replacement, less effective at finer contouring duration is unpredictable 6 months to 10 years	"Predictably unpredictable"
Silicone (Silicon 1000 and Adaptosil 5000)	Highly refined silicone oil is injected using microdroplet technique	Volume replacement and contouring	Permanent	Cannot be removed after being injected	Beware of black market non-medical silicone; off label cosmetic use
Poly(methyl methacrylate) (PMMA); Artecoll and Artefill	PMMA microspheres surrounded by collagen	FDA approved for nasolabial folds, deep wrinkles	Permanent	Numerous injections needed for volume; allergic reactions possible; requires 3 months for full effects; sometimes visible under skin	Because of the bovine collagen component, allergy skin testing is required; PMMA does not break down

Abbreviation: FDA, US Food and Drug Administration.
Adaptosil 5000 is manufactured by Bausch Lomb (Rochester, NY). Artecoll is manufactured by Artes (San Diego, CA). Captique, Cosmoderm, Cosmoplast, Hylaform, and Juvederm are manufactured by Allegan, Inc (Invine, CA). New-Fill is manufactured by Ashford Aesthetics (Brussels, Belgium). Perlane is manufactured by QMed (Eatontown, NJ). Radiesse is manufactured by Bioform Medical (San Mateo, CA). Restylane is manufactured by Medicis (Scottsdale, AZ). Sculptra is manufacutured by Sanofi-Aventis (Bridgewater, NJ). Silikon 1000 is manufactured by Alcon (Fort Worth, TX). Zyplast is manufactured by Inamed Aesthetics (Santa Barbara, CA).

2,000 kDa), found in all living organisms and identical in all species and tissue types.

Hyaluronic acid, when depleted with age, is being restored due to the material that is injected. These fillers imbibe water over time and give volume, hence the patient is advised to drink lots of water after filler injection. They prevent further degradation of the preexisting HA and also induce HA formation over time. The half-life of natural HA is 1–2 days, and thus, current HA for augmentation is the coupling fragmented product after chemical process (MW 250/400 kDa). Although insoluble in water, HA can attract large amounts of water molecules to form hydrogel. Therefore, HA gel, in theory, has the advantage of isovolumetric degradation as its ability to attract water molecules will maintain its original volume even after it has been degraded, until all HA is lysed, causing the entire gel structure to collapse. This is one of the reasons why HA has a longer therapeutic effect than collagen.

Hyaluronic acid products are a mainstay of dermal filler tissue augmentation. They vary in their concentration, gel particle size and hence indications. Different HA products available are shown in Table 3.[45,46]

Understanding the distinct physical characteristics of different HA dermal fillers and how these characteristics may predict their clinical behavior help clinicians in achieving the desired results in patients seeking facial rejuvenation.[47]

Table 3: Hyaluronic acid products[44]

Products	*Description*
Hylaform (Hylan B gel)	5.5 mg/mL extracted
Hylaform Plus (Hylan B gel)	from rooster combs
Restylane®	5.5 mg/mL HA from
Perlane	rooster combs
Restylane® Sub q	20 mg/mL NASHA
Juvederm® ultra	20 mg/mL NASHA
Juvederm® ultra Plus	20 mg/mL NASHA
Juvederm® Voluma	24 mg/mL NASHA
IAL system	24 mg/mL NASHA
	20 mg/mL NASHA
	18 mg/mL

Abbreviation: NASHA: non-animal stabilized hyaluronic acid.

Mechanism of Action of HA Dermal Fillers: A study was conducted to determine whether endogenous synthesis of new extracellular matrix might contribute to the degree and duration of clinical benefits derived from cross-linked HA dermal filler injections.[48] Immunostaining of skin receiving cross-linked HA injections revealed increased collagen deposition around the filler, as compared to control saline injection sites. Immunostaining of type I procollagen was enhanced at 4 weeks and 13 weeks after treatment as did gene expression for types I and III procollagen and several pro-fibrotic growth factors were also up-regulated at 4 weeks and 13 weeks as compared to controls. Fibroblasts in filler-injected skin demonstrated a mechanically stretched appearance and a biosynthetic phenotype. In vitro, fibroblasts did not bind the filler, suggesting that cross-linked HA is not directly stimulatory. In conclusion, injection of cross-linked HA stimulates collagen synthesis, partially restoring dermal matrix components that are lost in photodamaged skin. These findings imply that cross-linked HA may be useful for stimulating collagen production therapeutically, particularly in the setting of atrophic skin conditions.

In another study, injection of dermal filler, cross-linked HA, into the skin of individuals over 70 years old stimulated fibroblasts to produce type I collagen.[49] This stimulation was associated with localized increase in mechanical forces, indicated by fibroblast elongation/spreading, and mediated by upregulation of type II TGF-β receptor and connective tissue growth factor. Interestingly, enhanced mechanical support of the ECM also stimulated fibroblast proliferation, expanded vasculature, and increased epidermal thickness.

Autologous Fat Transplantation

Fat has the potential to be the ideal soft-tissue filler because it is abundant, easily accessible, inexpensive, host compatible and can be harvested repeatedly. It also offers a similar long-term durability with a low-cost compared to dermal fillers.[50] Autologous fat transplantation has a long history. Although there are now various other natural or synthetic materials available for tissue augmentation, fat transplantation still has undeniable advantage in shaping facial profile. Especially, when auto-transplantation with purified fat granules has become available the postoperative survival rate of fat has been greatly improved. Autologous fat grafting is still a prevailing method of aesthetic augmentation.

It has a wide range of clinical indications, such as depressed scar, facial depression, acne or varicellar scars, roughness in skin after liposuction, augmentation and plastic operation for buttock, facial wrinkles, augmentation for nasolabial folds, hemi-facial atrophy, deformity of small breast, and thickened penis.[51] Overall, auto-transplantation of fat, in comparison to collagen and HA, is more suitable for "crude" adjustment to facial profile.

The most common adverse reaction is continuous edema and ecchymosis for between few days and 2 weeks. Also, there may be sterile lipocyst, pigmentation, and fat necrosis. Infections following augmentation have been reported.[52] The survival rate of fat after transplantation varies according to body area, but it is generally believed that the survival rate is lower around lips and mouth.

To achieve the best result, at least four sessions of fat auto-transplantation are required with an interval of 1–3 months. Following each injection, some fat is partially absorbed, and the rate can reach as much as 1/3 of the transplanted.

Autotransplantation of fat involves two steps: liposuction and injection. It is worthy to note that fat for auto-transplantation is extracted using specific instrument because the fat granules are damaged under the negative pressure, mixed with swollen liquid or even blood, making these factors not beneficial to transplantation of adipocytes to survive and maintain the profile. Donor site for fat transplantation is generally the buttock or lateral femoral region. Either using special equipment or general injector for liposuction, sharp needle head must be replaced by a dull suction tube. Under general conditions, 50–100 mL of fat are sucked out.

Autologous dermal fillers: Use of autologous dermis as a filler substance for both esthetic and reconstructive procedures has been demonstrated to be a viable option. It could be advised for patients requiring filler correction who undergo concomitant procedures involving excision of potential donor dermis.[53]

Facial lipoatrophy is a common side effect of HIV treatment with highly active antiretroviral therapy. Dermal fillers and autologous fat transfer are effective treatment modalities for human immunodeficiency virus-associated facial lipoatrophy, with high rates of facial volume restoration and patient satisfaction. Autologous fat transfer may offer similar to superior long-term durability but with less of a financial burden compared with injectable fillers.[54]

Sharp-needle intradermal fat (SNIF) grafting technique can be used to achieve results lasting more than 1 year, which exceeds the expected duration for resorbable dermal fillers (typically 3–6 months). No major complications occurred, the most common minor complications being bruising and swelling. SNIF is a safe and effective alternative to classic resorbable dermal fillers for patients who can accept the minor discomfort involved in extracting fat from the donor site.[55]

Other Types of Dermal Fillers

Poly-L-Lactic acid: Injectable poly-L-lactic acid (PLA) is a synthetic, biodegradable polymer approved in the United States for use in immunocompetent patients as a single regimen of up to four treatment sessions for correction of shallow to deep nasolabial fold contour deficiencies and other facial wrinkles. Injectable PLA is also approved for restoration and/or correction of signs of facial lipoatrophy in individuals with HIV. Although the specific mechanisms remain hypothetical, injections of PLA are believed to cause a cascade of cellular events that lead to collagen repair and subsequent restoration of facial volume. Because the development of a response to injectable PLA is gradual and its duration of effect is long lasting, sufficient time between treatment sessions should be allocated to avoid overcorrection.[56]

Cross-linked carboxymethyl cellulose: Sodium carboxymethyl cellulose (CMC) has been chemically treated by the cross-linking process and thus used as a hydrogel for soft-tissue augmentation through injection with thin needles. Cross-linked CMC hydrogel proves to be useful for soft tissue augmentation with regard to safety and ease of application. It did not cause infection, extrusion, migration, or adverse reactions in the patients who have been followed for two years. Delayed aesthetic results on facial wrinkles were very satisfactory.[57]

Fillers and Dark-skinned Populations

The dark-skinned (skin types IV–VI) populations are increasingly concerned and the cosmetic industry is responding to the demand for dark skin targeted anti-aging treatments. Generally, there are two components of aging:

1. Extrinsic which is mostly caused by sunlight (photo-damage). In light skin individuals (individuals with Fitzpatrick skin types I–III), facial photo-aging effects are manifested as coarse and fine wrinkles, dyschromia, laxity, and an enormous amount of photo-damage, which can also cause swallowing, wrinkling, and laxity. But, due to the photoprotective effects of increased pigment in dark skin, the manifestations of photo-damage are often minimal or delayed as compared to their light skin counterparts.
2. Intrinsic or biologic aging, which affects all of us. Intrinsic aging involves loss of volume, laxity, and gravitational effects. The intrinsic process of losing volume and gravity effect cannot be stopped but is slower in dark skin as compared to light skin.[58,59]

There are many different soft-tissue fillers on the market, all of which having been safely used in darker-skinned patients. As with all procedures, there are risks of post-inflammatory pigmentary alteration even after minor injection related trauma. Dark skin aging face has a unique pattern that can be successfully augmented by dermal fillers. Though many subjects with dark skin are not typically included in the pre-market dermal filler clinical trials, some post-market studies have examined the safety and risks of adverse events in this population. Study results have demonstrated no keloidal scarring, but hyperpigmentation of the nasolabial folds and hypertrophic scars in a small number of patients.[60-64] Melanocytes in darker skin tend to be much more reactive and will respond to minimal traumatic influences. So, there is a greater incidence or risk for PIH or hypopigmentation. Developing a specific care plan and instituting close follow up is imperative when using dermal fillers in dark-skinned subjects.[65]

As indicated before, due to the photoprotective effects of increased pigmentation, the manifestations of aging in dark-skinned individuals are often delayed in comparison with their light skin counterparts. Unlike individuals of lighter skin tones, solar lentigines as well as fine and coarse wrinkles are not the major manifestations of aging. Rather, textural changes, uneven skin tone, loss of volume and the presence of laxity predominate. In overall, manifestations of aging result from the interplay of fat atrophy, soft-tissue redistribution due to gravity, bone remodeling and photo-damage.

Aging face can be divided into three areas: (1) upper, (2) mid, and (3) lower face. The upper area of the face of dark-skinned individuals displays brow ptosis, forehead rhytids and crow's feet (but often to a lesser extent than in light skin individuals), accentuated tear trough deformity, infraorbital hollowing and temporal depression. There may also be concerns about upper eyelid fullness and redundant skin as well as lower eyelid bags.

In dark-skinned individuals, treating surface lines and creases is less of a concern. However, volumizing with an array of dermal fillers can successfully address the loss of collagen, fat and bone in this population.

Based on the particular ethnic skin type, some soft-tissue fillers will achieve better results than others will. For example, volumizers are generally more effective in ethnic skin, caused by the presence of sagging skin. Histologically, there is less thinning of collagen bundles and elastic tissue in this skin type. As a result, fillers that stimulate collagen or elastin production or skin tightening are more effective in dark skin. In particular, soft tissue augmentation with HA filler injections showed good results on the treatment of nasolabial folds in Indian skin.[66-68]

REFERENCES

1. Sarkar R, Bansal S, Garg VK. Chemical peels for melasma in dark-skinned patients. J Cutan Aesthet Surg. 2012;5:247-53.
2. Clark E, Scerri L. Superficial and medium-depth chemical peels. Clin Dermatol. 2008;26:209-18.
3. Moy LS, Moy RL. Glycolic acid peels. Dermatol Surg. 1996;22:419.
4. Becker FF, Langford FP, Rubin MG, et al. A histological comparison of 50% and 70% glycolic acid peels using solutions with various pHs. Dermatol Surg. 1996;22:463-5.
5. Kupper TS. Immune and inflammatory processes in cutaneous tissues. Mechanisms and speculations. J Clin Invest. 1990;86:1783-9.
6. Coleman WP, Brody HJ. Advances in chemical peeling. Dermatol Clin. 1997;15:19-26.
7. Rendon MI, Berson DS, Cohen JL, et al. Evidence and considerations in the application of chemical peels in skin disorders and aesthetic resurfacing. Clin Aesthet Dermatol. 2010;3:32-43.
8. Yamamoto Y, Uede K, Yonei N, et al. Effects of alpha hydroxyacids on the human skin of Japanese subjects: the rationale for chemical peeling. J Dermatol. 2006;33:16-22.
9. Béchaux S. [Superficial peelings]. Ann Dermatol Venereol. 2009;136:S363-6.
10. Saint-Léger D, Lévêque JL, Verschoore M. The use of hydroxy acids on the skin: characteristics of C8-lipohydroxy acid. J Cosmet Dermatol. 2007;6:59-65.
11. Pierard G, Lévèque JL, Rougier A, et al. Dermo-epidermal stimulation elicited by a salicylic acid derivative: a comparison with salicylic acid and all trans-retinoic acid. Eur J Dermatol. 2002;12:XLIV-XLVI.

12. Oresajo C, Yatskayer M, Hansenne I. Clinical tolerance and efficacy of capryloyl salicylic acid peel compared to a glycolic acid peel in subjects with fine lines/wrinkles and hyperpigmented skin. J Cosmet Dermatol. 2008;7:259-62.
13. Monheit GD. The Jessner's trichloroacetic acid peel. An enhanced medium-depth chemical peel. Dermatol Clinics. 1995:13:277-83.
14. Salam A, Dadzie OE, Galadari H. Chemical peeling in ethnic skin: an update. Br J Dermatol. 2013;169:82-90.
15. Fischer TC, Perosino E, Poli F, et al. Chemical peels in aesthetic dermatology: an update 2009. J Eur Acad Dermatol Venereol. 2010;24:281-92.
16. Landau M. Chemical peels. Clin Dermatol. 2008;26(2):200-8.
17. Roberts WE. Chemical peeling in ethnic/dark skin. Dermatol Ther. 2004;17:196-205.
18. Khunger N. IADVL Task Force. Standard guidelines of care for chemical peels. Indian J Dermatol Venereol Leprol. 2008;74:S5-12.
19. Nikalji N, Godse K, Sakhiya J, et al. Complications of medium depth and deep chemical peels. J Cutan Aesthet Surg. 2012;5:254-60.
20. Sheth VM, Pandya AG. Melasma: a comprehensive update: part II. J Am Acad Dermatol. 2011;65:699-714.
21. Grimes PE. The safety and efficacy of salicylic acid chemical peels in darker racial-ethnic groups. Dermatol Surg. 1999;25:18-22.
22. Khunger N, Sarkar R, Jain RK. Tretinoin peels versus glycolic acid peels in the treatment of Melasma in dark-skinned patients. Dermatol Surg. 2004;30:756-60.
23. Safoury OS, Zaki NM, El Nabarawy EA, et al. A study comparing chemical peeling using modified Jessner's solution and 15% trichloroacetic acid versus 15% trichloroacetic acid in the treatment of melasma. Indian J Dermatol. 2009;54:41-5.
24. Sarkar R, Kaur C, Bhalla M, et al. The combination of glycolic acid peels with a topical regimen in the treatment of melasma in dark-skinned patients: a comparative study. Dermatol Surg. 2002 Sep;28(9):828-32; discussion 832.
25. Kim SW, Moon SE, Kim JA, et al. Glycolic acid versus Jessner's solution: which is better for facial acne patients? A randomized prospective clinical trial of split-face model therapy. Dermatol Surg. 1999;25:270-3.
26. Taub AF. Procedural treatments for acne vulgaris. Dermatol Surg. 2007;33:1005-26.
27. Briden ME. Alpha hydroxyacid chemical peeling agents: case studies and rationale for safe and effective use. Cutis. 2004;73:18-24.
28. Ahn HH, Kim IH. Whitening effect of salicylic acid peels in Asian patients. Dermatol Surg. 2006;32:372-5.
29. Rubin ME. Superficial and medium depth. Manual of chemical peels; Philadelphia: Lippincott; 1995. pp. 17-25.
30. Garg VK, Sarkar R, Agarwal R. Comparative Evaluation of Beneficiary Effects of Priming Agents (2% Hydroquinone and 0.025% Retinoic Acid) in the Treatment of Melasma with Glycolic Acid Peels. Dermatol Surg. 2008;34:1032-40.
31. Nanda S, Grover C, Reddy BS. Efficacy of hydroquinone (2%) versus tretinoin (0.025%) as adjunct topical agents for chemical peeling in patients of melasma. Dermatol Surg. 2004;30:385-8.
32. Salam A, Dadzie OE, Galadari H. Chemical peeling in ethnic skin: an update. Br J Dermatol. 2013;169:82-90.
33. Roguet R, Cohen C, Leclaire J, et al. Use of a standardized reconstructed epidermis kit to assess in vitro the tolerance and the efficacy of cosmetics. Int J Cosmet Sci. 2000;22:409-19.
34. Lelièvre D, Justine P, Christiaens F, et al. The EpiSkin phototoxicity assay (EPA): development of an in vitro tiered strategy using 17 reference chemicals to predict phototoxic potency. Toxicol in vitro. 2007;21:977-95.
35. Spielmann H, Hoffmann S, Liebsch M, et al. The ECVAM international validation study on in vitro tests for acute skin irritation: Report on the validity of the EPISKIN and EpiDerm assays and on the skin integrity function test. Selection of chemical. ATLA. 2007;35:559-619.
36. Goldberg DJ. Breakthroughs in US dermal fillers for facial soft-tissue augmentation. J Cosmet Laser Ther. 2009;11:240-7.
37. Li Hang. Series of Seminars for Dermatological Surgery (Tissue augmentation). Chin J Aesthetic Med. 2009;7:1024-6.
38. Billings E, May JW. History review and present status of free fat graft auto-transplantation in plastic and reconstructive surgery. Plast Reconstr Surg. 1989;83:368-81.
39. Wise JB, Greco T. Injectable treatments for the aging face. Facial Plast Surg. 2006;22:140-6.
40. Dayan SH, Bassichis BA. Facial dermal fillers: selection of appropriate products and techniques. Aesthet Surg J. 2008;28:335-47.
41. Sadick N, Khan MH, Rao BK. Skin fillers. In: Draelos Z (ed). Cosmetic Dermatology Products and Procedures, 1st edition. Oxford: Wiley-Blackwell; 2010. pp. 361-72.
42. He Li, Liu Wei. Augmentation with injection of collagen. Dermatological Aesthetic. Beijing: General People's Health Press. 2008;6:239-40.
43. Cassuto D. The use of Dermicol-P35 dermal filler for nonsurgical rhinoplasty. Aesthet Surg J. 2009;29:S22-4.
44. Bassetto F, Turra G, Salmaso R, et al. Autologous injectable dermis: a clinical and histological study. Plast Reconstr Surg. 2013;131(4): 589-96.
45. Vedamurthy M. Soft Tissue Augmentation: hyaluronic acid fillers. In: Textbook on cosmetic and aesthetic surgery. Venkataram M, (ed). New Delhi, India: Jaypee Brothers Medical Publishers; 2012. pp. 634-45.
46. Pallack SV. Some new injectable dermal filler materials: Hylaform, Restylane, and Artecoll. J Cut Med Surg. 1999;3:27-35.
47. Stocks D, Sundaram H, Michaels J, et al. Rheological evaluation of the physical properties of hyaluronic acid dermal fillers, J Drugs Dermatol. 2011;10:974-80.
48. Wang F, Garza LA, Kang S, et al. In vivo stimulation of de novo collagen production caused by cross-linked hyaluronic acid dermal filler injections in photodamaged human skin. Arch Dermatol. 2007;143:155-63.
49. Quan T, Wang F, Shao Y, et al. Enhancing structural support of the dermal microenvironment activates fibroblasts, endothelial cells, and keratinocytes in aged human skin in vivo. J Invest Dermatol. 2013;133:658-67.
50. Alexander RW. Liposculpture in the superficial plane: Closed syringe system for improvements in fat removal and free fat transfer. Am J Cosmet Surg. 1992;11:127-34.
51. Marwah M, Kulkarni A, Godse K, et al. Fat Fulfillment: A Review of Autologous Fat Grafting. J Cutan Aesthet Surg. 2013;6:132-8.
52. Obagi S. Autologous fat augmentation and periorbital laser resurfacing complicated by abscess formation. Am J Cosmet Surg. 2003;20:155-7.
53. Shuck J, Iorio ML, Hung R, et al. Autologous fat grafting and injectable dermal fillers for human immunodeficiency virus-associated facial lipodystrophy: a comparison of safety, efficacy, and long-term treatment outcomes. Plast Reconstr Surg. 2013;131:499-506.
54. Zeltzer AA, Tonnard PL, Verpaele AM. Sharp-needle intradermal fat grafting (SNIF). Aesthet Surg J 2012;32:554-61.
55. Bauer U, Gravier MH. Optimizing injectable poly-L-lactic acid administration for soft tissue augmentation: The rationale for three treatment sessions. Can J Plast Surg. 2011;19:22-7.
56. Leonardis M, Palange A, Dornelles RF, et al. Use of cross-linked

carboxymethyl cellulose for soft-tissue augmentation: preliminary clinical studies. Clinical Interv Aging. 2010;5:317-22.

57. Heath CR, Taylor SC. Fillers in the skin of color population. J Drugs Dermatol. 2011;10:494-8.
58. Talakoub L, Wesley NO. Differences in perceptions of beauty and cosmetic procedures performed in ethnic patients. Semin Cutan Med Surg. 2009;28:115-29.
59. Burgess C. Special Considerations in African American Skin. In: Alam M, Bhatia A, Kundu R,Chan H (eds). Cosmetic Dermatology for Skin of Color. New York: McGraw-Hill Professional; 2008. pp. 163-8.
60. Grimes PE, Thomas JA, Murphy DK. Safety and effectiveness of hyaluronic acid fillers in skin of color. J Cosmet Dermatol. 2009;8:162-8.
61. Taylor SC, Burgess CM, Callender VD. Safety of nonanimal stabilized hyaluronic acid dermal fillers in patients with skin of color: A randomized, evaluator-blinded comparative trial. Dermatol Surg. 2009;35:1653-60.
62. Marmur ES, Taylor SC, Grimes PE, et al. Six-month safety results of calcium hydroxylapatite for treatment of nasolabial folds in Fitzpatrick skin types IV to VI. I. Dermatol Surg. 2009;35:1641-5.
63. Narins RS, Baumann L, Brandt FS, et al. A randomized study of the efficacy and safety of injectable poly-L-lactic acid versus human-based collagen implant in the treatment of nasolabial fold wrinkles. J Am Acad Dermatol. 2010;62:448-62.
64. Narins RS, Brandt F, Leyden J, et al. A randomized, double-blind, multicenter comparison of the efficacy and tolerability of Restylane versus Zyplast for the correction of nasolabial folds. Dermatol Surg. 2003;29:588-95.
65. Vedamurthy M. IADVL Dermatosurgery Task Force. Standard guidelines for the use of dermal fillers. Indian J Dermatol Venereol Leprol. 2008;74:S23-7.
66. Sood V, Nanda S. Patient Satisfaction with Hyaluronic Acid Fillers for Improvement of the Nasolabial Folds in Type IV & V Skin. J Maxillofac Oral Surg. 2012;11:78-81.
67. Arsiwala SZ. Safety and persistence of non-animal stabilized hyaluronic acid fillers for nasolabial folds correction in 30 Indian patients. J Cutan Aesthet Surg. 2010;3:156-61.
68. Nanda S, Bansal S. Upper face rejuvenation using botulinum toxin and hyaluronic acid fillers. Indian J Dermatol Venereol Leprol. 2013;79:32-40.

Chapter 15

Natural Medicine with Proven Efficacy for Beauty of Skin and Hair

Mukta Sachdev, *Manipal Hospital, Bengaluru, India*
Amit Tewari, *L'Oréal Research and Innovation, Bengaluru, India*
Niti Khunger, *VM Medical College and Safdarjung Hospital, New Delhi, India*
Nita Roy, *L'Oréal Research and Innovation, Bengaluru, India*

INTRODUCTION

The word "Cosmetics" derives from the Greek "kosmein" which means "to adorn".[1] It refers to preparations that are used for enhancing the appearance of the skin or emphasizing features of the face. Ethnobotany, the study of the association between human cultures and the use of plants, bears testimony to the old age human fondness toward the use of botanicals for beautification purpose. As early as in 2000 BC, herbal products like wild oats were used for skin care in the middle and far-east countries like Egypt and Arabia. In India, the Ayurvedic system of medicine mentions numerous herbs that can be used to enhance beauty and treat skin diseases. Since the Aryan period, turmeric and *Chandan* or Indian sandalwood (*Santalum album*) have been used for beautification and *Mehndi* (henna) has been used for dyeing and conditioning hair in various Indian communities. In the early 19th century, Raja Serfoji of Tanjore studied and tested many of the ancient Indian herbal formulations and had them written by Tamil pundits. He recommended *Masoor* (brown-skinned lentils which are orange inside) and honey face pack to confer "the splendor of the petals of the white lotus flower" to the face.

Nowadays, there is an increasing inclination toward the use of botanical cosmetic ingredients inducing the general belief that these natural ingredients are devoid of any side effects. About 70 plant extracts find a place in present skin care products for their antioxidant, antiaging, fragrance, antibacterial, moisturizing and healing benefits. It is, therefore, essential for dermatologists to have a working knowledge upon botanicals to provide an optimal skin care.

NATURAL MEDICINE IN INDIA: THE AYURVEDIC SYSTEM

"Ayurveda" is the ancient Indian holistic medical system, based on achieving physical and mental harmony with nature, which has been practiced for more than 5,000 years. Ayurveda is the science of health, awareness and self-accomplishment.

Definition of Ayurveda

The word Ayurveda derives from two Sanskrit words, "Ayus" and "Veda", i.e. the knowledge of life. In the Vedic context, the definition of life encompasses broader aspects than chronological lifespan. *Ayus* is a combination of the body (*sarira*), senses (*indriya*), mind (*manas*) and soul (*atma*). Together, these four factors are responsible for sustaining the life, air or force (*prana*) in the body, and all must be present in order to produce *ayus*. If one of the above factors is absent, life/*ayus* cannot be reached. Everything on earth has a physical body and a soul, but whether it also has a mind and senses, determines whether it is alive.

"Veda" is a Sanskrit word which means "knowledge" or "science". Ayurvedic medicine has its roots in the Vedas, the oldest Hindu religious scriptures, comprising the four Vedas (the *Rigveda, Yajurveda, Samaveda* and *Atharvaveda*).

With the time course of Ayurveda, the way of life and its knowledge became the science of life, which roots in ancient Vedic literature and encompasses our entire life, body, mind and spirit.

In India, the history of health care dates back to 5,000 years BC, when health care needs and diseases were noted in ancient literatures like *Rigveda* and

Atharvaveda. Later, the texts like "Charak Samhita" and "Sushruta Samhita" documented (about 1,000 years BC) the use of plants, and polyherbal formulations were highlighted for health care.

With time, the principle of using natural resources for maintaining or improving health was developed through the experimentation and experiences of daily lifestyle of Indian people.

Fundamentals of Ayurveda

According to Ayurveda, life is considered as the union of body, sense, mind and soul. The five basic elements of life are earth, air, fire, water and ether (space). Interactions between these five elements give rise to all existing lives, creating the three *doshas* (forces), seven *dhatus* (tissues) and three *malas* (waste products).

Doshas

Ayurveda asserts that we are all born into an unchanging constitution known as *dosha*. The five universal elements combine in pairs to form three dynamic basic forces or interactions called *doshas*, namely *vata, pitta* and *kapha*, denoting respectively: kinetic energy, energy of transformation and cohesion energy. A person is characterized by his/her proportion of *doshas* present in the body. The *doshas* are constantly moving in dynamic balance, one with the others. An imbalance of one, two or all three *doshas* causes diseases that are indicated by an increase or decrease of one, two or all the three *doshas* (Table 1).

Vata: It means wind. *Vata* is a force made up of the two elements, ether and air, which controls motor and nervous function. The amount of ether affects the ability of air to gain momentum.

Disturbance in *vata* causes manifestations of gas and muscular or nervous energy, leading to pain. *Vata* is indeed related to movement of cells in the body and disturbance or vitiation of *vata* will influence conductivity of nerve impulses in the body. Increase in impulse results in deformity like tremors and on the other hand decrease (*shamana* of *vata*) will cause restricted movement of the particular part like muscles spasm of the body, e.g. frozen shoulder is due to "vata shamana".

Pitta: It is composed of fire and water, which control or modulate each other. It governs digestion, metabolism and production of energy. It is responsible for pigmentation, body temperature, hunger, thirst, sight, courage and mental activities.

Disruption of normal function causes imbalance of gastric juice (*pachak pitta*) and bile involved in digestion leading to inflammation. Inflammation is more enhanced in *pitta prakriti* due to "ushguna" (hot property) of *pitta dosha*.

Kapha: It represents earth and water, water being the main constituent. *Kapha* is responsible for passive energy and regulates the body's structural elements, cohesiveness, and biological strength. Like an emulsifying force, it promotes harmonious mixing, cements the elements in the body, provides lubricant to the joints and water to the skin. Regulating *vata* and *pitta*, it helps

Table 1: Doshas in summary

Vata	*Kapha*	*Pitta*
Skin type • People with *vata* skin have excessive movement by burning off all lubrication as well as constitutional deficiency of nourishing fluid (the *rasa*) • Skin has a tendency to be dry, rough and thin with visible veins • *Vata* individuals tan easily and their cold nature draws them toward sun	Skin type • Skin is easily aggravated and people with *kapha* skin cannot tolerate the sun exposures • Skin is thick, smooth and moist with few wrinkles. Complexion is usually clear, fair or pale • Skin is prone to inflammation, rashes and acne	Skin type • Skin appears thick, oily and smooth with a "pasty" look • Skin is soft and warm. *Pitta* subjects have a lot of body heat and often perspire excessively • Skin flushes easily and often presents many freckles and moles. Skin develops acne, rashes, bruises or get sunburnt easily • The cool nature of these individuals draws them to sun; the skin is prone to sunburn but will tan soon
Hair • Generally less hair on scalp • Dry, rough, smoky, thin and cracked hair, and less in number	Hair • Premature graying of hair • Baldness, pinkish or reddish, soft thin hair, and less in number	Hair • Sticky hair • Strong, thick, dark, long, dark blue, good growth, and good quality

keeping the body lubricated and maintains its solid nature, tissues, sexual activity and vigor.

Disruption causes its manifestation in liquid and mucus, leading to swelling with or without discharge.

Dhatus

The human body is a matrix of seven basic tissues (*dhatus*). *Dhatus* are the elements that build our body. *Dhatus* protect our body from external encounters. They are responsible for our immune mechanism. A waste of *dhatus* leads to body destruction and end of life.

Each *dhatu* "tissue" is related to a skin layer and governs a specific function as shown in Table 2.

Malas

Malas are the waste products of the *dhatus* produced during normal metabolic process. They primarily comprise urine, feces and sweat from digested foods and beverages. They also include products from skin, cerumen, nasal and mucous secretion, tears, saliva, sebum, etc. Hairs and nails are also considered as *malas*. Although being waste products, they all serve a role in maintaining health as long as they remain in normal amount (*pramana*), qualities (*gunas*) and function (*karma*). Balanced condition of *doshas*, *dhatus*, and *malas* is *arogya*, i.e. good health and being disease free.

Any imbalance or disturbance in these basic principles causes disease. In Ayurvedic medicine, the treatment of the disease aims at recovering the balance of the basic elements and functional principles of the body.

AYURVEDIC DERMATOLOGY AND NATURAL SKIN CARE TREATMENTS

Ayurvedic Dermatology

Ayurvedic dermatology is a mind-body combination medicine. Skin is a sensory organ, since ensuring the senses of touch, pain, temperature and pressure. According to Ayurveda, the skin has six layers, located not only superficially but extended to deeper levels of the body.

A skin disease is rooted deeply into various *dhatus* or tissues like fat, muscles, blood, etc. Most skin treatments are generally external applications through creams or oils. These never reach the deeper layers of the skin. As a result, the symptoms disappear temporarily and the disease is not eradicated.

Ayurveda always tries to eliminate the disease by treating it specifically according to its cause. Fixing the problem rapidly is difficult when the disease is deep-rooted. Ayurvedic skin treatments may take a few weeks to remove the symptoms, but the disease remains permanently treated.

Skin diseases comprise dermatitis (*Sarumap-pun*), abscess (*katti*), tumor (*hazhalai*), leprosy (*kuttum*) and cancer (*putru*).

Ayurvedic Perspectives on Skin

Skin care in Ayurveda brings beauty from the inside out. The balance of our inner health controls the vitality and luster of our skin. This includes the roles of plasma tissue, blood tissue, *pitta, dosha* and the strength of digestive

Table 2: The seven *dhatus* and their functional significance

Dhatu	*Skin Layer*	*Functional Significance*
Rasa (plasma, lymph and tissue fluids)	Stratum corneum	Makes skin smooth and soft
Rakta (blood)	Stratum lucidum	Maintains color of skin and lips
Mamsa (muscles)	Stratum granulosum	Skin provides protection
Meda (fat and fatty tissue)	Stratum spinosum	Lubricates body, maintains water balance and provides sebaceous secretion
Asthi (bone)	Stratum germinosum	Gives support and firmness
Majya (marrow)	Papillary dermis	Lubricates eyes and skin
Shukra (male and female sexual fluids)	Reticular dermis	Produces *ojas* (vigor, essential energy), provides immunity

Note: This approach, also being very sophisticated, could be a source of inspiration to specific products tract. The theory of Ayurveda describes how someone can easily take control of her/his skin health and keep it glowing and lustrous.

Rasa Dhatu (Plasma Tissue)

Plasma is the first tissue being nourished by ingested food. Plasma tissue is a sweet, transparent, sticky liquid that flows within blood. Along with other blood tissue components, i.e. lymphatic fluid nourishing all the mucus membranes of the body, the plasma tissue also makes skin. A healthy plasma tissue leads to a glowing and healthy skin—smooth, soft and beautiful skin—free from moles or pimples and also of a uniform color.

Pitta Dosha (Fire Principle)

This is the functional principle responsible for regulating all hormonal cycles in the body. It is also responsible for the body metabolism and its imbalance frequently brings heat, redness and inflammation; a too elevated pitta which, in turn, heats blood which, in turn, creates flushed skin, redness, pimples, inflammations as well as anger and irritability.

Digestive System

In Ayurveda, all diseases root in the digestive system and a perfect digestion keeps the basis of a complete body health, including skin.

Causes of Skin Diseases

In Ayurveda, a wrong diet and lifestyle cause diseases. The factors of different dermatoses range from dietary practices, daily activities, climatic conditions up to sexual activities. Following a diet or lifestyle that is opposed to season or the *prakriti* (nature) of a person, creates an imbalance in the *doshas*, thus contaminating the body tissues to induce a skin disease. Skin diseases are caused due to imbalance of all three *doshas*; the prime *dosha* involved being *pitta*.

Ayurvedic Skin Treatment

Treating skin diseases includes both external application and internal intake of different herbal and/or mineral preparations. The latter include healing plants, tinctures, pastes, pills, salves, emulsions, suppositories, plasters, oils, lotions and liniments. Mineral substances, such as gold, silver, copper, tin, lead, zinc, mercury, borax, sulfur, alum, iron sulfate and zinc carbonate are indicated in the treatment of skin diseases.

The first step in the holistic Ayurvedic approach to skin care is finding out the Ayurveda skin type of the subject.

Vata skin is in general dry, thin, cool to touch, easily gets dehydrated and is very vulnerable to dry windy weather. The imbalance in *vata* skin makes it prone to premature aging. A lack of sebum relates to less present and sluggish sebaceous glands. The small pores characteristic of this type of skin lose water quickly; thanks to a surface phenomenon rather than a biological one, water loss from bigger surface area will be faster than with a smaller surface area. This leads in turn to tiny superficial wrinkles. Signs of aging, therefore, appear much faster in *vata* constitutions than in other types of skin.

Pitta is mostly associated with fire, therefore, more prone to breakouts, increased photosensitivity and less tolerant to hot and fiery food. It looks reddish and is warm at touch. *Pitta* skin imbalance makes it sensitive, with blotchy red patches, medium to large pores present in the T-zone, and prone to blackheads and allergic reactions.

Kapha skin gathers all the qualities of water and earth. It can be greasy, "bouncy", thicker and more tolerant to sun rays. Its imbalances bring out the following characteristics: cool, fair, oily and thick skin, with large pores with proneness to cystic acne, and deep wrinkles.

Vata skin: Dry
Pitta skin: Sensitive
Kapha skin: Oily

Ayurvedic skin care theory states that seven different types of constitutions govern our skin and hair types: *Vata, Pitta, Kapha, Vata-Pitta, Vata-Kapha, Pitta-Kapha*, or *Vata-Pitta-Kapha*. Most people combine two of the above three principles.

Recommendations for Care of the Doshas

Herbal/Home Remedies

Triphala: "three fruits" is a well-known traditional herbal combination that works well in all types of skin. Its cleansing action leads to replenishing instead of draining and since nutritive, *triphala* is an excellent skin tonic. *Triphala* being convenient to *vata, pitta* and *kapha doshas*, it is of a useful help to all skin types.

- *Vata* skin contains little moisture and preventing it from drying is a major consideration. With regard to food, warm, unctuous diet, sour, salty and sweet tastes balance *vata*. Avoiding dried foods like crackers, drinking 6–8 glasses of warm water throughout the day and sweet juicy fruits as well are recommended. Going to bed early (before 10 PM) soothes *vata* and will positively impact your skin. Avoid cleansing products that dry the skin (like alcohol-based cleansers) and perform Ayurvedic oil massage to your whole body before shower
- The use of nurturing skin care products helps to sustain youth. These products include some essential oils or herbs in combination, which can nourish the skin and rehydrate it, otherwise susceptible to wrinkling and premature aging
- *Pitta* skin should avoid excessive sunlight, tanning treatments, and highly heating therapies, such as facial or whole body steams. Hot, spicy foods should be avoided. Astringent,, bitter and sweet foods which balance *pitta* should be favored instead. Sweet juicy fruits (especially melons and pears), cooked greens and rose petal preserves are especially good. Drinking plenty of water helps wash out impurities from a sensitive pitta skin. Reduce external or internal contact with synthetic chemicals to which *pitta* skin is especially prone to react. Avoid skin products that are abrasive, heating or contain artificial colors or preservatives. The *pitta* skin type needs both cooling and nurturing. Use of skin care products that enhance resistance to sun is highly recommended. Avoid tanning treatments and therapies that expose this delicate sensitive skin to steam for extended periods of time
- *Kapha* skin is more prone to clogging and needs more cleansing than other skin types, carefully avoiding greasy, clogging creams. As for food, fatty meats, fried food, cheeses and rich desserts must be avoided. Light, easy to digest, astringent, bitter and pungent (well-spiced) foods should be privileged since these foods help in balancing *kapha*. Olive oil is the best cooking oil and a little ginger and lime juice can be taken before meals to increase this characteristically sluggish digestive fire. Frequent warm baths and use of gentle cleansers to open the skin pores are suggested. Avoiding constipation and exercising every day to increase circulation and help purify the skin through the sweating process are recommended. Scrubbing the skin with gently exfoliating clay can help external cleansing, combined with herbal formulations.

Daily Face Care Routine

The Indian woman starts and ends her day with a skin cleansing routine. This routine is a three-step (cleansing, nourishing and moisturizing) procedure. Herbs and oils used in the daily skin care routine, as well as the methods of application, differ with type of complexion.

A typical Indian cleansing regime includes the following steps:

To begin, a muslin cloth is applied to the face with hot water to soften the skin using a circular motion for stimulation. Then a mixture of yogurt, turmeric paste and lentil flour are applied to the face as a moisturizing exfoliant using the same circular motions, allowing the finger tips to massage the facial muscles to soothe and tone sagging muscles that progressively come with aging. After several minutes, the face is rinsed with the muslin cloth dipped into icy cold water that helps sealing pores, improving the skin's overall condition. After cleansing, a freshly made toner consisting of cucumber juice, elderflower water or orange flower water along with a few drops of tincture benzoin is used each morning for further tightening of the pores. At night, the skin is left alone to "breathe" after cleansing.

In the northern regions of India and for more mature skin types, moisturizers consist of coconut or mustard oil infused with herbs like bergamot, jasmine or sandalwood which allow the skin to absorb vitamins A and E to keep skin of youthful aspect.

Skin Care Tips

Ayurveda recommends a daily oil massage using sesame, coconut or almond oils (persons with *pitta* constitution may opt for safflower oil for its cooling properties). The oils are lightly warmed and used to massage the whole body, leaving the oil on for 20 minutes and then washed off in a warm shower. Skin then feels soft, supple and nourished, absorbing the oils.

An intake of organic aloe vera every morning on an empty stomach is recommended since it is known to help staying young and healthy. It helps to clear excess *pitta*, to nourish the plasma tissue and clean the liver.

Skin is a protective barrier between inner and outer worlds. The quality of the skin reflects inner vitality and health. A look at skin implies self and outer-world protections.

Ayurveda in Hair Care: Herbal and Home Remedies

Hair is a vital parameter of beauty making everyone concerned about its appearance and its disorders. Ayurveda has specific treatments for maintaining healthy and beautiful hair free from problems. According to Ayurveda, the health of hair depends on proper functioning of *dhatus* or the tissues. The nutrient plasma produced from the digestion of food nourishes the *dhatus*; so healthy nutrient plasma will therefore produce healthy hair. Poor diet, illness, lack of proper hygiene, and nutritional deficiencies can affect the hair and cause various problems.

Massaging the scalp and hair with warm oil, preferably infused with hair-friendly herbs (*Amla, Brahmi*), is the best way to nourish them, topically. The process of massage helps to increase blood circulation to the hair follicles and supports the growth of healthy hair. It is especially beneficial for dry hair as the increased circulation facilitates production of natural oil thus restoring lost luster. The oil from *Amla* (Indian gooseberry), prepared by boiling dry pieces of *Amla* in coconut oil, is a hair tonic for stimulating hair growth and preventing hair loss.

An effective remedy for fighting dandruff involves Fenugreek (*methi*) seeds (two tablespoons) soaked overnight in water. The softened seeds are ground to a fine paste at morning and applied over the scalp, left for half an hour and then washed thoroughly. A handful of fresh neem (*Azadirachta indica*) leaves are boiled in water for nourishing hair.

APPLICATION OF NATURAL MEDICINE AND PLANTS IN MODERN COSMETICS

From a cosmetic point of view, Ayurvedic theories previously exposed such as balance, holism, analysis of syndromes and treatment selection, prescription rules and specificities of traditional Indian herbs are really meaningful and applicable to cosmetic product development. Herbal cosmetics, referred as "products", are formulated using various permissible cosmetic ingredients to form the base in which one or more herbal ingredients can be integrated to provide strictly defined cosmetic benefits.

Clinical Issues

- *Lack or scarcity of clinical trials:* There is a paucity of human clinical studies on the potency, efficacy, side effects and interactions of topically applied plant products, with often a lack of sound scientific rationale. The maximal concentration of botanical ingredients in commercial products is not subject to any regulation.
- *Efficacy:* It is believed by practitioners of alternative medicine that a naturally occurring mixture of active ingredients in plant extracts is more effective than individual molecules or their synthetic counterparts.[2] However, since clinical studies are lacking to support the effects of most of the herbal ingredients, the certainty of a real efficacy, topically, at the concentrations used appears rather fuzzy. Moreover, both the concentration and nature of active principles in plant extracts are not harmonized and depend upon many external factors, i.e. seasonal and climatic growing conditions of the plants, the availability of water, harvesting and storage conditions.[2,3] The plant material used must be grown under controlled optimized environmental conditions, handled and processed properly to maintain the activity of the extract, and further should be added in proper concentration into the final formulation. Besides, to ensure proper delivery of the product into the desired strata of skin through the stratum corneum, the use of a proper vehicle is of utmost importance. The raw materials derived in the form of natural extracts in a formulation should be standardized.
- *Side effects:* The belief that herbal medicines are not associated with adverse effects is clearly a false testimonial. Topical herbal medicines are well described as causes of contact dermatitis.[3] In a study, 12 of 106 allergic patients showed positive patch test reaction to tea tree oil with positive reactions to other natural products like lavender.[4] In an Indian study, a significant number of subjects showed positivity to turmeric through patch testing.[5] In a study on

pigmented dermatosis in south India, the major sensitizer was found being *kumkum*, a constituent of groundnut oil and *haldi* (turmeric) of cosmetic products.[6]

Major Natural Ingredients

A number of plant products are used in cosmetics today and the most common ones are listed in Table 3.

Natural Extracts in Present Skin Care Products

Since long, most botanicals used in folk medicine proved to be effective in treating dermatological ailments. In patients unwilling to use chemical drugs or in skin conditions where no effective treatment is available, botanical based cosmetics provide an alternative. They may also be used as adjuncts to prescription medications to improve the efficacy of the latter.

Antiaging

Free radicals generated in the skin, degrade collagen, elastin and also cause inflammation. Vegetable oils particularly wheat germ oil and palm oil are rich in tocopherols and tocotrienols, and can be utilized as effective antioxidants. Carotenoids such as beta carotene

Table 3: The most common plants used in cosmetics

S. No.	*Botanical Name*	*Common Name*	*Chemical Constituents*	*Cosmetic Uses*	*References*
1	*Persea americana*	Avocado	Oleic acid, linoleic acid and tocopherols	Protects against skin aging by inhibiting matrix metalloproteinases gelatinase and stomalysine	7
2	*Phoenix dactylifera*	Date palm	Proanthocyanidins, phytohormones and piperidine derivatives	Used in Asian medicine for wound healing. Has wrinkle reducing properties	8,9
3	*Punica granatam*	Pomegranate	Tannins, polyphenols, ascorbic acid, niacin and piperidines	Used in Asian and folk medicine to treat skin inflammation and to strengthen vessel wall. Potent antioxidant, has antimicrobial and astringent properties. Induces photoprotection when administered systemically or applied topically in clinicals	10–14
4	*Glycine soja*	Soy	Phytoestrogens, genistein	Stimulates fibroblasts and induces collagen synthesis. Soy was found to improve skin tone and texture when applied to the face. Protects skin against photocarcinogenesis	15,16
5	*Camellia sinensis*	Tea (black, green, oolong, and white)	Epigallocatechin gallate, methylxanthines, flavonoids and saponins	Green tea is anticarcinogenic in mice and modulates wound healing. Topically applied green tea provides photoprotection to the human skin and prevents skin from psoralen-induced photodamage. It is used in skin care products to soothe sunburn and reduce baggy eyelids	13,17,18
6	*Actaea racemosa*	Black cohosh	Triterpene glycosides	It has anti-inflammatory properties. Visible improvement in skin texture and wrinkles were noted in a clinical trial when a combination formulation with vitamin C and transforming growth factor β was applied	7,14,19

Contd...

Contd...

S. No.	*Botanical Name*	*Common Name*	*Chemical Constituents*	*Cosmetic Uses*	*References*
7	*Symphytum officinale*	Comfrey root	Allantoin	It is an antioxidant and has antitrichomonal properties. It is used in the treatment of burns, ulcers, dermatitis, psoriasis, scars, keloids, acne, onychomycosis and impetigo. It is also used in hand sanitizers. It is carcinogenic and contraindicated in pregnancy and lactation	13,20,21
8	*Aloe barbadensis, A. capensis, A. vera*	Aloe	Aloesin	Aloe vera is a competitive tyrosinase inhibitor and inhibits melanogenesis. It reduces skin pigmentation in a dose dependent manner and is more effective when combined with arbutin. Aloe inhibits *Staphylococcus aureus, H. pylori,* dermatophytes, herpes simplex and varicella zoster viruses. It inhibits ultraviolet B-induced photoimmunosuppression. The health concerns of aloe vera use are cutaneous eruptions and mutagenicity	13,14,22-27
9	*Curcuma domestica*	Turmeric	Curcumin, tumerone, curcuminoids and heptanoids	Curcumin derived from the root and tuber of the plant exerts antioxidant, antitumor, antimicrobial, antiscabietic, anti-inflammatory and wound healing actions	28-32
10	*Vitis vinifera*	Grape seed	Proanthocyanidins, kaempferol, quercetin, resveratrol, viniferins and tocopherols	The pharmacological effects of grape seed extract are mostly attributable to proanthocyanidins as potent antioxidants. It protects keratinocytes from ultraviolet B-induced photodamage and inhibits collagen and elastin degeneration. It is, therefore, included in various antiaging formulations	33-35
11	*Melaleuca alternifolia*	Tea tree	Terpenes	Tea tree oil exhibits activity against *M. furfur*, dermatophytes, *Candida, Propionibacterium acnes, E. coli,* Sarcoptes scabiei, etc. It has been effectively used in the treatment of acne, dermatophytosis and yeast infections. The use of tea tree oil is not advised in burns and sunexposed skin as it interferes with healing and has strong sensitizing potential	36,37
12	*Avena sativa*	Wild oats	Phenolic alkaloids like avenanthramides	Colloidal oatmeal is one of the few FDA regulated biological products as it is considered an effective skin protectant. It protects skin and hair from the damaging effects of smoke, UV radiation, bacteria and free radicals and ameliorates cutaneous irritation and inflammation. Recent studies show the presence of phenolic alkaloids like avenanthramides in oats, which possess antioxidant and anti-inflammatory properties	38-42

Contd...

Contd...

S. No.	*Botanical Name*	*Common Name*	*Chemical Constituents*	*Cosmetic Uses*	*References*
13	*Olea europaea*	Olive oil	Polyphenols	The polyphenols in olive oil are well-known antioxidants and anti-inflammatory compounds. Topically applied extra virgin olive oil has shown antitumor properties and inhibitory effects on UV-induced photocarcinogenesis in murine experiments. A topical formulation combining olive oil, beeswax and honey has been found effective in the treatment of tinea cruris, tinea corporis, psoriasis, eczema, diaper dermatitis, fissure and hemorrhoids	43–48
14	*Lavandula officinalis*	Lavender	Pinene, limonene, 1,8-cineole, cis-ocimene and trans-ocimene	This plant is extensively used for its fragrance. It also has promising medicinal potential. It has shown success in the treatment of alopecia areata	49–51
15	*Grifola frondosa, Ganoderma lucidum*	Mushrooms	Polysaccharides	Mushroom has been used in traditional medicine as a medicinal flora to treat major illnesses like bronchitis, arthritis, hepatitis, nephritis, scleroderma and cancer since time immemorial. Mushroom extract, especially from *Grifola frondosa*, has been shown to confer photoprotection to UV-irradiated human fibroblasts. Used for wound healing and treating inflammation	52–55
16	*Coffea arabica*	Coffee	Polyphenols, caffeine	The antioxidant property chiefly lies in the polyphenols. It is used in several botanical antiaging formulations as cleansers and creams which have shown to reduce wrinkles and pigmentation of photoaged skin. Used topically to treat cellulite	56–58
17	*Arnica montana*	Arnica	Sesquiterpene lactones	Made popular by the homeopaths for treating inflammatory conditions, topical arnica finds a place in modern cosmetology in reducing bruising following procedures like rhytidectomy, soft tissue augmentation, Botox injections, fat transfer and liposuction. The anti-inflammatory action of the dried flower heads is conferred by sesquiterpene lactones	59
18	*Matricaria recutita, Chamomilla recutita*	Chamomile	Apigenin and alpha-bisabolol	It has both anti-inflammatory and antioxidant properties. The skin benefits offered by chamomile are improvement of skin texture and elasticity and reduction of pruritus and signs of photodamage. It is also an effective soothing agent. It is commonly included in skin formulations to enhance their emollient and anti-inflammatory actions	60,61

Contd...

Contd...

S. No.	Botanical Name	Common Name	Chemical Constituents	Cosmetic Uses	References
19	*Glycyrrhiza glabra, G. inflata*	Licorice	Liquiritin, licochalcone A	Liquiritin, an active ingredient of the root extract, is effective in the treatment of melasma. Licochalcone A extracted from *Glycyrrhiza inflata* has been incorporated in a product to treat rosacea	62–65
20	*Rosemarinus officinalis*	Rosemary	Rosmarinic acid, carnosic acid	A food spice in wide use in the west for its aroma, rosemary has also been traditionally used as an antispasmodic, tonic and hair growth stimulant. Nowadays, it is incorporated in hair care products as a hair conditioner and an antidandruff agent. Rosemary has a good prospect in the times to come because of its antioxidant, anti-inflammatory, antimicrobial and anticarcinogenic properties which are being extensively studied	66–69
21	*Polypodium leucotomos*	Golden serpent fern		It is a fern with anti-inflammatory, immunomodulatory and photoprotective actions. Recent research advocates its inclusion in sunscreens	70–73
22	*Azadirachta indica*	Neem	Bioflavonoids such as quercetin, carotenes and ascorbic acid, limonoids	Neem leaf and its constituents have been demonstrated to exhibit immunomodulatory, anti-inflammatory, antihyperglycemic, antiulcer, antimalarial, antifungal, antibacterial, antiviral, antioxidant, antimutagenic and anticarcinogenic properties. Neem juice has been used topically for acne for its antibacterial properties. A shampoo made from neem seed extract has also shown efficacy in head lice. Of particular interest are the strong antimelanogenic properties and anti-inflammatory properties of the seeds. A recent report from Japan states that salanin and other limonoids of the N-hexane extract and defatted alcoholic extract of the neem could be valuable skin whitening and anti-inflammatory agents	74–76
23	*Cucumis sativus*	Cucumber		Used as home remedy for skin lightening	77

are also well-known antioxidants. Ascorbic acid,[78] flavonoids such as extracts from *Gingko*, *Fagopyrum* (buckwheat), *Eucalyptus sambucus* (European elder), or *Sophora japonica* are used for their antioxidant and anti-free radical properties.[79] Blackcurrant (*Ribes nigrum*), *Centella asiatica* (rich in Asiatic acid and madecassoside, a growth factor) supports the synthesis of type I collagen fibers and protects collagen fibers from enzymatic degradation. A facial cream containing 0.1% madecassoside and 5% vitamin C demonstrated a significant increase in skin smoothness, dermal thickness and skin elasticity after 6 months of use.[80]

Plant extracts used in antiaging arsenal in cosmetics include polyphenols from green tea, isoflavones from soy or red clover, pycnogenol from French pine bark extract, emblica from *Phyllanthus emblica*, silymarin, ectoin, *Fucus vesiculosus* extracts, white grape seed extracts containing polyphenols, *Cimicifuga racemosa* extracts or maritime plant extracts like those from algae or microalgae. Apigenin, extracted from chamomile and its derivatives, and rutin from *Fagopyrum* protect mucopolysaccharides from degradation. Other extracts rich in polyphenols such as tannins also have antihyaluronidase activity. Alpha- or beta-hydroxyacids are common in the botanical extracts either from fruits such as bilberry, apple, lemon, orange, *Kalanchoe*, tamarind (*Tamarindus indica*), *Hibiscus*, sugarcane (*Saccharum officinalis*), *Acer saccharum* (sugar maple), *Salix, Betula* (sweet birch) or *Gaultheria procumbens* (American wintergreen), they are efficacious in smoothing, brightening, and sloughing skin of dead cells from the skin surface, thus, favoring epidermal cell renewal at a natural younger pace, as well as moisturizing. The topical use of fruit extracts may be superior to single topical antioxidants such as vitamin C, vitamin E, or α-lipoic acid because they serve as a rich source of different antioxidants. The use of date seed oil on human skin showed that the extract contained a mixture of polyphenols and tocopherols with antioxidant properties.[81] Another study using lemon peel oil on human volunteers; reported that the peel extract was superior to α-tocopherol (vitamin E) in reducing ultraviolet (UV)-induced erythema and oxidative stress over 7 days.[82]

Photoprotection

The addition of botanical antioxidants and vitamins C and E to a broad-spectrum sunscreen appears to enhance its protective efficiency by further decreasing UV-induced damage compared with sunscreen alone.[83,84] These agents have been shown to enhance protection against UV-induced epidermal thickening, overexpression of matrix metalloproteinase 1 (MMP-1) and matrix metalloproteinase 9 (MMP-9), and depletion of CD1a(+) Langerhans cells.[85] Tea extract contains polyphenols such as epigallocatechin-3-gallate (EGCG) and was shown to protect against UV-induced DNA damage and immune suppression, by its ability to reduce oxidative stress and inhibit NF-kB.[86] Caffeine has been shown in animal models to provide some protection against UVB-induced erythema and act as a photoprotective agent.[87] A study showed that combining sunscreens with *Cassia alata* leaf extract, that contains anthraquinones, flavonoids and their glucoside derivatives, result in superior photoprotection.[88]

Few phytoconstituents, that can add some photoprotection to sunscreen are curcumin, resveratrol, tea polyphenols, silymarin, quercetin and ascorbic acid. They can be included in herbal cosmetic formulations to contribute to the reduction of the induction of skin cancer and delay the process of photoaging.[89]

Skin Lightening Agents

Botanicals are widely used as skin-lightening agents. They are considered safer and less irritating as compared to hydroquinone, the negative reference. Arbutin derived from bearberry (*Arctostaphylos uva-ursi*) is a skin-lightening agent that acts by competitively inhibiting tyrosinase and is now incorporated in most skin-lightening creams. Kojic acid from mushrooms, licorice derived from the root of *Glycyrrhiza glabra* plant, mulberry leaves (*Morus alba*), Pycnogenol (*Pinus pinaster*), hesperidin from the peel of citrus fruits and *Gingko* are some botanicals claimed having skin-lightening properties.

Moisturizers

Oil and butters from rice, wheat, coffee, mango, sorgho, corn and soya are rich in essential fatty acids such as oleic and linoleic acids. Plant waxes from sugarcane, *Camauba, Ceroxylon*, jojoba and rose are used to protect lips, hands, or face from dehydration. Certain plants like wheat, apple, potatoes, rice bran, *Agaricus, Morus alba*, or white mulberry that are rich in ceramides and glycosylceramides can be incorporated in cosmetics for skin or hair care to provide hydration or reconstitute epidermal barrier function or hair cuticle condition.

Acne

A recently published double-blind, vehicle-controlled trial performed on 60 age-matched participants with mild acne for 8 weeks showed a beneficial effect of a seaweed-derived oligosaccharide associated with 0.1% zinc pyrrolidone as compared to the vehicle alone, without any irritation.[90] The authors attribute this effect through a combination of anti-inflammatory and anti-*P. acnes* properties as shown by reduction in the number of papules, pustules and comedones.

CONCLUSION

Plants and plant products are the most common nonprescription formulations used in skin care.

Botanicals play an increasingly important role in the activity and safety of cosmetics. Many botanical extracts which were used in traditional medicine are being rediscovered by companies and marketed as cosmetic products. However, few works remain available to sustain their contribution, implying that more research and investigations are needed. Less adverse and beneficial effects make them ideal for use as topical maintenance or adjuvant therapy in skin treatment. A better knowledge of their active ingredients and more clinical studies with larger populations for assessing the specific effects of botanicals are needed to enlighten on their values.

REFERENCES

1. Wikipedia Cosmetics. Available from: en.wikipedia.org/wiki/Cosmetics.
2. Thornfeldt C. Cosmeceuticals containing herbs: fact, fiction, and future. Dermatol Surg. 2005;873-80; discussion 880.
3. Allemann IB, Baumann L. Botanicals in skin care products. Int J Dermatol. 2009;48:923-34.
4. Jancin B. Cross-sensitivity in tea tree oil allergy. Skin & Allergy News. 2002;33:38.
5. Nath AK, Thappa DM. Kumkum-induced dermatitis: an analysis of 46 cases. Clin Exp Dermatol. 2007;32:385-7.
6. Shenoi SD, Rao R. Pigmented contact dermatitis. Indian J Dermatol Venereol Leprol. 2007;73:285-7
7. LaGow B. PDR for Herbal Medicines, 3rd edition. Montvale, NJ: Thomson PDR; 2004.
8. Bauza E, Dal Farra C, Berghi A, et al. Date palm kernel extract exhibits antiaging properties and significantly reduces skin wrinkles. Int J Tissue React. 2002;24:131-6.
9. Ghosh DK, Murthy UV. Antiaging benefits of a topical formulation containing coenzyme Q10: results of 2 clinical studies. Cosmet Dermatol. 2002;15:55-60.
10. Baumann LS. Cosmeceutical critique: pomegranate. Skin & Allergy News. 2004;35:42.
11. De M, Krishna De A, Banerjee AB. Antimicrobial screening of some Indian spices. Phytother Res. 1999;13:616-8.
12. Murad H, Shellow VRW. Pomegranate extract both orally ingested and topically applied to augment the SPF of sunscreens. Cosmet Dermatol. 2001;14:43-5.
13. PDR for herbal medicines, second edition. Montvale (NJ): Thomson Medical Economics; 2000.
14. Jellin JM, Gregory P, Butz F, et al. Natural medicines comprehensive database, third edition. Stockton (CA): Therapeutic Research Facility; 2000.
15. Wu J, Liu JC, Kollias N, et al. The effect of total soy on combination skin. Poster 0473 presented at: 20th World Congress of Dermatology; July 1-5, 2002; Paris, France.
16. Weil H, Spencer JM, Gelfand J, et al. The soy isoflavone genistein: a new agent in dermatology. Cosmet Dermatol. 2001;14:13-9.
17. Spencer JM. Chemoprevention of skin cancer and photoaging. Cosmet Dermatol. 2001;14:25-8.
18. Zhao JF, Zhang YJ, Jinx XH, et al. Green tea protects against psoralen plus ultraviolet A-induced photochemical damage to skin. J Invest Dermatol. 1999;113:1070-5.
19. Pinnell SR. Cutaneous photodamage, oxidative stress and topical antioxidant protection. J Am Acad Dermatol. 2003;48:1-19.
20. Baumann LS. Cosmeceutical critique: allantoin. Skin & Allergy News. 2003;34:10.
21. Clark LF, Baker B, Trahan C, et al. A prospective double blinded study of Mederma skin care versus placebo for traumatic scar reduction. Cosmet Dermatol. 1999;12:19-26.
22. Jones K, Hughes J, Hong M, et al. Modulation of melanogenesis by aloesin: a competitive inhibitor of tyrosinase. Pigment Cell Res. 2002 Oct;15: 335-40.
23. Choi S, Lee SK, Kim JE, et al. Aloesin inhibits hyperpigmentation induced by UV radiation. Clin Exp Dermatol. 2002;27:513-5.
24. Klein AD, Penneys NS. Aloe vera. J Am Acad Dermatol. 1988;18:714-20.
25. Syed TA, Ahmad SA, Holt AH, et al. Management of psoriasis with aloe vera extract in a hydrophilic cream: a placebo-controlled, double-blind study. Trop Med Int Health. 1996;1:505-9.
26. West DP, Zhu YF. Evaluation of aloe vera gel gloves in the treatment of dry skin associated with occupational exposure. Am J Infect Control. 2003;31:40-2.
27. Wasserman L, Avigad S, Beery E, et al. The effect of aloe emodin on the proliferation of a new Merkel carcinoma cell line. Am J Dermatopathol. 2002;24:17-22.
28. Ruby AJ, Kuttan G, Babu KD, et al. Anti-tumor and antioxidant activity of natural curcuminoids. Cancer Lett. 1995;94:79-83.
29. Huang MT, Lysz T, Ferraro T, et al. Inhibitory effects of curcumin on in vitro lipoxygenase and cyclooxygenase activities in mouse epidermis. Cancer Res. 1991;51:813-9.
30. Limtrakul P, Lipigorngoson S, Namwong O, et al. Inhibitory effect of dietary curcumin on skin carcinogenesis in mice. Cancer Lett. 1997; 24;116:197-203.
31. Srimal RC, Dhawan BN. Pharmacology of diferuloyl methane (curcumin), a non-steroidal anti-inflammatory agent. J Pharm Pharmacol. 1973;25:447-52.
32. Maheshwari RK, Singh AK, Gaddipati J, et al. Multiple biological activities of curcumin: a short review. Life Sci. 2006;78:2081-7.
33. Carando S, Teissedre P-L. Catechin and procyanidin levels in French wines: contribution to dietary intake. In: Gross GG, Hemingway RW, Yoshida T (Eds). Plant Polyphenols 2: Chemistry, Biology, Pharmacology, Ecology. New York: Kluwer Academic/ Plenum Publishers;1999. p. 725-37.
34. Waterhouse AL, Walzem RL. Nutrition of grape phenolics. In: Rice-Evans CA, Packer L (Eds). Flavonoids in Health and Disease. NewYork: Marcel Dekker;1998. pp.359-85.
35. Mittal A, Elmets CA, Katiyar SK. Dietary feeding of proanthocyanidins from grape seeds prevents photocarcinogenesis in SKH-1 hairless mice: relationship to decreased fat and lipid peroxidation. Carcinogenesis. 2003;24:1379-88.
36. Walton SF, McKinnon M, Pizzutto S, et al. Acaricidal activity of Melaleuca alternifolia (tea tree) oil: in vitro sensitivity of sarcoptes scabiei var hominis to terpinen-4-ol. Arch Dermatol. 2004;140: 563-6.
37. Baumann LS. Cosmeceutical critique: tea tree oil. Skin & Allergy News. 2002;33:14.
38. US Food and Drug Administration. Title 21: Food and Drugs, Chapter 1: Food and Drug Administration Department of Health and Humans Services, Subchapter D: Drugs for Human Use, Part 347: Skin Protectant Drug Products for Over-the-Counter Human Use. Washington DC: US Department of Health and Human Services, Food and Drug Administration, April 1, 2007:21 CFR347.
39. Aburjai T, Natsheh FM. Plants used in cosmetics. Phytother Res. 2003;17:987-1000.

40. Vie K, Cours-Darne S, Vienne MP, et al. Modulating effects of oatmeal extracts in the sodium lauryl sulfate skin irritancy model. Skin Pharmacol Appl Skin Physiol. 2002;15:120-4.
41. Tsao R, Akhtar MH. Neutraceutical and functional foods. I. Current trend in phytochemical antioxidant research. J Food Agric Environ. 2005;3:10-7.
42. Saeed SA, Butt NM, McDonald-Gibson WJ, et al. Inhibitors of prostaglandin biosynthesis in extracts of oat (Avena sativa) seeds. Biochem Soc Trans. 1981;9:444.
43. de la Puerta R, Martinez-Dominguez E, Ruíz-Gutiérrez V. Effect of minor components of virgin olive oil on topical antiinflammatory assays. Z Naturforsch C. 2000;55:814-9.
44. Owen RW, Giacosa A, Hull WE, et al. Olive-oil consumption and health: the possible role of antioxidants. Lancet Oncol. 2000;1: 107-12.
45. Budiyanto A, Ahmed NU, Wu A, et al. Protective effect of topically applied olive oil against photocarcinogenesis following UVB exposure of mice. Carcinogenesis. 2000;21:2085-90.
46. Ichihashi M, Ahmed NU, Budiyanto A, et al. Preventive effect of antioxidant on ultraviolet-induced skin cancer in mice. J Dermatol Sci. 2000;23:S45-50.
47. Al-Waili NS. An alternative treatment for pityriasis versicolor, tinea cruris, tinea corporis and tinea faciei with topical application of honey, olive oil and beeswax mixture: an open pilot study. Complement Ther Med. 2004;12:45-7.
48. Al-Waili NS, Saloom KS, Al-Waili TN, et al. The safety and efficacy of a mixture of honey, olive oil, and beeswax for the management of hemorrhoids and anal fissure: a pilot study. Scientific World Journal. 2006;6:1998-2005.
49. Cornwell S, Dale A. Lavender oil and perineal repair. Mod Midwife. 1995;5:31-3.
50. Hay IC, Jamieson M, Ormerod AD. Randomized trial of aromatherapy. Successful treatment for alopecia areata. Arch Dermatol. 1998;134:1349-52.
51. Evandri MG, Battinelli L, Daniele C, et al. The antimutagenic activity of Lavandula angustifolia (lavender) essential oil in the bacterial reverse mutation assay. Food Chem Toxicol. 2005;43:1381-7.
52. Sliva D. Ganoderma lucidum (Reishi) in cancer treatment. Integr Cancer Ther. 2003;2:358-64.
53. Wasser SP, Weis AL. Therapeutic effects of substances occurring in higher Basidiomycetes mushrooms: a modern perspective. Crit Rev Immunol. 1999;19:65-96.
54. Lakshmi B, Ajith TA, Sheena N, et al. Antiperoxidative, anti-inflammatory, and antimutagenic activities of ethanol extract of the mycelium of Ganoderma lucidum occurring in South India. Teratog Carcinog Mutagen. 2003;1:85-97.
55. Bae JT, Sim GS, Lee DH, et al. Production of exopolysaccharide from mycelial culture of Grifola frondosa and its inhibitory effect on matrix metalloproteinase-1 expression in UV-irradiated human dermal fibroblasts. FEMS Microbiol Lett. 2005;251:347-54.
56. Charurin P, Ames JM, del Castillo MD. Antioxidant activity of coffee model systems. J Agric Food Chem. 2002;50:3751-6.
57. Farris P. Idebenone, green tea, and Coffeeberry® extract: new and innovative antioxidants. Dermatol Ther. 2007;20:322-9.
58. Hexsel D, Orlandi C, Zechmeister do Prado D. Botanical extracts used in the treatment of cellulite. Dermatol Surg. 2005;31:866-72; discussion 872.
59. Wagner S, Suter A, Merfort I. Skin penetration studies of Arnica preparations and of their sesquiterpene lactones. Planta Med. 2004;70:897-903.
60. Lee KG, Shibamoto T. Determination of antioxidant potential of volatile extracts isolated from various herbs and spices. J Agric Food Chem. 2002;50:4947-52.
61. Craig WJ. Health-promoting properties of common herbs. Am J Clin Nutr. 1999;70:491S-499S.
62. Amer M, Metwalli M. Topical liquiritin improves melasma. Int J Dermatol. 2000;39:299-301.
63. Tsukiyama R, Katsura H, Tokuriki N, et al. Antibacterial activity of licochalcone A against spore-forming bacteria. Antimicrob Agents Chemother. 2002;46:1226-30.
64. Shibata S, Inoue H, Iwata S, et al. Inhibitory effects of licochalcone A isolated from Glycyrrhiza inflata root on inflammatory ear edema and tumour promotion in mice. Planta Med. 1991;57:221-4.
65. Friis-Møller A, Chen M, Fuursted K, et al. In vitro antimycobacterial and antilegionella activity of licochalcone A from Chinese licorice roots. Planta Med. 2002;68: 416-9.
66. al-Sereiti MR, Abu-Amer KM, Sen P. Pharmacology of rosemary (Rosmarinus officinalis Linn.) and its therapeutic potentials. Indian J Exp Biol. 1999;37:124-30.
67. Aburjai T, Natsheh FM. Plants used in cosmetics. Phytother Res. 2003;17:987-1000.
68. Larrondo JV, Agut M, Calvo-Torras MA. Antimicrobial activity of essences from labiates. Microbios. 1995;82:171-2.
69. Darshan S, Doreswamy R. Patented antiinflammatory plant drug development from traditional medicine. Phytother Res. 2004;18:343-57.
70. González S, Pathak MA, Cuevas J, et al. Topical or oral administration with an extract of Polypodium leucotomos prevents acute sunburn and psoralen-induced phototoxic reactions as well as depletion of Langerhans cells in human skin. Photodermatol Photoimmunol Photomed. 1997;13:50-60.
71. Middelkamp-Hup MA, Pathak MA, Parrado C, et al. Oral Polypodium leucotomos extract decreases ultraviolet-induced damage of human skin. J Am Acad Dermatol. 2004 Dec;51(6):910-8.
72. Piñeiro Alvarez B. [2 years personal experience in anapsos treatment of psoriasis in various clinical forms]. Med Cutan Ibero Lat Am. 1983;11: 65-72.
73. Capote R, Alonso-Lebrero JL, García F, et al. Polypodium leucotomos extract inhibits trans-urocanic acid photoisomerization and photodecomposition. J Photochem Photobiol B. 2006;82:173-9.
74. Subapriya R, Nagini S. Medicinal properties of neem leaves: a review. Curr Med Chem Anticancer Agents. 2005;5:149-6.
75. Abdel-Ghaffar F, Al-Quraishy S, Al-Rasheid KA, et al. Efficacy of a single treatment of head lice with a neem seed extract: an in vivo and in vitro study on nits and motile stages. Parasitol Res. 2012;110:277-80.
76. Akihisa T, Takahashi A, Kikuchi T, et al. The melanogenesis-inhibitory, anti-inflammatory, and chemopreventive effects of limonoids in n-hexane extract of Azadirachta indica A. Juss. (neem) seeds. J Oleo Sci. 2011;60:53-9.
77. Gandía-Herrero F, Jiménez M, Cabanes J, et al. Tyrosinase inhibitory activity of cucumber compounds: enzymes responsible for browning in cucumber. J Agric Food Chem. 2003;51:7764-9.
78. Humbert PG, Haftek M, Creidi P, et al. Topical ascorbic acid on photoaged skin. Clinical, topographical and ultrastructural evaluation: double-blind study vs placebo. Exp Dermatol. 2003;12:237-44.
79. Leung AY, Foster S. Encyclopedia of Common Natural Ingredients Used in Food, Drugs and Cosmetics, second edition. New York: John Wiley & Sons, Inc.; 1996.

80. Haftek M, Mac-Mary S, Le Bitoux MA, et al. Clinical, biometric and structural evaluation of the long-term effects of a topical treatment with ascorbic acid and madecassoside in photoaged human skin. Exp Dermatol. 2008;17: 946-52.
81. Dammak I, Abdallah FB, Boudaya S, et al. Date seed oil limit oxidative injuries induced by hydrogen peroxide in human skin organ culture. Biofactors. 2007;29:137-45.
82. Calabrese V, Scapagnini G, Randazzo SD, et al. Oxidative stress and antioxidants at skin biosurface: A novel antioxidant from lemon oil capable of inhibiting oxidative damage to the skin. Drugs Exp Clin Res. 1999;25:281-7.
83. Lin JY, Selim MA, Shea CR, et al. UV photoprotection by combination topical antioxidants vitamin C and vitamin E. J Am Acad Dermatol. 2003;48:866-74.
84. Oresajo C, Stephens T, Hino PD, et al. Protective effects of a topical antioxidant mixture containing vitamin C, ferulic acid, and phloretin against ultraviolet-induced photodamage in human skin. J Cosmet Dermatol. 2008;7:290-7.
85. Wu Y, Zheng X, Xu XG, et al. Protective effects of a topical antioxidant complex containing vitamins C and E and ferulic acid against ultraviolet irradiation-induced photodamage in Chinese women. J Drugs Dermatol. 2013;12:464-8.
86. Elmets CA, Singh D, Tubesing K, et al. Cutaneous photoprotection from ultraviolet injury by green tea polyphenols. J Am Acad Dermatol. 2001;44:425-32.
87. Lu YP, Lou YR, Xie JG, et al. Caffeine and caffeine sodium benzoate have a sunscreen effect, enhance UVB-induced apoptosis, and inhibit UVB-induced skin carcinogenesis in SKH-1 mice. Carcinogenesis. 2007;28:199-206.
88. Oresajo C, Yatskayer M, Galdi A, et al. Complementary effects of antioxidants and sunscreens in reducing UV-induced skin damage as demonstrated by skin biomarker expression. J Cosmet Laser Ther. 2010;12:157-62.
89. Saraf S, Kaur CD. Phytoconstituents as photoprotective novel cosmetic formulations. Pharmacogn Rev. 2010;4:1-11.
90. Capitanio B, Sinagra JL, Weller RB, et al. Randomized controlled study of a cosmetic treatment for mild acne. Clin Exp Dermatol. 2012;37:346-9.

Chapter 16

Dermatology, Cosmetics and Well-being: Current Status of Research

Claire Battie, *L'Oréal Research and Innovation, Asnières, France*
Nina Madnani, *P.D. Hinduja National Hospital and Medical Research Centre, Mumbai, India*
Narasimha Rao P, *Bhaskar Medical Colleges, Hyderabad, India*

INTRODUCTION

The World Health Organization (WHO) has defined health as "a state of complete physical, mental and social well-being and not merely the absence of disease or infirmity." Such a definition has given a strong impulsion to quality of life (QoL) studies. Quality of life was defined as "individuals' perception of their position in life in the context of the culture and value systems in which they live and in relation to their goals, expectations, standards and concerns."[1] It is a broad ranging concept affected in a complex way by the person's physical health, psychological state, personal beliefs, social relationships and their relationship to salient features of their environment. "Quality of life" or QoL is a wide concept that incorporates all aspects of life and has been used in a variety of fields.

In medicine, specific grading scales have been developed, in part to fill the gap between the different perception of diseases by medical doctors and patients, the severity and duration of the disease being not the only predictors of psychosocial consequences. QoL impairment is very important to consider since it may affect the outcome of therapies and alter both satisfaction in and compliance to treatment. Health-related quality of life (HRQoL) is the patient's perception of his/her physical, mental and social health.

A multitude of methods and QoL scales have been developed and validated to objectively show the impact of some diseases and their treatments on the psychological and social status of individuals. Measuring QoL is now increasingly included in the management of diseases, the objective being not only to evaluate the improvement of clinical signs but also to consider the real impact of a treatment upon the patient's everyday life.

Measuring QoL is pertinent in dermatology since dermatological diseases are visible and often chronic, and therefore of high impact on patients' life. Validated scorings of QoL have also been used to assess the contribution of a complementary use of cosmetics in improving the well-being of these patients, a role now abundantly recognized in the global management of skin diseases.

MEASURING QUALITY OF LIFE IN DERMATOLOGY

Why?

In dermatology, the evaluation of QoL is very important since many skin diseases, such as atopic eczema, psoriasis, vitiligo and leg ulcers, although not life-threatening, are recognized as a considerable burden upon health status and QoL.[2,3] "In 20–50% of patients with skin diseases in secondary care, this impairment may be severe enough to classify the patient at risk of severe psychosocial impairments such as clinical depression or psychiatric morbidity."[4]

Dermatological skin disorders affect a patient's mental condition, self-acceptance, social relations and adaptability; and especially for visible skin disorders—they reduce self-esteem and induce poor body image and low sense of self-worth. In this context, specific QoL scales have been developed to better understand and evaluate the "patient's side" and to reduce the psychosocial burden and the QoL impairment caused by skin diseases and their treatments. Clinical research has traditionally put emphasis on clinical signs as outcome data but QoL measurement affords an additional and patient-oriented outcome assessment, which does not necessarily parallel changes in clinical signs. This was recently emphasized by a work on psoriasis[5] which clearly demonstrated that measurement techniques cluster into two groups: one formed by clinical severity measurements, and the other comprising QoL and psychological indexes, stressing the need for more comprehensive assessment. In routine practice, clinicians assess how severely individual patients' lives are affected by their skin disease. These assessments are used in the risk/benefit considerations relating to treatment decisions. Additional measurement of QoL would be useful to objectively inform patients about some critical decisions, for example, where systemic drugs with significant side effects are being considered. Although QoL questionnaires are now widely used in dermatology, they are not yet regularly used in routine clinical work either as outcome measures or to support a clinical decision-making. It is necessary that QoL scores and changes in QoL score be easily understood by clinicians before these instruments become of any help and widely used. This issue is being addressed[6] but remains an important research challenge in the development of QoL assessment in dermatology.

Available Scales

Quality of life is assessed by standardized and validated questionnaires, of variable specificity.

General QoL assessments allow the major effects of skin diseases to be compared to the effects of other nonskin diseases. Specific QoL scales have been validated to evaluate the impact of some specific skin conditions upon patients' psychosocial state and everyday activities. Over the last 20 years, a very wide range of questionnaires have been developed for patients with skin disease. Table 1, although not fully comprehensive, includes the most widely used techniques.

The most commonly used QoL scales in dermatology remain the Dermatology Life Quality Index (DLQI), Skindex and Dermatology Quality of Life Scales (DQOLS).

Dermatology Life Quality Index

It was developed and validated by Finlay in 1994,[14] and is the first dermatology-specific QoL instrument evaluating functional, psychological and social aspects. This simple 10-item validated questionnaire can be applied to 33 different skin conditions and has been widely used

Table 1: Most widely used quality of life (QoL) measures

QoL Measures	*Source*
General measures	
Medical Outcome Study 36-item Short Form Health Survey (SF-36)	Brazier et al., 1992[7]
Nottingham Health Profile (NHP)	Hunt et al., 1981,1985,1986[8-10]
Sickness Impact Profile (SIP)	Bergner et al., 1981[11]
World Health Organization Quality of Life assessment (WHOQOL)	The WHO Group, 1995, 1998[12,13]
Dermatology-specific measures: adults	
Dermatology Life Quality Index (DLQI)	Finlay and Khan, 1994;[14] Lewis and Finlay, 2004[15]
Skindex	Chren et al., 1996[16]
Dermatology-Specific Quality of Life (DSQL)	Anderson and Rajagopalan, 1997[17]
Dermatology Quality of Life Scales (DQOLS)	Morgan et al., 1997[18]
Freiberg Life Quality Assessment (FLQA)	Augustin et al., 2004[19]
Dermatology-specific measures: children	
Children's Dermatology Life Quality Index (CDLQI)	Lewis-Jones and Finlay, 1995[20]
Children's Dermatology Life Quality Index (CDLQI) (Cartoon version)	Holme et al., 2003[21]
Disease-specific measures	
Psoriasis	
Psoriasis Disability Index (PDI)	Finlay and Kelly, 1987[22]; Lewis and Finlay, 2005[23]
Psoriasis Life Stress Inventory (PLSI)	Gupta and Gupta, 1995[24]
Salford Psoriasis Index (PSI)	Kirby et al., 2000[25]
PSORIQoL	McKenna et al., 2003[26]
Atopic dermatitis	
Infant's Dermatitis QoL Index (IDQOL)	Lewis-Jones et al., 2001[27]
Dermatitis Family Impact (DFI) Questionnaire	Lawson et al., 1998[28]
QoL Index for Atopic Dermatitis (QoLIAD)	Whalley et al., 2004[29]
Acne	
Acne Disability Index	Motley and Finlay, 1989[30]
Cardiff Acne Disability Index	Motley and Finlay, 1992[31]
Assessment of the psychological and social effects of acne	Layton, 1994[32]
Acne-Specific Quality of life Questionnaire (Acne-QoL)	Girman et al., 1996;[33] Martin et al., 2001[34]
Acne Quality of Life Scale	Gupta et al., 1998[35]

Contd...

Contd...

QoL Measures	*Source*
Other disease-specific measures	
Chronic venous insufficiency (FLQA)	Augustin et al., 1997[36]
Skin disease in human immunodeficiency virus (HIV)-infected patients (HIV-DERMDEX)	Aftergut et al., 2001[37]
Melasma (MELASQOL)	Balkrishnan et al., 2003[38]
Vitiligo (Vitiligo Impact Scale)	Krishna et al.,2013[39]
Alopecia (WAA-QOL)	Dolte et al., 2000[40]
Scalp dermatitis (Scalpdex)	Chen et al., 2002[41]

(over 500 publications). The higher the DLQI score the lower the QoL. Since its introduction in 1994, the DLQI has played an important role in assessing dermatology-specific HRQoL and has contributed to several medical decision-making processes. It is reliable, valid and easy to use. The DLQI has been used to determine the HRQoL in patients with skin problems and has been considered to be superior, in terms of reliability, to general (nondermatological) measurements in dermatological patients.[42]

Skindex

It is a reliable and validated measure[16] which, originally, was a 61-item self-administered survey instrument. Skindex had eight scales, each of them addressing a different component, in a comprehensive conceptual framework: cognitive effects, social effects, depression, fear, embarrassment, anger, physical discomfort and physical limitations. Item responses are standardized from 0 (no effect) to 100 (maximal effect). A 29-item derived version has been created, Skindex-29. Skindex is also available in a 16-item version, Skindex-16. The latter, brief single-page version of Skindex accurately and sensitively measures how much patients are bothered by their skin condition. This brief QoL outcome measure is useful for studies of dermatologic care.

QUALITY OF LIFE IN SOME DERMATOLOGICAL DISEASES

Quality of Life and Vitiligo

Vitiligo is a chronic skin affection concerning approximately 1% of total population. The prevalence is often said to be higher in India ranging from 0.46% to 8.8%.[43]

Although the disease does not produce direct health impairment, it considerably influences the psychological well-being of the patients[44,45] (Fig. 1). It is an important skin disease having major impact on QoL of patients, many of whom feel distressed and stigmatized by their condition. These patients often develop negative feelings about it, which are reinforced by their experiences over a number of years. Most patients with vitiligo report feelings of embarrassment, which can lead to low self-esteem and social isolation. The chronic nature of disease, its long-term treatment, a lack of uniform effective therapy and an unpredictable course of disease are serious demoralizing and/or distressing causes to patients suffering from vitiligo.

Vitiligo is a much dreaded disease in India with social stigma and ostracization. Dermatology Life Quality Index scores of Indian patients with vitiligo appeared higher as compared to other countries. Parsad et al. found a mean DLQI of 10.67 in India,[46] compared to 4.82 in UK,[47] 4.95 in Belgium,[44] 5.9 in the US,[48] 6.40 in Malaysia,[49] 7.05 and 8.16 in Iran.[50,51]

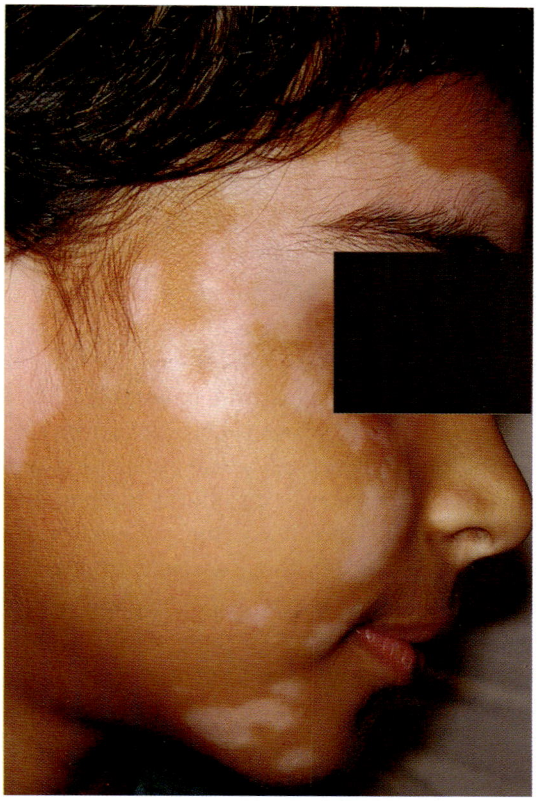

Figure 1: A young patient with facial vitiligo
Courtesy: Dr Nina Madnani, Mumbai, India

The impact of the disease upon the psychosocial and HRQoL is evaluated based on several parameters, including country of origin, skin type, gender, age, marital status and involved body site.[51,52] In particular, Dolatshahi et al. showed a relationship between DLQI score and skin phototype: the mean DLQI scores in individuals with phototype V were statistically higher than those of other types, indicating that darker phenotypes are more affected by discoloring diseases such as vitiligo. Interestingly, married women had significantly higher DLQI scores than single women, while single and married men showed no significant difference ($p = 0.801$).

It is therefore important to recognize and deal with psychological components of this disease to improve QoL of patients and to obtain a better response to treatment. Recently, Krishna et al. from the All India Institute of Medical Sciences (AIIMS), New Delhi, India, developed the Vitiligo Impact Scale (VIS) based on 27 items.[39] The need to develop a new scale arose from the severe stigmatization faced by patients, where the intense psychological trauma could not be correlated with the extent of disease. Very often, a few spots on face could psychologically traumatize a patient more than an extended vitiligo on unexposed areas. VIS scale correlated well with that of DLQI, and Skindex-16.

Quality of Life and Psoriasis

Psoriasis is a chronic inflammatory skin condition of physical impact on skin, but it also has a profound influence on a patient's QoL. It equally affects both genders, arises at all ages and concerns 2.5% of the world's population. It brings social stigmatization, pain, discomfort, physical disability and psychological stress. Psoriasis is a disease with profound impact upon the psychophysiological profile of the patient, particularly since highly visible.[53-55] Thus, assessment by a health professional of the extent of apparent disease in terms of clinical severity alone may not suffice, and a more holistic approach to the QoL becomes mandatory. An improvement in the overall psychosocial morbidity associated with the disease is an important associated part of a favorable treatment outcome.[56,57]

Very few studies have examined this aspect in Indian patients with psoriasis. Using Psoriasis Area Severity Index (PASI), Psoriasis Disability Index (PDI), and Psoriasis Life Stress Inventory (PLSI), a study. showed that daily activities, employment and treatment were the most affected factors in these patients with psoriasis[58] who are also most likely to feel self-conscious, disturbed or inconvenienced by the abnormal shedding of the skin, live in a constant fear of relapse, and avoid social interactions. A recent study using the QoL and PDI in psoriatic patients attending a South Indian Medical College Hospital, showed that QoL was affected in 75% of the patients, daily activities being the most affected.[59]

Quality of Life and Acne

Acne is a very common dermatological condition, strongly linked to sexual puberty. Although it does not cause direct physical impairment, it can produce a significant psychosocial burden and has a substantial impact upon patients' QoL. Face is one of the privileged sites of acne, and facial appearance is a major component of one's perception of body image (Fig. 2). It is not surprising therefore that an individual whose face is spoiled with acne develops significant psychosocial disability. As part of the emotional impact, increased levels of anxiety,

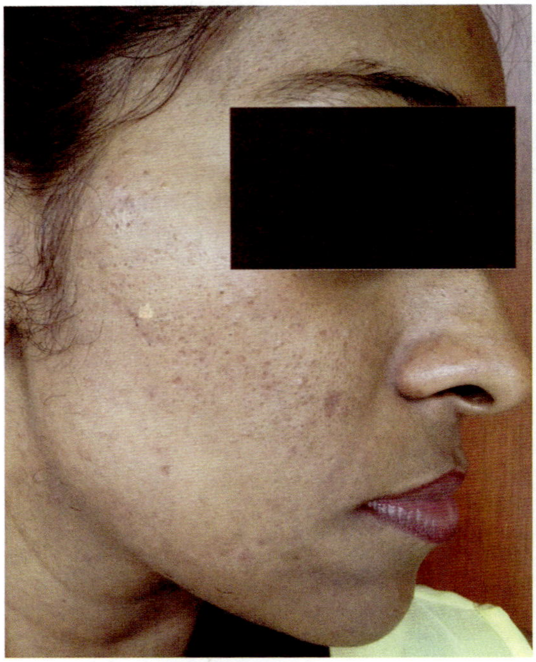

Figure 2: Acne with scarring with pigmentation
Courtesy: Dr Nina Madnani, Mumbai, India

anger, depression and frustration are observed in patients with acne.[60-63] The onset of acne, mainly during teen-ages coincides, in addition, to a period of life where psychosocial balance is naturally fragile.

Most studies on the psychosocial impact of acne have been conducted among patients from the US and Europe, very few being available among other population groups. A study conducted by Pruthi et al.[64] focused on acneic adult females in India (acne can persist much beyond teen years). Using a semi-structured clinical interview of the Skindex, they showed a higher level of emotional and social impairment, in terms of physical discomfort, anger, and the intermingling impact of these, among the 11 women with mild-to-moderate acne. The consensus of the Indian Acne Alliance (IAA) members, on Indian patients with acne is that the negative impact is lower in Indians as they accept acne more easily, as an unavoidable part of life.[65]

IMPACT OF COSMETICS ON QUALITY OF LIFE

Since cosmetics strongly contribute to improve the appearance, they are prone to affect our relationship with ourselves and with others, thereby contributing to improved QoL. Many studies have been conducted using QoL objective measures to assess the effects of cosmetics in various situations. In pathological conditions, during which the physical and mental conditions are altered and for which self-reconciliation is important, cosmetic treatments are sought to help rebuilding self-image. Besides the obvious benefit in these pathological conditions that alter the appearance, a growing number of studies illustrate the beneficial effects of cosmetics upon well-being in normal physiological conditions. The relationship between QoL, health and wellness becomes closer, all three aspects being strongly influenced by the use of cosmetics.

Benefits of Cosmetics in Pathological Conditions

The importance of cosmetic and esthetic care is particularly pertinent in chronic dermatological conditions such as vitiligo, lichen planus, rosacea, atopic dermatitis, and also in nondermatological diseases like systemic cancers, whose treatment often induces numerous skin and hair disorders. In this context, evaluating the role of cosmetics in some diseases may provide help to their better medical management.

Dyspigmentary Disorders and Other Facial Disfigurements—Major Role of Cosmetic Camouflage

As previously shown, hypopigmented as well as hyperpigmented lesions have severe psychological consequences and the lack of efficacious treatment contributes to the burden of these frequent diseases, particularly in India. For many, it goes far beyond a cosmetic problem, i.e. it is a major social dysfunction that seriously curtails their ability to lead normal, professional, social or married lives.[66] The use of corrective makeup being obvious in such cases (Fig. 3), an increasing number of studies now attempt to demonstrate its beneficial impact by using QoL scales.

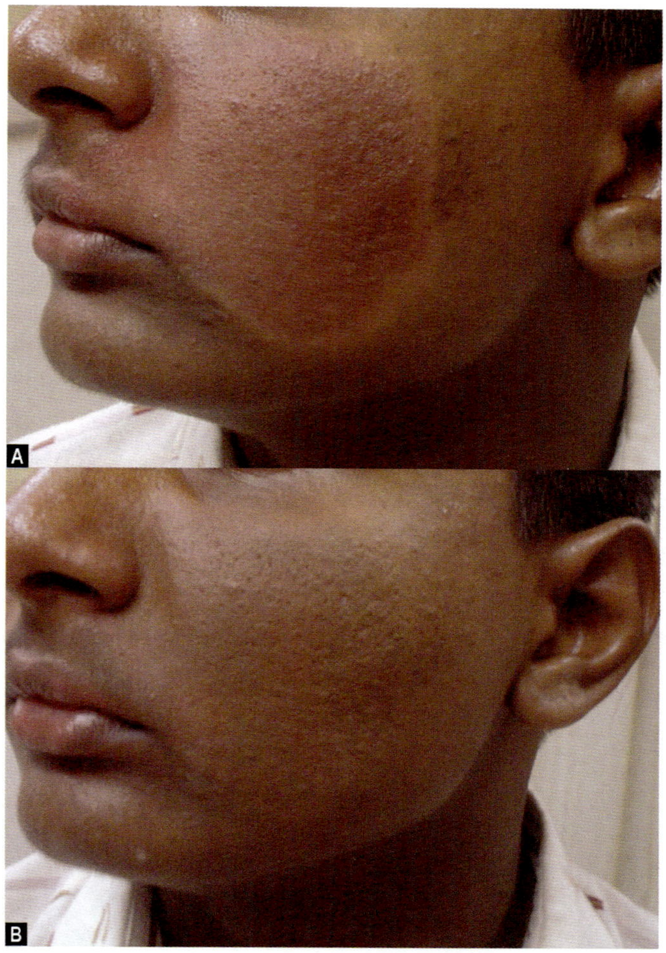

Figure 3: Photographs of before and after camouflage in a patient with hypopigmented patch of leprosy on the face. **A,** Before **B,** After
Courtesy: Dr K Udaya Kiran, Hyderabad, India

Several clinical studies have thus addressed the question how cosmetics may influence the perception of skin dyspigmentation. In a study of vitiligo affected patients, Ongenae et al. showed that the DLQI improved after the use of cosmetic camouflage and hence, recommended the use of camouflage in patients with higher DLQI scores.[67] Using the DLQI scoring system, Holme et al.[68] studied the effect of cosmetic camouflage on 82 patients from the UK suffering from pigmentary disorders, scarring or port-wine stains, before and after applying cosmetic advices, measuring the impact on QoL. DLQI was evaluated before and 1 month after their first visit to a cosmetic camouflage clinic. Results showed a significant improvement in QoL, with a mean DLQI dropping from 9.1 to 5.8, after 1 month of use. The mean scores of all 10 DLQI questions fell following camouflage advice, suggesting a benefit from attendance at a cosmetic camouflage clinic. Interestingly, the greatest overall improvements as compared to the initial score were related to sexual and other interpersonal relationships.

Other studies evaluated the effect of corrective cosmetics on facial pigmentary disorders, with another validated QoL scoring called Skindex.[69,70] The significant benefit on the psychological impact of the disease was demonstrated in 73 women at various times, i.e. 2, 4 and 12 weeks after starting the use of the product.[69] This study could check and confirm both the immediate self-perceived improvement and the long-term effect, where the cosmetic qualities of the corrective makeup and its tolerance are pivotal for QoL.

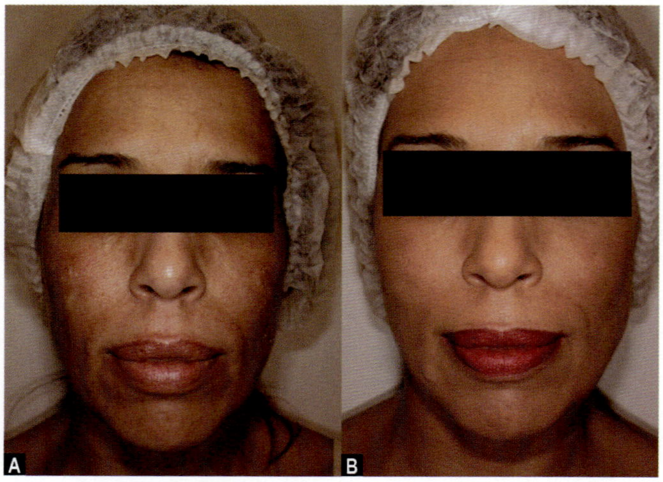

Figure 4: A patient with a resistant melasma before and after a cosmetic camouflage (Unifiance, La Roche Posay). **A,** Before **B,** After
Courtesy: Dr Fernando Stengel, Buenos Aires, Argentina

Another recent study focused upon the impact of skin conditions of patients with various skin diseases on their QoL and the improvement afforded by the use of a corrective makeup.[71] A group of 129 patients with various skin diseases affecting their face (acne, rosacea, angioma, melasma, vitiligo, hypo- or hyperpigmentation) were enrolled in the study and were instructed on how to adequately use corrective makeup. DLQI was evaluated before and after 1 month of makeup use (Fig. 4). The results showed that the mean DLQI score dropped significantly from 9.9 to 3.5.

Cancer and Side-effects of its Treatment—Role of Cosmetics in Self Mental Reconstruction

In more severe chronic conditions, the impact of appearance and body image has also been studied. Breast cancers affect women emotionally and physically. The meaning of body in breast cancer female patients is complex and can be viewed as involving three aspects:[72] (i) the body as a symbol of social expression; (ii) the body as a way of feeling sensations and symptoms (including the side effects of treatments); and (iii) the body as a means of expressing existence. It is suggested that any appropriate intervention on each of these three aspects will be very helpful for the comfort and the prognosis of female cancer patients. The program "Look Good Feel Better" is a dedicated service which has been developed to help women for cancer and cancer treatment side effects upon their appearance. Reconstruction of body image and improving appearance with cosmetic care will help these patients to recover feminity and feel physically attractive. This program established the significant improvement in body image and self-esteem using cosmetics.[73-75] Validated scales for evaluation of self-image, social interactions, and anxiety confirmed the significant improvement ($p < 0.05$) in self-image and social interactions emphasizing the influence of appearance on the mood in this particularly serious condition.

An increasing number of studies are currently carried out worldwide to illustrate the effect of cosmetics care on the mood of cancer patients. For example, the positive influence of cosmetics in the management of this disease was evaluated in a randomized study involving 27 women with breast cancer treated with chemotherapy and radiotherapy.[76] One group, the "cosmetic group" received specific wig advice, body moisturizing massages with oils and creams, camouflage when needed, manicure, pedicure and makeup. The control group did not receive any specific care and advice. Psychosocial modifications were evaluated. Patients from the "cosmetic group" were significantly less discouraged ($p < 0.032$) and more self-confident ($p < 0.032$) than patients from the control group.

In addition, the evidence of improved biological parameters is now demonstrated. In a study involving 39 patients with cancer, massages with oil or aromatherapy were randomly allocated and compared to control group with no massage.[77] A significant drop of cortisol and prolactin levels was found in the massaged groups. This physiological response to aromatherapy and massage was accompanied by a feeling of relaxation and a significant reduction in the "need to stay in bed" item. The improvement in well-being can, therefore, be attributed to massages and aromatherapy, such study clearly supporting the link between physiological responses and psychological improvement.

Benefits of Cosmetics on Quality of Life in Healthy Population

Besides the obvious benefits of cosmetics and appearance improvement in some pathological conditions, more studies now focus upon the beneficial effects of cosmetics in normal physiological states and how this improvement impacts self-esteem and social life.

Positive Sensorial and Social Effects of Cosmetics

Since 1985, in their Magnum opus *Psychology of Cosmetic Treatments*, Graham and Kligman were explaining the emotional and social benefits of using cosmetics.[78] Women appeared more self-confident and more positive after the utilization of cosmetics.

In a large study performed on 359 women,[79] aged 15 to over 56 years, a questionnaire of "Mood Adjective Check List" was filled up by individuals before and after hair care performed by professionals in hair salons. Psychological mood significantly improved by the hair care procedure, irrespective of the type of hair care received. The scores for joy in living, energy and sociability increased together with a drop in stress, anxiety and aggressiveness scores (Fig. 5). Interestingly, the major improvements in sociability were mostly found in the populations aged 46–55.

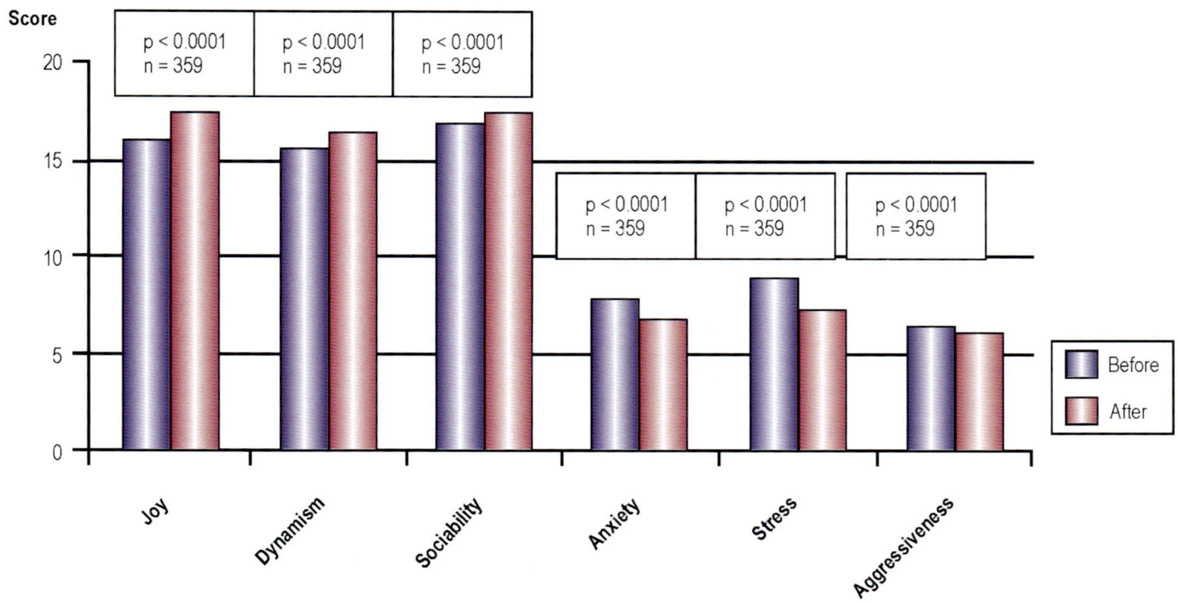

Figure 5: Variations of the positive and negative dimensions of mood after hair-dressing (mean ± 95% confidence interval of the mean)[79]

In another study, it has been demonstrated that a lipohydroxyacid-containing shampoo enhances both scalp condition and QoL in patients with seborrheic dermatitis and light-to-moderate scalp psoriasis.[80]

Makeup plays an oblivious role in altering appearance and its importance in the management of disfiguring diseases has already been stressed above. In normal conditions, embellishing or masking minor cutaneous defects is a daily routine for many women. The first demonstration of the psychoimmunological benefits of cosmetics came from Kimura et al.,[81] who showed an activation of positive immune response, thus demonstrating the connection between mind and body benefits. The controlled clinical study included two trials—one experiment tested a perfume, and the other tested a makeup. The authors demonstrated on 10 healthy subjects an improvement of psychological health evaluated with a mood check sheet, as well as an increase in the immunoglobulin A (IgA) level in the saliva, i.e. an activation of the immune response following psychological changes induced by the cosmetic product. IgA plays an important role in bacterial defenses, creating a first line of immune defense against bacterial action. This study enlightened subtle functionality of cosmetics and opening the door to a better understanding of the relationship between skin and brain. In a more recent study,[82] it was shown that use of makeup reduced mental stress, decreased anxiety state and induced psychological benefits. As for physiology, it induced a decrease in serum cortisol and an increase in superoxide dismutase and catalase levels in saliva.

Fragrances contained in cosmetic creams as well as perfumes also impact the physiology of mood, thus linked to pleasure perception.[83-85] Reliable measurements of such effects were developed and tested in various physiological states. A Mood Mapping method was recently established[83] and showed the moody associations of aromas contained in cosmetic products or in fragrances. The mood profile of each aroma can be multi-dimensionally mapped from emotional scores or through principal component analysis (PCA). For example, comparison of clementine aroma to vanilla bean aroma showed the major effect of clementine on happiness and stimulation, whereas vanilla induced a more relaxed mood. These findings were later confirmed using psychophysiological methods. Measurable muscle relaxation can be induced when smelling specific fragrances. It has been demonstrated for visual and olfactory stimuli that an increase in heart rate, skin conductance, facial electromyogram activity and respiratory rate correlates with negative and/or excited emotional states whereas a decrease correlates with positive and/or relaxed emotional states. Based on this concept, a study looked at the psychophysiological status of emotional moods associated with use of a men's skincare range.[84] Physiological measurements were performed on 19 men before and after smelling different fragrances contained in a shaving product. Recorded data was correlated with the results obtained from a general mood estimate questionnaire.

Effects of Cosmetics in Improving Quality of Life in Certain Physiological Conditions

Some particular physiological conditions can also induce some undesired alterations of skin appearance and thereby can have a negative psychological impact. For example, oily skin is a cosmetic skin problem that women often describe as "invalidating". Oily skin can indeed negatively affect the psychological status of an individual. This was demonstrated in a controlled study performed on 200 women of 26 years in average.[86] Two groups were formed according to a standardized evaluation of sebum levels: one group with oily skin versus one group with normal skin (control group). A specific validated questionnaire: Oily Skin Self Image Questionnaire (OSSIQ) was used to assess the psychological impact of a cosmetic product against oily skin. The study confirmed that women with oily skin presented an altered psychological status compared to the control group. Following a 35 day use of specific care, the results showed a strong improvement in psychological profiles, with clear benefits on self-perception and self-confidence, correlated with a significant improvement in skin appearance.

Aging is also a physiological process leading to conspicuous skin changes. Besides diseases specific to an aging skin, elderly people suffer from age-related conditions such as xerosis, skin fragility, sagging and wrinkling, and at a sensorial level—itching. All these conditions make skin less comfortable, induce deterioration of skin appearance and decreased self-esteem. By enhancing appearance and comfort, cosmetics improve psychological and physical health.[87-89] The degradation of tactile spatial acuity with age was confirmed in one study using the Two Point Gap Discrimination method on 13 elderly people.[90] Discriminative function was partially restored after hydration of the skin with a moisturizer. In another study involving 24 elderly subjects affected by depression, physical touch was evaluated for its effects on different validated scales of depression: Geriatric Depression Scale, Life Satisfaction Scale, Rosenberg Self-Esteem Scale and Locus of Control Scale.[91] Significant differences were found between pre-test and post-test scores of depression scales. The most comfortable areas of the subjects' body when touched were arms, hands, shoulders and back.

This study confirms the important link between depression, self-esteem, life satisfaction and expressive touch on the body. The social consequences are major. Improving skin texture and smoothness with adapted cosmetic care can echo far beyond than clinical and measurable effects on skin. In brief, by enhancing appearance and comfort, cosmetics improve psychological and physical health.

CONCLUSION

A multitude of methods and QoL scales have been developed and validated to objectively show the impact of some diseases and their treatments on the psychological and social status of individuals. Measuring QoL should be considered as a full part of the management of diseases: it allows to rationalize the individual impact of a disease but also to better evaluate the benefit of a treatment with regard to the difficulty of processing.

The very visibility of skin, the emotional significance of cutaneous disturbances, the symbolic meaning of hair and skin, and sense of touch are paramount in the everyday life of humans. Taking care of appearance is consequently crucial worldwide. Attractiveness influences self-esteem, social relationships and ultimately sexual behavior.

Today, many studies illustrate, with measurable parameters, the influence of appearance upon physiological parameters in both normal health condition and pathological situations, such as dyspigmentation or breast cancers. Cosmetics may increase well-being as they can indirectly influence some important physiological mechanisms through their impact upon mental status. The Indian culture, since long, integrated the link between beauty and health. Cosmetic care and esthetics appear inseparable from well-being and health. Methods for quantitative assessment of well-being are now available to demonstrate how taking care of appearance in both normal and disordered/diseased states both subtly and profoundly reverberates.

REFERENCES

1. WHOQOL Group. Development of the WHOQOL: Rationale and current status. Int J Mental Health. 1994;23:24-56.
2. Finlay AY. Quality of life measurement in dermatology: a practical guide. Br J Dermatol. 1997;136(3):305-14.
3. Jowett S, Ryan T. Skin disease and handicap: an analysis of the impact of skin conditions. Soc Sci Med. 1985;20(4):425-9.
4. Basra MK, Shahrukh M. Burden of skin diseases. Expert Rev Pharmacoecon Outcomes Res. 2009;9(3):271-83.
5. Sampogna F, Gisondi P, Melchi CF; et al. IDI Multipurpose Psoriasis Research on Vital Experiences Investigators. Prevalence of symptoms experienced by patients with different clinical types of psoriasis. Br J Dermatol. 2004;151(3):594-9.
6. Hongbo Y, Thomas CL, Harrison MA, et al. Translating the science of quality of life into practice: What do dermatology life quality index scores mean? J Invest Dermatol. 2005;125(4):659-64.
7. Brazier JE, Harper R, Jones NM, et al. Validating the SF-36 health survey questionnaire: new outcome measure for primary care. BMJ. 1992;305(6846):160-4.
8. Hunt SM, McKenna SP, McEwen J, et al. The Nottingham Health Profile: subjective health status and medical consultations. Soc Sci Med A. 1981;15:221-9.
9. Hunt SM, McEwen J, McKenna SP. Measuring health status: a new tool for clinicians and epidemiologists. J R Coll Gen Pract. 1985;35(273):185-8.
10. Hunt SM. Cross-cultural issues in the use of socio-medical indicators. Health Policy. 1986;6(2):149-58.
11. Bergner M, Bobbitt RA, Carter WB, et al. The Sickness Impact Profile: development and final revision of a health status measure. Med Care. 1981;19(8):787-805.
12. The World Health Organization Quality of Life assessment (WHOQOL): position paper from the World Health Organization. Soc Sci Med. 1995;41(10):1403-9.
13. The WHOQOL Group. Development of the World Health Organization WHOQOL-BREF quality of life assessment. Psychol Med. 1998;28(3):551-8.
14. Finlay AY, Khan GK. Dermatology Life Quality Index (DLQI)-a simple practical measure for routine clinical use. Clin Exp Dermatol. 1994;19(3):210-6.
15. Lewis V, Finlay AY. 10 years experience of the Dermatology Life Quality Index (DLQI). J Investig Dermatol Symp Proc. 2004;9(2): 169-80.
16. Chren MM, Lasek RJ, Quinn LM, et al. Skindex, a quality-of-life measure for patients with skin disease: reliability, validity, and responsiveness. J Invest Dermatol. 1996;107(5):707-13.
17. Anderson RT, Rajagopalan R. Development and validation of a quality of life instrument for cutaneous diseases. J Am Acad Dermatol. 1997;37(1):41-50.

18. Morgan M, McCreedy R, Simpson J, et al. Dermatology quality of life scales—a measure of the impact of skin diseases. Br J Dermatol. 1997;136(2):202-6.
19. Augustin M, Lange S, Wenninger K, et al. Validation of a comprehensive Freiburg Life Quality Assessment (FLQA) core questionnaire and development of a threshold system. Eur J Dermatol. 2004;14(2):107-13.
20. Lewis-Jones MS, Finlay AY. The Children's Dermatology Life Quality Index (CDLQI): initial validation and practical use. Br J Dermatol. 1995;132(6):942-9.
21. Holme SA, Man I, Sharpe JL, et al. The Children's Dermatology Life Quality Index: validation of the cartoon version. Br J Dermatol. 2003;148(2):285-90.
22. Finlay AY, Kelly SE. Psoriasis—an index of disability. Clin Exp Dermatol. 1987;12(1):8-11.
23. Lewis VJ, Finlay AY. Two decades experience of the Psoriasis Disability Index. Dermatology. 2005;210(4):261-8.
24. Gupta MA, Gupta AK. The Psoriasis Life Stress Inventory: a preliminary index of psoriasis-related stress. Acta Derm Venereol. 1995;75(3):240-3.
25. Kirby B, Fortune DG, Bhushan M, et al. The Salford Psoriasis Index: an holistic measure of psoriasis severity. Br J Dermatol. 2000;142(4):728-32.
26. McKenna SP, Cook SA, Whalley D, et al. Development of the PSORIQoL, a psoriasis-specific measure of quality of life designed for use in clinical practice and trials. Br J Dermatol. 2003;149(2):323-31.
27. Lewis-Jones MS, Finlay AY, Dykes PJ. The Infants' Dermatitis Quality of Life Index. Br J Dermatol. 2001;144(1):104-10.
28. Lawson V, Lewis-Jones MS, Finlay AY, et al. The family impact of childhood atopic dermatitis: the Dermatitis Family Impact Questionnaire. Br J Dermatol. 1998;138(1):107-13.
29. Whalley D, McKenna SP, Dewar AL, et al. A new instrument for assessing quality of life in atopic dermatitis: international development of the Quality of Life Index for Atopic Dermatitis (QoLIAD). Br J Dermatol. 2004;150(2):274-83.
30. Motley RJ, Finlay AY. How much disability is caused by acne? Clin Exp Dermatol. 1989;14(3):194-8.
31. Motley RJ, Finlay AY. Practical use of a disability index in the routine management of acne. Clin Exp Dermatol. 1992;17(1):1-3.
32. Layton A. Psychological assessment of skin disease. Interfaces Dermatol. 1994;1:9-11.
33. Girman CJ, Hartmaier S, Thiboutot D, et al. Evaluating health-related quality of life in patients with facial acne: development of a self-administered questionnaire for clinical trials. Qual Life Res. 1996;5(5):481-90.
34. Martin AR, Lookingbill DP, Botek A, et al. Health-related quality of life among patients with facial acne—assessment of a new acne-specific questionnaire. Clin Exp Dermatol. 2001;26(5):380-5.
35. Gupta MA, Johnson AM, Gupta AK. The development of an Acne Quality of Life scale: reliability, validity, and relation to subjective acne severity in mild to moderate acne vulgaris. Acta Derm Venereol. 1998;78(6):451-6.
36. Augustin M, Dieterle W, Zschocke I, et al. Development and validation of a disease-specific questionnaire on the quality of life of patients with chronic venous insufficiency. Vasa. 1997;26(4):291-301.
37. Aftergut K, Carmody T, Cruz PD. Use of the HIV-DERMDEX quality-of-life instrument in HIV-infected patients with skin disease. Int J Dermatol. 2001;40(7):478-81.
38. Balkrishnan R, McMichael AJ, Camacho FT, et al. Development and validation of a health-related quality of life instrument for women with melasma. Br J Dermatol. 2003;149(3):572-7.
39. Krishna GS, Ramam M, Mehta M, et al. Vitiligo impact scale: An instrument to assess the psychosocial burden of vitiligo. Indian J Dermatol Venereol Leprol. 2013;79(2):205-10.
40. Dolte KS, Girman CJ, Hartmaier S, et al. Development of a health-related quality of life questionnaire for women with androgenetic alopecia. Clin Exp Dermatol. 2000;25(8):637-42.
41. Chen SC, Yeung J, Chren MM. Scalpdex: a quality-of-life instrument for scalp dermatitis. Arch Dermatol. 2002;138(6):803-7.
42. McCombs K, Chen SC. Patient preference quality of life measures in dermatology. Dermatol Ther. 2007;20(2):102-9.
43. Shah H, Mehta A, Astik B. Clinical and sociodemographic study of vitiligo. Indian J Dermatol Venereol Leprol. 2008;74(6):701.
44. Ongenae K, Van Geel N, De Schepper S, et al. Effect of vitiligo on self-reported health-related quality of life. Br J Dermatol. 2005;152(6):1165-72.
45. Sehgal VN, Srivastava G. Vitiligo: Compendium of clinico-epidemiological features. Indian J Dermatol Venereol Leprol. 2007;73(3):149-56.
46. Parsad D, Dogra S, Kanwar AJ. Quality of life in patients with vitiligo. Health Qual Life Outcomes. 2003;1:58.
47. Kent G, al-Abadie M. Factors affecting responses on Dermatology Life Quality Index items among vitiligo sufferers. Clin Exp Dermatol. 1996;21(5):330-3.
48. Silverberg JI, Silverberg NB. Association between vitiligo extent and distribution and quality-of-life impairment. JAMA Dermatol. 2013;149(2):159-64.
49. Wong SM, Baba R. Quality of life among Malaysian patients with vitiligo. Int J Dermatol. 2012;51(2):158-61.
50. Aghaei S, Sodaifi M, Jafari P, et al. DLQI scores in vitiligo: reliability and validity of the Persian version. BMC Dermatol. 2004;4:8.
51. Dolatshahi M, Ghazi P, Feizy V, et al. Life quality assessment among patients with vitiligo: comparison of married and single patients in Iran. Indian J Dermatol Venereol Leprol. 2008;74:700.
52. Bhandarkar SS, Kundu RV. Quality-of-life issues in vitiligo. Dermatol Clin. 2012;30(2):255-68.
53. Ginsburg IH. Psychological and psychophysiological aspects of psoriasis. Dermatol Clin. 1995;13(4):793-804.
54. de Arruda LH, De Moraes AP. The impact of psoriasis on quality of life. Br J Dermatol. 2001;144:33-6.
55. Kirby B, Richards HL, Woo P, et al. Physical and psychological measures are necessary to assess overall psoriasis severity. J Am Acad Dermatol. 2001;45(1):72-6.
56. Fortune DG, Main CJ, O'Sullivan TM, et al. Quality of life in patients with psoriasis: the contribution of clinical variables and psoriasis-specific stress. Br J Dermatol. 1997;137(5):755-60.
57. Prins M, Krabbe PF, Swinkels QO, et al. The effect of treatment on quality of life in psoriasis patients. Acta Derm Venereol. 2005;85(4):304-10.
58. Rakhesh SV, D'Souza M, Sahai A. Quality of life in psoriasis: a study from south India. Indian J Dermatol Venereol Leprol. 2008;74(6):600-6.
59. Manjula VD, Sreekiran S, Saril PS, et al. A study of psoriasis and quality of life in a tertiary care teaching hospital of Kottayam, Kerala. Indian J Dermatol. 2011;56(4):403-6.
60. Koo J. The psychosocial impact of acne: patient's perceptions. J Am Acad Dermatol. 1995;32:S26-30.
61. Thomas DR. Psychosocial effects of acne. J Cutan Med Surg. 2004;8 (Suppl 4):3-5.
62. Smithard A, Glazebrook C, Williams HC. Acne prevalence, knowledge about acne and psychological morbidity in mid-adolescence: a community-based study. Br J Dermatol. 2001;145(2):274-9.
63. Walker N, Lewis-Jones MS. Quality of life and acne in Scottish

adolescent school children: use of the Children's Dermatology Life Quality Index (CDLQI) and the Cardiff Acne Disability Index (CADI). J Eur Acad Dermatol Venereol. 2006;20(1):45-50.

64. Pruthi GK, Babu N. Physical and psychosocial impact of acne in adult females. Indian J Dermatol. 2012;57(1):26-9.
65. Kubba R, Bajaj AK, Thappa DM, et al. Acne and quality of life. Indian J Dermatol Venereol Leprol [serial online] 2009 [cited 2013 May 23];75:4-5.
66. Sarveswari KN. Cosmetic camouflage in vitiligo. Indian J Dermatol. 2010;55(3):211-4.
67. Ongenae K, Dierckxsens L, Bronchez L, et al. Quality of life and stigmatization profile in a cohort of vitiligo patients and effect of the use of camouflage. Dermatology. 2005;210(4):279-85.
68. Holme SA, Beattie PE, Fleming CJ. Cosmetic camouflage advice improves quality of life. Br J Dermatol. 2002;147(5):946-9.
69. Balkrishnan R, McMichael AJ, Hu JY, et al. Corrective cosmetics are effective for women with facial pigmentary disorders. Cutis. 2005;75(3):181-7.
70. Tanioka M, Yamamoto Y, Kato M, et al. Camouflage for patients with vitiligo vulgaris improved their quality of life. J Cosmet Dermatol. 2010;9(1):72-5.
71. Seité S, Deshayes P, Dréno B, et al. Interest of corrective makeup in the management of patients in dermatology. Clin Cosmet Investig Dermatol. 2012;5:123-8.
72. Cohen MZ, Kahn DL, Steeves RH. Beyond body image: the experience of breast cancer. Oncol Nurs Forum. 1998; 25(5):835-41.
73. Anderson MS, Johnson J. Restoration of body image and self-esteem for women after cancer treatment: a rehabilitative strategy. Cancer Practice 2. 1994;2(5):345-9.
74. Kendrick K. Normalizing female cancer patients: Look good, feel better and other image programs. Disability & Society. 2008;23: 259-69.
75. Taggart LR, Ozolins L, Hardie H, et al. Look Good Feel Better Workshops: "a big lift" for women with cancer. J Cancer Educ. 2009;24(2):94-9.
76. Titeca G, Poot F, Cassart D, et al. Impact of cosmetic care on quality of life in breast cancer patients during chemotherapy and radiotherapy: an initial randomized controlled study. J Eur Acad Dermatol Venereol. 2007;21(6):771-6.
77. Stringer J, Swindell R, Dennis M. Massage in patients undergoing intensive chemotherapy reduces serum cortisol and prolactin. Psycho-Oncology. 2008;17(10):1024-31.
78. Graham JA, Kligman AM. The psychology of cosmetic treatments. New-York: Prager;1985.
79. Picot-Lemasson A, Decocq G, Aghassian F, et al. Influence of hairdressing on the psychological mood of women. Int J Cosmet Sci. 2001;23(3):161-4.
80. Seité S, Paries J, Reygagne P, et al. A lipohydroxyacid-containing shampoo improves scalp condition and quality of life in patients with seborrheic dermatitis and light-to-moderate scalp psoriasis. J Cosmet Dermatol. 2009;8(2):108-13.
81. Kan C, Kimura S. Psychoneuroimmunological benefits of cosmetics, in Proceedings of the IFSCC meeting, Venezia, 769-784 (1994).
82. Tochio T. Makeup inhibits reduction of reactive oxygen scavenging enzyme activity induced by mental stress. Int J Cosmet Sci. 2008;31:159-61.
83. Warrenburg S. Effects of fragrance on emotions: moods and physiology. Chem Senses. 2005;30:i248-9.
84. Abriat A, Barkat S, Bensafi M, et al. Emotional and psychological effects of fragrance in men's skin care. Int J Cosmet Sci. 2005;27: 299-300.
85. Abriat A, Barkat S, Bensafi M, et al. Psychological and physiological evaluation of emotional effects of a perfume in menopausal women. Int J Cosmet Sci. 2007;29(5):399-408.
86. Segot-Chicq E, Compan-Zaouati D, Wolkenstein P, et al. Development and validation of a questionnaire to evaluate how a cosmetic product for oily skin is able to improve well-being in women. J Eur Acad Dermatol Venereol. 2007;21(9):1181-6.
87. Kligman AM. Psychological aspects of skin disorders in the elderly. Cutis. 1989;43(5):498-501.
88. Graham JA, Kligman AM. Cosmetic therapy for the elderly. J Soc Cosmet Chem. 1984;35:133-45.
89. Koblenzer CS. Psychologic aspects of aging and the skin. Clin Dermatol. 1996;14(2):171-7.
90. Buschmann MT, Hollinger-Smith LM, Peterson-Kokkas SE. Implementation of expressive physical touch in depressed older adults. Journal of Clinical Geropsychology. 1999;5:291-300.
91. Lévêque JL, Dresler J, Ribot-Ciscar E, et al. Changes in tactile spatial discrimination and cutaneous coding properties by skin hydration in the elderly. J Invest Dermatol. 2000;115(3):454-8.

Index

Page numbers followed by *f* refer to figure and *t* refer to table

D

E

F

G

H

I

J

K

L

M

T

U

V

W

X

Y

Z